Medieval Medicine

Advisory Board

Renate Blumenfeld-Kosinski
Professor of Romance Languages and Literature, University of Pittsburgh

Barbara Hanawalt
King George III Professor of British History, Ohio State University

E. Ann Matter
William R. Kenan, Jr. Professor of Religious Studies and Associate Dean of Arts and Letters, College of Arts and Sciences, University of Pennsylvania

Marilyn J. Stokstad
Judith Harris Murphy Distinguished Professor of Art History Emerita, University of Kansas

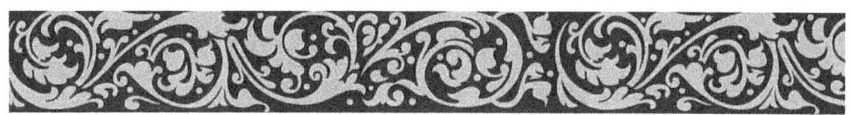

Medieval Medicine

The Art of Healing, from Head to Toe

Luke Demaitre

Praeger Series on the Middle Ages
Jane Chance, Series Editor

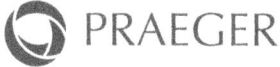

AN IMPRINT OF ABC-CLIO, LLC
Santa Barbara, California • Denver, Colorado • Oxford, England

Copyright 2013 by Luke Demaitre

All rights reserved. No part of this publication may be reproduced, stored in a retrieval system, or transmitted, in any form or by any means, electronic, mechanical, photocopying, recording, or otherwise, except for the inclusion of brief quotations in a review, without prior permission in writing from the publisher.

Library of Congress Cataloging-in-Publication Data

Demaitre, Luke E., 1935–
  Medieval medicine : the art of healing, from head to toe / Luke Demaitre.
    p. cm. — (Praeger series on the Middle Ages)
  Includes bibliographical references and index.
    ISBN 978-0-275-98485-4 (hardcopy : alk. paper) — ISBN 978-0-313-03842-6 (ebook)
I. Title. II. Series: Praeger series on the Middle Ages.
[DNLM: 1. History of Medicine.   2. History, Medieval. WZ 54]
LC Classification not assigned
610.938—dc23   2012043760

ISBN: 978-0-275-98485-4
EISBN: 978-0-313-03842-6

17 16 15 14 13   1 2 3 4 5

This book is also available on the World Wide Web as an eBook.
Visit www.abc-clio.com for details.

Praeger
An Imprint of ABC-CLIO, LLC

ABC-CLIO, LLC
130 Cremona Drive, P.O. Box 1911
Santa Barbara, California 93116-1911

This book is printed on acid-free paper ∞

Manufactured in the United States of America

Contents

Illustrations	vii
Introduction	ix
1. Learning to Heal	1
2. Paradigms of Disease: Fever, Pestilence, and Poison	35
3. The Body Surface; Tumors and Trauma	77
4. Head Problems, from Hair Loss to Epilepsy	111
5. The Face and the Senses	153
6. Uvula to Diaphragm and *Passiones Spirituales*	197
7. From Gullet to Gut: *Passiones Nutritivorum*	239
8. From the Haunches to the Heels, and *Passiones Membrorum Generationis*	283
Chronology of the Collated Latin Medical Manuals	325
Glossary	329
Bibliography of Sources	333
Selected Bibliography	337
Index	341

Illustrations

Plates

Bernard de Gordon, *Lilium medicine*	x
Bernard de Gordon, *Lilium*	xi
Galen in a magisterial chair, instructs an assistant compounding a medicine, while a scribe records the recipe	7
Theory and Practice: A Master of Medicine, holding a book, points from a student to a patient	14
Constantinus Africanus collecting authoritative texts, in conference with Haly Abbas and Isaac Judeus	27
A Master of Medicine, with an open book at hand, teaches about interpreting urine	46
A clinic with a surgeon-physician performing a phlebotomy on one patient and a physician examining the urine of another, and two more patients waiting in line	60
A man covered with spots (likely smallpox or measles), and a woman with inflamed eyes	85
"The Royal Touch": King Edward the Confessor touching for scrofula	97
A woman brushes lice out of a boy's hair	118

Map of the brain, faculties, and senses	128
A manic patient does cartwheels and, restrained, is treated with sprigs of peony	144
The physician Rhazes, in the gown and cap of a 15th-century physician, with a book and spectacles	176
A healer brings herbal medicines for "ailments or pains of the eyes" and "ailments and pains of the ears" to a patient in agony	182
A lay healer treats a patient's nose, with hematite for bleeding	190
Anatomy of the head, thorax, and torso, including the *membra spiritualia* (left margin), and showing one lung (*pulmo*) wrapped around the heart (*cor*)	206
Syncope. Valesco's patient and patron, Gaston de Foix, dying of a heart attack	236
General anatomy, with arteries and intestines; and diagrams of the stomach, liver, and other organs of digestion	254
A practitioner administers an enema to a kneeling patient	269
"The master extracts a stone" in "the Celsan operation" for bladder stone, performed from the rear	289
The correlation of *Physionomie,* complexion, temperament, and the planets with sexual function and dysfunction	307

Tables

2.1	Organization of chapters on fevers	42
3.1	Avicenna's humoral scheme of tumors	81
7.1	Bleeding hemorrhoids, in the *Canon* and the *Lilium*	270
8.1	Contents of sections on the (male) reproductive organs	304
8.2	Chapters on female reproductive organs (*muliebria*)	314

Introduction

The subtitle of this book combines the historic name of medicine with a common phrase that has replaced the classical expression. The combination, while the result of editorial give-and-take, opens two principal perspectives for this study. Hippocrates and Galen devoted their writings to "The Art of Healing." Their characterization highlights a dimension that is crucial to an understanding of medieval learning and practice, while it is easily overlooked in the modern celebration of science and technology. From Greek antiquity to 15th-century Europe, medicine as "The Art" consisted of knowledge *and* skill, logic *and* intuition, and tradition *and* observation. The Art was both the transcendent cause and the daily practice that inspired authors to write the manuals for physicians that will be examined in these pages. For the second part of the subtitle, my original choice was "from head to heel." The choice of the idiomatically off-key expression troubled several editors, but it sprang from historical fact and semantic fancy. First, our common expression, "from head to toe," is unmatched in Latin where, in fact, the same word, *digitus,* referred both to "toe" and "finger." A Latin equivalent existed for "head to foot," but the classic phrase was "from head to heel" or *a capite ad calcem.* This was the phrase that for centuries graced the cover of medical manuals.

One such manual, and the seed of this study, was the *Practica sive Lilium medicine,* completed by Bernard de Gordon in 1305. A particularly inspiring exemplar has been a version, printed at Paris in 1542, that bears the solemn title, *B. Gordonii Omnium Aegritudinum a vertice ad calcem opus praeclarissimum quod Lilium medicinae appellatur*—note the subtle emendation—or "from the crown of the head to the heel." A remarkable copy is among the Vaulted Treasures in the Historical Collections of the Claude Moore Health Sciences Library in the School of Medicine at the University of Virginia. A practitioner and professor at one of the oldest universities of medicine, in Montpellier, Bernard de Gordon wrote treatises

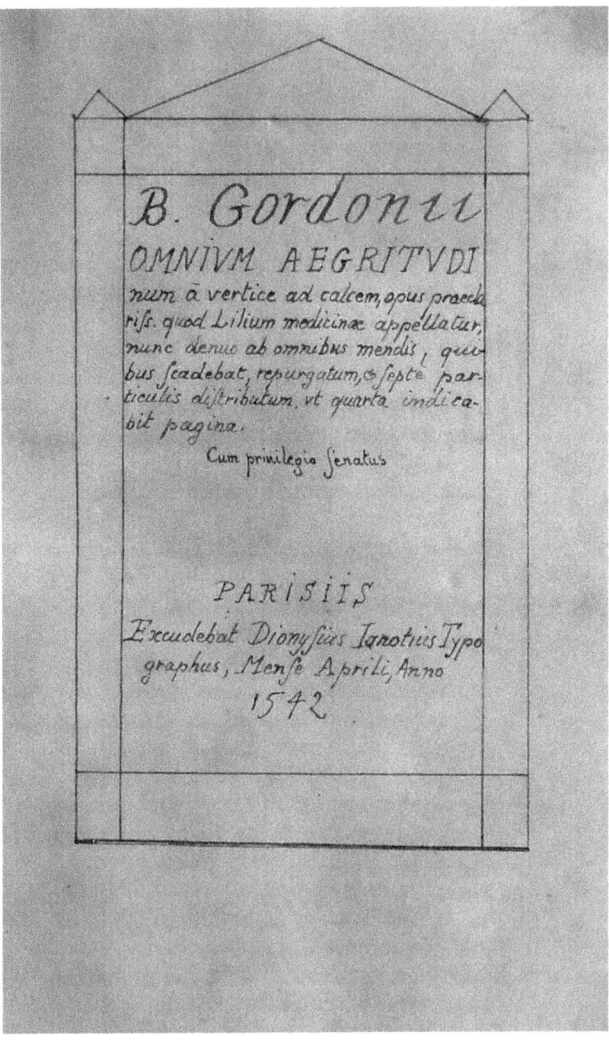

Bernard de Gordon, *Lilium medicine,* frontispiece of *B. Gordonii Omnium Aegritudinum a vertice ad calcem opus praeclarissimum* (*The Most Distinguished Work of B[ernard] Gordon on All Diseases from the Top of the Head to the Heel*). Handwritten title page, copied by a modern (18th century?) owner to replace the original title page printed in Paris in 1542. (Courtesy of Historical Collections & Services, Claude Moore Health Sciences Library, University of Virginia. http://exhibits.hsl.virginia.edu/treasures/bernard-de-gordon-1260-ca-1318/)

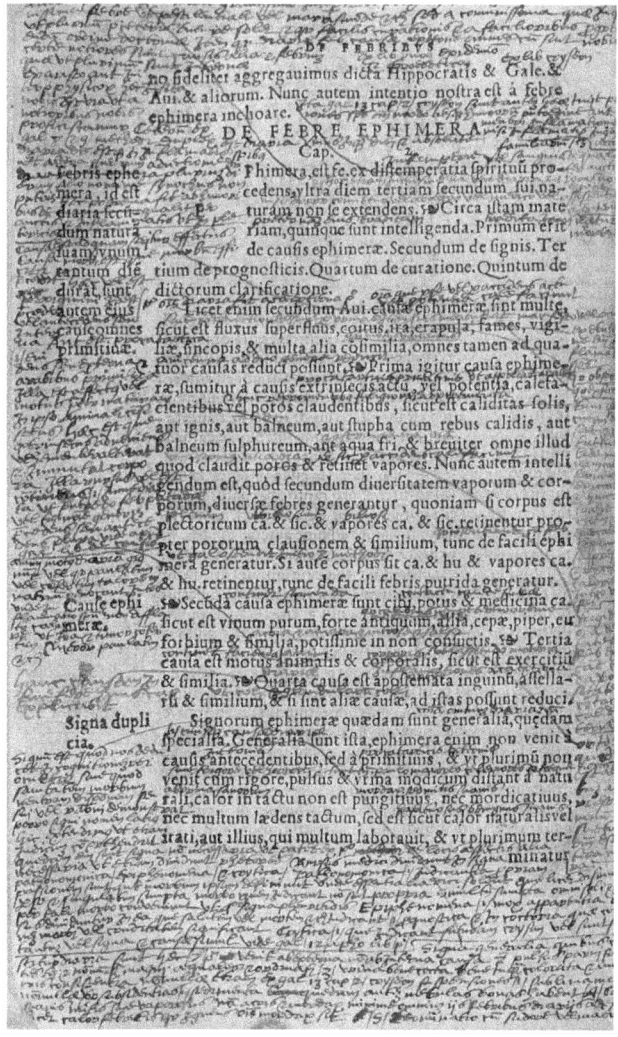

Bernard de Gordon, *Lilium,* page on "ephemeral fever" with copious notes in Latin by a late-16th-century reader. *B. Gordonii Omnium Aegritudinum a vertice ad calcem,* Paris, 1542, fol. 3v. (Courtesy of Historical Collections & Services, Claude Moore Health Sciences Library, University of Virginia)

on diet, diagnosis, prognostication, and therapeutics. The "Lily of Medicine" was his most celebrated work. It enjoyed a wide and long circulation in Latin; it was translated into Castilian, English, French, Gaelic, and Hebrew; and it was still printed in Madrid in 1697, almost four centuries after it was written. The copious and sophisticated marginal notes in the volume at the University of Virginia attest to an enduring and active interest.

INTRODUCTION

In addition to sounding too incongruous in a subtitle, the phrase "head to heel" might, at first sight, have appeared as a frivolous attempt at punning. The serious intent, however, was to project, even before a reader opens this book, my strong conviction that the wish *to heal* was the raison d'être of the medieval physician's manuals. The ultimate objective of the authors was neither the pursuit of profit nor the contemplation of metaphysical verities but the health of patients. Their concentration was evident in a title that several of them gave to their manual, *Practica de egritudinibus* or "practical matters about diseases." The focus of this survey, too, is on diseases, rather than on health and its maintenance (*regimen*) or on medical methodology (*ingenium*) and theory (*doctrina*). This is not a lexicon or inventory of medieval diseases, however, and even less a dictionary with modern equivalents, which would rely on retrospective diagnosis and ample anachronisms. The expression "from head to foot" might raise expectations of exhaustive coverage. Such expectations would be misdirected at an introductory survey that lays no claim to a definitive assessment. At the outset, therefore, I should alert the reader that, rather than promising completeness, the title refers to the organization and the structure of the handbooks.

I may also (try to) prevent disappointment by pointing out some of the limitations in this survey. The greatest challenge, which also faced the authors cited in this book, was finding a balance between inclusiveness and brevity. The great number and diversity of medical encyclopedias made it necessary to carve out a manageable group and, thereby, to leave aside a considerable number of very rich and relevant sources. This meant, first of all, bypassing the surgical manuals by Theodoric Borgognoni, Henri de Mondeville, Guy de Chauliac, and others; for these manuals, however, we are fortunate to have an enlightened and indispensable appraisal in Michael R. McVaugh's *The Rational Surgery of the Middle Ages*. Another group of encyclopedic documents, which awaits a synthesis, was excluded as closer to the classroom than to the bedside. This group includes a vast body of scholastic commentaries on authoritative texts that range from the Hippocratic *Aphorisms* and Galen's *Art of Medicine* to Avicenna's *Canon of Medicine* and Rhazes's *Book for Al-Mansuri*. At the opposite end of the spectrum, recipe books without reference to theory fall short of being true manuals, although many of them bear the title *Practica*. A further narrowing, to manuals that addressed neophyte physicians and schooled practitioners, entailed the exclusion of such popular health guides as the 13th-century *Treasure of the Poor* by Peter of Spain. Practical limitations forced omissions even within the tightened ambit, of several significant manuals, including the "Practice" (*Practica*) of Petrus Musandinus, the "Mild Book" (*Liber mitis*) of Guido d'Arezzo Junior, and the "Medical Compendium" (*Summa medicinalis*) by Tommaso Del Garbo.

The dozen compendia selected for this book were compiled between the 11th and 15th centuries. I hope that the selection has yielded a reasonably reliable image of the medieval physician's manual. In addition to comparing the works as methodically as time and energy allowed, I have correlated significant propositions with their classic sources. As a general result, it has been refreshing to discover how much the authors varied in their personalities, views, and responses to tradition. This variety, together with the dynamic developments in the form and content of the manual, should contradict—as still seems necessary—the stereotypical image of medieval stagnation and derivativeness. We should keep in mind, nevertheless, that the compilers did not intend to be scientific pioneers and that their readers were not members of a Royal Society or Academy of Sciences.

It may be a relief to know that the contents of this book evolve gradually, from an inevitably didactic beginning to a more impressionistic narrative. The first chapter introduces the learned, indeed bookish, tradition that formed the foundation and context of the medical manual. The second chapter mines the manuals themselves for the framework of general and generic concepts of diseases. After a chapter on external ailments, the remaining pages closely follow the head-to-heel order, as it was perceived in medieval medicine. Most of the compilers attached some appendix to their *practica*, with material that they were unable to accommodate within the body, or which they considered of separate significance. The contents of these attachments range from antidotaries to dietetics and surgical procedures, and from cosmetics to guidelines for travel. They are so miscellaneous that they will be ignored as too distracting. For the same reason, I recount fewer details about treatments than some readers may wish: hundreds of recipes and procedures and, in fact, thousands of ingredients and steps would greatly overburden a survey, whereas general therapeutic guidelines and individual observations afford a better insight into the physician's application of learning to care.

Even on their own, independent of the compendia context, the guidelines and observations weave a rich tapestry of medieval lore and practices. They supply a wealth of quotations that are interspersed (and, wherever possible, set off as blocks of text) in my discussion, not only for the sake of illustration but also because almost nothing of this material is available in English. All the translations from the Latin are my own. In translating,

I have aimed for clarity rather than literalness. When a term was interesting or a translation open to debate, I have supplied the Latin in parentheses. I have consciously limited the use of technical jargon and listed the most crucial terms in an appended glossary. Nevertheless, a study of this kind will inevitably contain some unfamiliar words, from "anfractuous" to "zedoary," which may prove the value of a dictionary (as they did to the writer). The woeful dearth of translated material is evident in the appended Bibliography of Sources, which identifies the texts on which my survey is based, and which, it is hoped, will serve as a plea for more translations. A separate appendix presents these texts in a chronological arrangement, which highlights the major phases in the evolution of the medical manual.

While working on this book, I have been animated by the fourth-year medical students at the University of Virginia who for more than 15 years have joined me in a History of Medicine elective, a few weeks before obtaining their MD degree. They have thrilled me with their old-fashioned love for written sources, taught me more about the science and practice of medicine than I ever found in books, stimulated me with their inquisitiveness, and inspired me with their dedication to Hippocratic ideals. As icing on the cake, I have enjoyed the warm friendship, beyond mere collegiality, of two colleagues at the University of Virginia, Marcia Childress, director of the Programs in Humanities at the Center for Biomedical Ethics, and Joan Echtenkamp Klein, curator for Historical Collections in the Claude Moore Health Sciences Library. I am also most deeply grateful to the close friends and the caring clinicians who, each in their way, healed me and thus gave me the chance to complete this labor of love.

Last not least,
as the heart beats through the body, head to toe,
so Dominique is the heartbeat of this book, cover to cover.

Learning to Heal

> Life is short, the Art long, opportunity fleeting, experience misleading, and judgment difficult. [The healer] must be prepared not only for doing what is necessary but also for making the patient, the bystanders, and the circumstances cooperate.

This is the first item in the *Aphorisms,* a collection of pithy observations by Hippocrates of Kos (460–377 BCE), who has been called the father of medicine. The *Aphorisms* were at the core of more than 50 Greek writings that, by the beginning of the fourth century BCE, coalesced into a body of instructions for maintaining health and treating disease. This body or Hippocratic Corpus stands in contrast with many other responses to disease by favoring natural over supernatural explanations, holistic over narrow assessments, and conservative over drastic measures. In addition, the writings emphasize the role of diet and lifestyle, the value of prognostication, and the sacredness of the healer's duties. The Hippocratic outlook exerted a deep influence on the development of medical teaching in the Roman Empire, in the monastic and other schools across Christendom, and in the emerging universities. The *Aphorisms,* together with commentaries, constituted the nucleus of the curriculum at the first faculties of medicine.

The first *Aphorism,* with a catchy opening phrase that has become famous in the Latin version, "Vita brevis, ars longa," has spawned countless interpretations and profound commentaries. A simple interpretation, one of several that are possible, will guide us through much of this chapter. A single lifetime is no match for the Art of medicine. Mastering this vast and complex art requires the combination of knowledge with skill, reason with experience, and method with intuition. This combination lies beyond the careers of many medical practitioners, through the ages and around the world. Instead, a majority of practitioners attract and retain the patient by claiming to have innate and seemingly superhuman healing powers and by demonstrating their acquired and impressively advanced expertise. The claimed supernatural ability may be an individual gift or an inherited trait. More significantly, the superior expertise is likely to transcend one person's life span by drawing on cumulative tradition. Medical lore and methods are passed on from generation to generation, most commonly by means of apprenticeships. Apprentice healers, like their counterparts in carpentry and other crafts, entrust themselves to a master (or, more frequently, to a wise woman). They learn about diseases and treatments by observing and assisting the master, and by gradually trying their own hand. This process, however, has built-in weaknesses. Observation and perception are "misleading," particularly in matters of disease, as Hippocrates warns in the *Aphorisms*. Moreover, learning by trial and error makes the patient a guinea pig, and it is especially risky in urgent cases. Learning is also hampered when pressures make, in the words of Hippocrates, "judgment difficult" and offer only "fleeting opportunity" for reflection and correction.

A few healers realized, early on, that they might reduce the risk by anchoring the transmission process more firmly. They stabilized the fleeting experience of separate cases by drawing generalized conclusions, and they remedied the deceptiveness of sense perception by positing principles that were objective or, at least, rational. The conclusions and principles were formulated in such itemized guidelines as the *Aphorisms,* to be transmitted vocally and committed to memory. To secure continuity, beyond the already considerable strength of oral transmission—which we tend to underestimate—the acquired knowledge was increasingly recorded in writing. This made it also more readily available for consultation. Scribes recorded recipes on clay tablets in Mesopotamia and on papyrus in the Nile Valley. One of the most impressive records is now known as the *Edwin Smith Papyrus*: it contains 4,000-year-old case descriptions with instructions for surgeons. This historic document (pristinely preserved at the New York Academy of Medicine) suggests a school setting, with broader interaction and reflection than in conventional apprenticeships. The case histories reflect methodical observation, and the lesson learned from each is constructed with an almost mathematical logic. The *Smith Papyrus* might be called the oldest medical textbook, if it were not limited to surgical cases, to the exterior of the body, and to injuries. Manual interventions did not include diseases, so that the teaching of surgery covered only a part of the developing Art of Healing.

In the Hippocratic tradition, learning to heal involves understanding the nature (definition) of diseases and their causes (etiology), identifying their signs (diagnosis) and foreseeing their course (prognosis), and managing their treatment (therapeutics). The treatment proceeds from prevention and management to the application of medicines and then to manual intervention (surgery). The scope of the Art, as skill and knowledge, never ceased to grow. In a bird's-eye view and at the risk of oversimplification, we may mark several stages in this growth, from ancient Greece to the early 14th-century university. At first, the practitioner was designated in general as one who makes the patient whole, a "healer" (*iatros*)—the Greek word for "healing" (*iatria*) became incorporated in such modern terms as "psychiatry" and "pediatrics." The designation of a healer was quite fluid, and it could extend to a shaman or to anyone who treated the sick with charms and incantations—a similarly broad range characterized the title of *tabib* in early Arabic usage and of *laece* in Old English (which became "leech"). In the Roman world, the Latin title of *medicus* indicated a narrower field. The term implied privileged knowledge, as is suggested by its derivation from the Sanskrit *madh,* which is the root both of "mathematics" and "magic" and of "medicine." The nomenclature gained further precision in the Middle Ages, with the idea that healing depended on the knowledge of nature (*physica* and *phusis,* see "physics"). Together with others who understood the complexions and workings of nature, the healer was called *physicus,* which is the origin of "physician." This label reflects an overlap with the philosophical study of nature, which was rooted in the works of Aristotle (384–322 BCE).

In the nascent universities, medical teaching built on the foundation of the seven arts. The three basic arts of the trivium (grammar, rhetoric, and logic), together with the four arts of the quadrivium (arithmetic, geometry, astronomy, and music theory), were indispensable for any advanced study, and much of their relevance to medicine should become evident in these pages. The "liberal arts"—liberal or free in contrast with such utilitarian and vocational arts as agronomy, architecture, and even medicine—supplied the principal constituency as well as the administrative framework of the university. From the 13th century on, the new faculties of medicine attached themselves to this framework, while organizing their own graduate education in their charters. Moreover, the faculty members underscored their academic standing by appropriating the title of "master" (*magister*) from the schools of liberal arts and even, eventually, of "teacher" (*doctor*) from the preeminent graduate disciplines of law and theology.

Medicine by the Book

From the 13th century on, the university teaching of medicine became increasingly structured, with lectures and disputations, curriculums and examinations, degrees and licenses. The elaboration of this structure was both a result of and a stimulus for the idea that the highest learning made the best doctor. University-trained practitioners liked to underscore the contrast with their nonprofessional or "lay" (*laici*) and "unlearned" (*idioti*) counterparts, even though they often admitted adopting folk wisdom, ironically, from illiterate "old wives" (*vetule*) in particular. Literacy, which had long been viewed as one of several assets in medicine, now rose to preeminence as distinguishing the elite healer. This rise dovetailed with the intensifying appreciation of books, which peaked in medieval and Renaissance Europe, and even with the rising reverence for the Bible as *the* "Book" (*biblios*). For a broad perspective, it is helpful to contrast the longtime primacy of the book, in medicine and in general culture, with the mounting dominance of electronic media in the 21st century—when websites serve as libraries, screens count as pages, and terabytes replace aphorisms.

For a growing segment of medieval society, books were valued depositories of information. Many were also precious and precarious objects, and it is sobering to realize how little it took to destroy them and, often with them, the knowledge that had been entrusted to them with uncommon effort and at considerable expense. All books were written by hand (*manu*, hence "manuscripts"). This greatly slowed their production and multiplication until printing began to gain ground late in the 15th century. Since scribes produced manuscripts one at a time, the number of copies of a work was severely limited until schools stimulated the reproduction of texts by teams of scribes in "workshops" (*scriptoria*). The writing materials, parchment or vellum, were laboriously produced from the skins of calves and other animals. As a result, books were expensive commodities, at least until paper became available as an alternative from the 14th century on. Sheets and inks, moreover, while more durable than modern writing materials, were vulnerable to damage and destruction by the elements, animals, and—arguably worst—humans.

Books figure prominently among the treasured possessions of early physicians and among the distinctive attributes of their social status. Thus, in a relief sculpture on a tomb monument from Imperial Rome, a learned practitioner displays his privileged and ample knowledge by reading from a scroll, in front of a cabinet that contains more scrolls; in addition, a kit with surgical instruments atop the cabinet testifies to his practical experience. While instruments remained emblematic of medical practice, books were more often depicted as the tools of elite healers. The depiction of some instruments faded because these, particularly the scalpel, were deemed too reminiscent of manual procedures by cutters, barbers, and bonesetters. Other implements, most notably the urine flask (and, later, the stethoscope), gained visibility because of their dual symbolism: they signified both the active intervention and the privileged knowledge of diagnostics. The book, on the other hand, unequivocally signified that learning was the highest asset, and literacy the minimum qualification, for practicing the Art. The most striking celebration of this idea, and of the vital link between book and bedside, is the "trademark," as we might call it, of one of the greatest medical libraries in the world—and no doubt the most consulted. The National Library of Medicine (NLM) of the United States has chosen an image from a priceless 13th-century manuscript in its collection as the icon for its History of Medicine Division. This choice is especially remarkable if we keep in mind that the NLM, on the campus of the National Institutes of Health in Bethesda, Maryland, is recognized as a leading source of current medical information. In the manuscript illumination, a historiated letter O, the clearly authoritative doctor (whose tonsured head also distinguishes him as a member of the literate clergy) prominently wields a book while telling the bedridden patient what ails him and what is to be expected.

The significance of the book as the mark of a genuine doctor was reinforced by a public awe of letters, words, formulas, and pages, even as tangible objects. This awe was easily exploited by quacks, as we see in a London court case of 1382. On May 13, Roger Clerk was summoned before the mayor and aldermen to answer a charge of "deceit and falsehood." While Clerk "knew nothing" of the Art of medicine "nor understood anything of letters," he had promised to cure Johanna, the ailing wife of Roger atte Hacche. After the latter paid part of the fee in advance, Roger Clerk gave him

> an old parchment, a leaf of some book, and rolled it up in a piece of cloth of gold, asserting that it would be very good for Johanna's fever and ailments; and he put this parchment about her neck, but it did not profit her at all. And so, falsely and maliciously, he deceived Roger atte Hacche, who brought the said parchment here in court, in proof of the said matters.

When the court interrogated Roger Clerk about the virtue of the parchment, he claimed that "upon it was written a good charm for fevers."

Upon examination, however, the parchment contained no such charm. The court reached a firm verdict.

> Whereas this man was in no way literate and altogether ignorant of the art of physic; Whereas the people should not be deceived by such ignorant persons, *etc.* [sic]; It was adjudged that said Roger Clerk should be led through the middle of the City, with trumpets and pipes, riding a horse without a saddle, the parchment being hung about his neck, also with a urinal hanging on his chest and another on his back.

Authors and the Authority of Tradition

For the literate practitioner, the prestige of books was paralleled by the stardom of their writers. The greatest stars were the authors who were seen as heirs to Hippocrates. These authors acquired a status that approached—but upon careful inspection and contrary to some modern critics, did not equal—infallibility. Their teachings made such an impression of learnedness that they exerted the highest authority, sometimes at the expense of observation and reason, the two other pillars of science. Moreover, they were quoted so pervasively, and so often without attribution, that the modern reader can hardly ever be sure that an idea or experience reported in a medieval text originated with its writer. This derivativeness, however, should not lead us to underestimate the originality of the writer's selection, interpretation, and application. In any event, personal observation was likely to yield to traditional authority when an author remembered that Hippocrates himself had called "experience misleading." New reasoning, in addition, might look naive, arrogant, or akin to an attempt to reinvent the wheel, to anyone who revered tradition and was dazzled by the rhetoric of the classic authors.

Geoffrey Chaucer cataloged the most authoritative writers in the late 1300s, when he drew a poetic portrait of the "Doctor of Physic" in his prologue to the *Canterbury Tales*. The most distinctive and detailed feature in this sketch is the physician's familiarity with the voluminous yet standard medical literature of the day.

> Well knew he the old Esculapius,
> And Deiscorides and eek Rufus,
> Old Ypocras, Hali, and Galien,
> Serapion, Razis, and Avicen,
> Averrois, Damascien, and Constantin,
> Bernard, and Gatesden, and Gilbertin.

The 15 authors, whom Chaucer lists with limited regard for chronology, represent four or five major phases in the rise of the Western medical tradition. The phases span more than one-and-a-half millennium, from Classical and Hellenistic Greece (400 BCE–200 CE) to the apex of Islamic culture (900–1100 CE) and to the beginning of Chaucer's own century. His list omits the names of some important ancient authors who had slipped into obscurity by his time, most notably, the Roman encyclopedist Aulus Cornelius Celsus (ca. 25 BCE–ca. 50 CE), whose treatise "On Medicine" (*De Medicina*) encapsulates much of the medical learning that preceded the Common Era. Some of the authors listed by Chaucer will make an appearance in later pages, as historic contributors to one or other subject. Two call for immediate attention, however, namely Galen and Avicenna, both of whom joined "Old Ypocras" as supreme luminaries and, in some ways, came to eclipse him in authority.

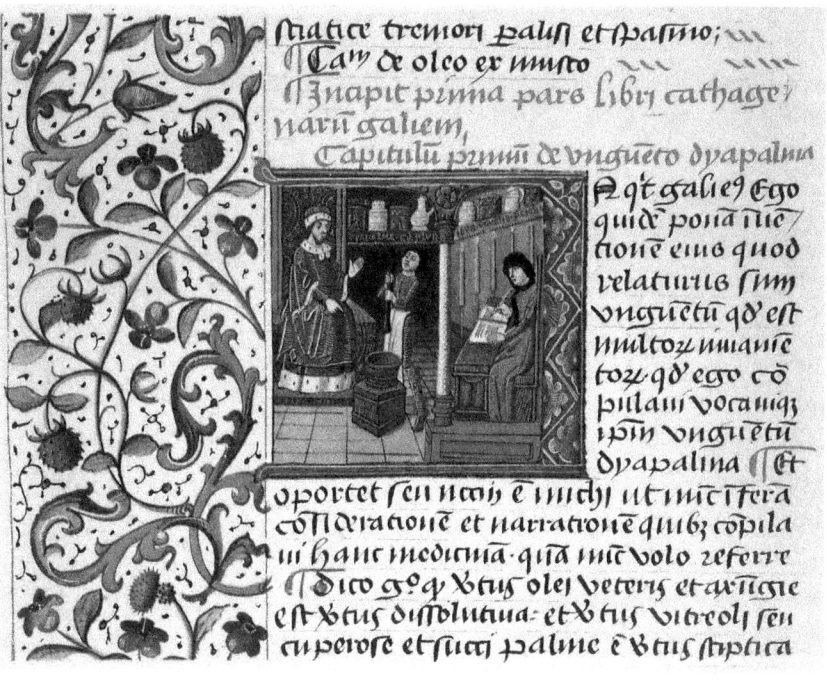

Galen in a magisterial chair, instructs an assistant compounding a medicine, while a scribe records the recipe. Miniature from a 15th-century manuscript (Dresden 37.181) now destroyed, of Galen, *Liber cathagenarum* [on the different kinds of medicines]. (Wellcome Library, London. Wellcome Images L0025921)

No writer projected a more authoritative aura than the Greek physician Galen, who appears as "Galien" in the *Canterbury Tales* and as "the author of truth" in an 11th-century manuscript, well before he reached the pinnacle of his commanding presence. Born and raised in the vibrant city of Pergamum—the origin of the word "parchment"—in Asia Minor, Galen (d. ca. 200 CE) received part of his medical formation in Alexandria, Egypt. The city of Alexandria, the center of Hellenistic culture, served as a crossroads between the predominantly eastern Mediterranean of Greek antiquity and the westward expanding Roman Empire. When Galen settled in Rome, his keen sense of observation, gift for arresting pronouncements, and success in difficult cases gained him a celebrity that he was fond of flaunting to contemporaries and for posterity. His patients included emperors and imperial notables, and he prided himself on his bedside skills, particularly on his extraordinary diagnostic discernment. He frequently sparred with colleagues and eagerly criticized the opinions of predecessors.

With a demonstrative flourish steeped in the art of rhetoric, Galen documented much of his discourse, even his most theoretical theses, with personal anecdotes. Equally well versed in Greek philosophy and in accumulated medical lore, he was a prolific writer on a wide variety of subjects, ranging from anatomy to therapeutics. He composed commentaries on the *Aphorisms* and other principal Hippocratic texts. Among Galen's many seminal works, one stands out because it became familiar to countless generations of physicians. His *Technē iatrikē*, or "The Medical Art," acquired the title *Tegni* (a transliteration of the Greek term *technē*) when it entered Latin medical literature. This title mutated, in turn, into *Microtegni* or "The Little Art," in order to avoid confusion with a larger (*macro-* or, as we will see, *mega-*) composition. The transformation continued when the work served as the basic textbook for medical students, under the title of *Ars parva*. In a long-range consequence of this metamorphosis, by the 13th century, the core readings of the syllabus became collectively known as "the little art" or *Articella*.

Connecting with the Textual Tradition

More than a thousand years passed between Galen and the development of a medical syllabus around his teachings. It took a long time for most of his works to find their way into the Western regions of the declining Roman Empire, where levels of literacy were uneven, centers of learning sporadic, and the classical legacy largely confined to monasteries. On the southern and eastern shores of the Mediterranean, by contrast, Greek civilization endured in a wide area, long after the conquests of Alexander the Great (356–323 BCE) and in spite of—or, rather, favored by—the subjugation of Asia Minor by Rome. The sway of Hellenistic culture fostered the dissemination of Hippocratic–Galenic medicine eastward, across Syria and Mesopotamia, and across regions as diverse as Byzantium and Egypt. Scholars from various places flocked to Alexandria to advance themselves in disciplines as varied as rhetoric and philosophy, which formed the background for the study of medicine. In this study, reverence for the book was matched by a curiosity about the body that manifested itself in dissections—to the disapproval of the Christian philosopher Augustine of Hippo (354–430 CE).

For a long time after Galen's prolific career, writers in the Eastern Roman Empire, and in Alexandria in particular, endeavored to preserve and pass on the medical writings bequeathed by antiquity. The available material was already considerable, as we may gather from the dual approach of the imperial physician Oribasius, who was probably born in Pergamum around 325. First, when Emperor Julian ordered him to assemble the existing texts, he compiled an anthology (*Synagogae* or *Collecta*) of the most important ones, rather than attempting to capture everything. In a second undertaking that suggests a relative abundance of material, Oribasius presented his son Eustachius with a summary (*Synopsis*). In the sixth and seventh centuries, Byzantine authors and alumni of Alexandrian schools produced several multivolume compilations, from the *Tetrabiblos* in four "books drawn from the Ancient Masters of Medicine" by Aetius of Amida to "Twelve Books on the Subject of Medicine" by Alexander of Tralles.

In the second century, when Galen moved from Alexandria to Rome, he attested to the unity of the Mediterranean world and to the continuing magnetism of the Eternal City. Political imbalances and cultural divisions, however, were permanent threats to the empire. Soon, growing alienation from old Rome opened the provinces to initially very different cultures. Two centuries after migrations of unshaven barbarians ended Roman control over the Western provinces, Muslims swept from the Arabian Peninsula into the Eastern territories. In little more than a decade after the death of the Prophet Muhammad (632 CE), caliphs conquered a large portion of the former empire. By the mid-eighth century, Islam ruled from the Indus to the Pyrenees. After initial hesitation, the conquerors adopted much of the Hellenized culture, which they then adapted, cultivated, and disseminated. By 1000 CE, the study and practice of medicine flourished, together with the creative arts, successively in the new capitals of Damascus, Baghdad, and Córdoba. Medicine and other branches of learning continued to thrive in the venerable centers of Alexandria and Gundishapur. Scholars expanded the influence of Gundishapur, in the Persian province of Khuzestan, when they codified Arabic grammar in the mid-ninth century.

Persia was the home of several authors of encyclopedic works on medicine in Arabic. The author who gained the most widespread and durable fame was Abu Ali al-Husayn ibn Abd Allah ibn Sina (980–1037). Claimed by modern Uzbeks as the greatest sage in their history, ibn Sina became known in the Latin West as Avicenna. From his youth, he dazzled the fabled courts of Samarkhand, Astrakhan, and Isfahan with his medical skills and intellectual acumen. The Persian tale of King Bedreddin, which originated in the era and milieu of "A Thousand and One Nights," eternalized him as having a perfect knowledge of all the secrets of nature. Ibn Sina might not have become so celebrated if he had lived in another place or age, which might not have tolerated his disregard of Muslim orthodoxy: he denied life after death, for example, and he prescribed drunkenness as therapeutic. His chief contributions lay in the elucidation of Aristotelian philosophy and the organization of Galenic medicine. He was a true polymath, however, who held forth on areas from astronomy to zoology. This range earned him a place in the First Circle of Dante's *Inferno* (IV.143), among The Great Pagans.

By the wide sweep of his learning, Avicenna emulated and surpassed a Persian predecessor named Muhammad ibn Zakariya ar-Razi (865–925). Ar-Razi, whom Latins called "Rhazes" or "Rasis"—and Chaucer "Razes"—attempted to summarize all medical knowledge in a nine-part book, which he dedicated to Prince Abu Salih al-Mansur ibn Ishaq. In addition, he left copious notes, which were bundled as *al-Hawi* or "the comprehensive book." By the standards of Avicenna, however, Rhazes's "Book for al-Mansur" (Latinized as *Liber ad Almansorem*) was too basic, and his "Comprehensive Book" (*Liber continens*) too disorganized. In the 1020s, Avicenna set out to assemble fundamental theories, practical guidelines, personal observations, and pharmaceutical information in a true medical encyclopedia. In a massive volume, titled *Al-Qanun fi 'l-Tibb,* he compiled and arranged the entire canon of the subject matter, which had grown rather chaotically around the Hippocratic corpus and the writings of Galen. The compilation, which incorporated not only Greco-Roman and Arabic-Persian but also Far Eastern teachings, is the basis of Unani healing as it is still taught in Indian medical colleges. Gerard of Cremona (d. 1187) and his associates translated the *Canon of Medicine* into Latin in the 12th century, and it became the most widely consulted medical encyclopedia in Christendom. "Avicen," as Chaucer called him, joined Hippocrates and Galen in the trinity that governed the first medical curriculum. It took more than one-and-a-half century, however, for Avicenna to reach this status in European schools.

Between Avicenna's career and his entry into Europe lay a momentous period of intensifying relations between East and West, and of shifting geographical balances around the Mediterranean. After 1100, ibn Zuhr (Avenzoar, 1091–1161) and his disciple ibn Rushd (Averroes, 1126–1198) still personified the dynamism of Arabic science, but their roots—and those of the great Rabbi Moshe (Maimonides, 1135–1204)—were in Córdoba rather than in Baghdad. Well before 1100, Europe manifested a surge in energy, inquisitiveness, and extroversion. The most notorious manifestation came with the Crusades. Less aggressive and more fruitful contacts, in Sicily, southern Italy, and the Iberian Peninsula, revealed the cultural splendor of the world of Islam. Latin scholars, keenly aware of the riches that lay waiting in Arabic, created an insistent demand for translations. In addressing this demand, no figure was more pivotal than a merchant who was probably born in the North African intellectual center of Kairouan (near modern Tunis) around 1020 and who entered history as Constantinus Africanus (Chaucer's "Constantin"). He gained the friendship of two leading churchmen. One of them was Desiderius, the abbot of Monte Cassino, which was the heart of Benedictine monasticism; the other, Alfanus, was the archbishop of Salerno, Italy, which was the flourishing commercial and health center southeast of Naples, Italy. At the request of these friends, Constantine brought a load of books across the Mediterranean. In response to the interest shown by practitioners and teachers in Salerno, he made at least three dozen Arabic books available in Latin translations or arrangements before his death, as a monk at Monte Cassino, in 1087.

Constantine the African's single most significant contribution was his interpretation of a work by the 10th-century author Ali Ibn al-Abbas al-Majusi, because it gave Christendom the first comprehensive view of medicine in Islam—and of the Greek legacy embedded in Arabic writings. In "The Complete Book of the Medical Art," the Persian physician whom Latins called Haly Abbas (and whom Chaucer inserted as "Hali" between Hippocrates and Galen) compiled information from more than a hundred sources. In 10 tractates on theory and 10 on practice, he covered the material more systematically than Rhazes and less speculatively than Avicenna. This made for an authoritative encyclopedia that became known as "the complete art" (*Pantegni*), when Constantine presented his very free and, ironically, incomplete adaptation. A second and more faithful Latin version appeared 40 years later, with the title *Liber regalis dispositionis* or "The Book of Royal Discourse" because the original had been dedicated to an emir. It is worth mentioning that the translator of this version, Stephen of Antioch, lived successively in Pisa, Salerno (both in Italy), and Syria, thus personifying the fruitful interaction around the Mediterranean.

Constantine contributed interpretations of three other texts that became a staple of the medieval curriculum. He made a summary of Galen's "Method of Healing" (*Medendi methodus*) available in the *Megategni*, the third work we encounter with "tegni" in the title. While in this work Constantine laid out procedural principles, he offered more directly practical advice in the *Viaticum* that, while an adaptation of the "Provisions for the Traveler and Nourishment for the Sedentary," by Ibn al-Jazzar (d. 980; a student of Haly Abbas), was often attributed to Isaac Judeus (a.k.a. Ysaac or Isaac Israeli, ca. 832—ca. 932). A third arrangement by Constantine was appropriately called "Introduction" (*Isagoge*) because it purportedly introduced the novice to Galen's *Tegni*. It was actually excerpted from the "Questions on Medicine" by Hunayn ibn Ishaq, a ninth-century Assyrian scholar whom Latin scribes named Johannitius. The *Isagoge Ioannitii*, a concise text on fundamental categories, became the standard primer in medical education. It was an ideal pedagogical tool because it condensed more than a millennium of teaching into relatively few pages, which were composed in question-and-answer format. The text enjoyed a special prestige beyond its scholastic usefulness, as we may gather from some copies that were produced with unusual care. One of these copies is part of the exquisitely illuminated 13th-century *Articella* manuscript from Oxford, from which the NLM adopted its logo, as we have seen. In the same manuscript, a historiated initial M graces the beginning of the *Ysagoge iohannicii id est introductiones*. The illustration on p. 14 shows a bearded and tonsured master pointing at a passage in the book from which he is lecturing to a young student. The obviously awed student, also tonsured, is holding a book or, more likely, wax tablets for taking notes. The reverential illumination reflects the special place that the *Isagoge Ioannitii* occupies in the history of medicine. For centuries, the *Isagoge* guided the initiation of students into an awe-inspiring art and science, through successive waves of accumulating information.

The Structure of Learning as Foundation of Practice

The *incipit* or opening sentence of the *Isagoge Ioannitii,* "Medicina dividitur in duas partes, id est, in theoricam et practicam," was copied with special care in such *Articella* manuscripts as the one with the initial M in the following illustration. Though less seminal than the famous first Hippocratic *Aphorism,* the *Isagoge* was hardly less consequential. The maxim, "Medicine is divided in two parts, that is, theoretical and practical," firmly established the twin pillars of teaching when faculties of medicine began to organize in the 12th century. By accurately recognizing the adjectives, *theorica* (not to be confused with *theoria,* the noun for "theory") and *practica,* we should avoid the impression that the statement demonstrates the dichotomy between theory and practice that is often seen as the greatest fault of all Scholasticism. This was, rather, a primary division of medical science that, in the *Isagoge* and many other sources, branched out into a logical framework for the curriculum. The celebrated Catalan physician Arnau de Vilanova (1235–1311) demonstrated the inherent practical thrust of theoretical foundations in his "Mirror (*Speculum*) of Medicine," a lucid synopsis of *theorica.* These foundations comprised the naturals, contra-naturals, and nonnaturals—three categories that will be explained anon. Instruction in *practica* covered the three phases of treatment, namely, dietary, medicinal, and surgical. The authors of the most widely used manuals organized their material on the same didactic framework.

The naturals in the first category of theoretical medicine were the essential components and factors of life, health, and disease. Knowledge of these was fundamental to the physician's practice as well as to the student's learning. The link between medicine and traditional natural philosophy or *physica* is evident in the presence of the elements, qualities, and humors. The four other naturals are associated with anatomy and, more predominantly, with Galenic physiology. Anatomical aspects were relatively underrepresented and, in a sense, almost limited to abstractions until dissection began to play a greater role in medical education in the 14th century. Even then, and well into modern times, didactic anatomy tended to concentrate on the skeleton rather than on perishable flesh and unsightly organs, and on the structure of the human body rather than on the complex operations inside.

Scholastic anatomy was deeply rooted in Aristotle, particularly in the metaphysics of potency and act, the ontology of matter and form, and the natural philosophy of elements and qualities. At best, it incorporated

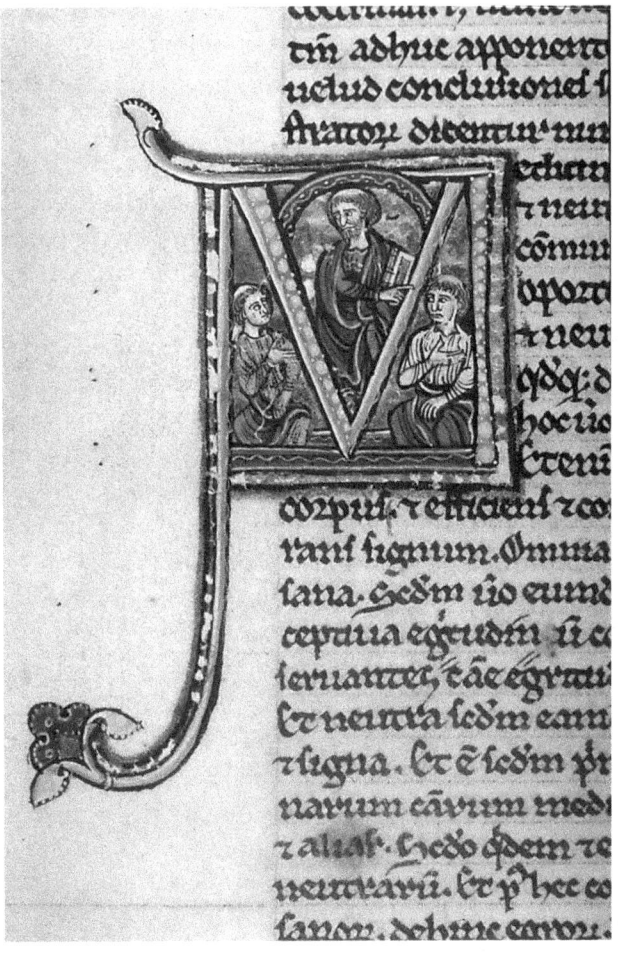

Theory and Practice: A Master of Medicine, holding a book, points from a student (left) to a patient (right). Initial "M" (for *Medicina*) in a manuscript of *Isagoge Johannitii*, written in Oxford, 13th century. (National Library of Medicine, MS 78, fol.61v. Images from the History of Medicine, # A027137)

insights that Aristotle, Galen, and some other authors had drawn from observing human corpses and from comparing human and animal anatomies. In the setting of the medieval classroom, anatomy was subservient to physiology. *Anatomia* referred less to the human anatomy than to a didactic demonstration, less to a physical activity than to a mental exercise (as in the cognate Greek term, "analysis"), and less to the cutting apart than to the logical division of the body. The organs appeared less as objects of examination than as conceptual entities, which could be represented schematically. They were viewed as mere instruments of the humors, faculties, and spirits. Hence, familiarity with the shape and substance of the organs was less important than an understanding of their functions in the larger scheme of nature.

Nature and the Naturals

Ever since late antiquity, the physician was characterized as "the servant of nature" (*minister naturae*). In the compound tradition of Hippocratic healing, Aristotelian philosophy, and Galenic rhetoric, nature (Latin *Natura*, Greek *physis*) was enthroned as the source of life, the measure of health, and the key to understanding. The concept injected an element of personification into the term that denoted, simply and universally, the way everything is made or born (*natus*), grows, and functions. Close to being deified, nature was considered intelligent, purposeful, almost omnipresent (with allowance for the realm of the supernatural), and near-perfect (with allowance for such errors of nature as certain birth defects). Today's yearning for things organic, together with alarm about tensions between mankind and the environment, may help us to appreciate the holistic outlook of earlier times. Everything, including the human body, was connected in the vastness of the universe and in the cycle of life. Awareness of the connection was—and, in large areas of today's world, remains—intensified by dependence on the weather, limited options for shelter and clothing, lack of reliable forecasts, narrow geographical and cultural horizons, and so on. This awareness inspired the Hippocratic insistence that the healer must consider not only the seasonal and regional setting of each case, but also the influences of the moon, planets, and stars.

The macrocosm of universal nature was reflected in the microcosm of the body. Physicians treated health as the natural human condition. They were largely silent, it may be noted, on any radical alienation between humanity and nature. This silence stands in contrast with the position of theologians who blamed illness on original sin—after all, the doctor's "study was but litel on the Bible" according to Chaucer. Doctors defined the natural human condition of health as an internal equilibrium and harmony with the environment. The most basic criterion was a balanced distribution and interaction of the four primary qualities, namely, dry, moist, cold, and warm. The role of these qualities overshadowed that of the elements to which they corresponded, namely, earth, water, air, and fire. While the four elements answered an ancient quest for the constituents of living matter, the primary qualities were more in tune with questions about human life and death. Much of medical rationalization was qualitative, showing markedly greater interest in the condition ("how?") and the purpose ("why?") of bodies and phenomena than in their composition ("what?") or quantity ("how much?").

Nature's timeless and beneficial purpose determined the shape and function—the "usefulness," in Galen's term—of the healthy body and every part. Teleology, the belief that everything has a preordained goal, may be characterized as the reverse of adaptive evolution. Thus Galen, building on Aristotle, rejected and inverted the proposition that hands played a role in the development of human intelligence: invoking Aristotle, he argued that, since humans are the most intelligent of animals and since hands best serve intelligent beings, they were given hands as instruments of their intelligence. A vertical perspective of individuality matched this horizontal perspective of teleology. The mixture and proportion of qualities accounted for the makeup or complexion of each person and, in fact, of almost everything. The natural complexion of an infant, for instance, was moist and warm; pepper, understandably, was of a hot and dry complexion; the moon was cold and moist, which may seem surprising until one thinks of the lunar influence on ocean tides. In sum, many daily observations seemingly confirmed the pairing of primary qualities—even if Hippocrates deemed "experience misleading." The scheme of complexions brought order into complex natural phenomena, as the Ptolemaic system did for the heavens. Both constructs, however, required further adjustments and elaborations.

The elements took organic form and the qualities materialized in the humors. Four humors constituted the living body, and each incorporated a distinct combination of primary qualities. Air prevailed in the blood that, as the essential vital constituent, was warm and moist, the ideal qualities for life. Fire resided, in some form, in the warm (or hot) and dry yellow or red bile, which was also known as choler. The two opposite humors are more difficult to recognize from a modern angle. Phlegm, cold and moist, was a watery and mucous substance, which we might visualize as similar to the slime of uncooked okra. Melancholy or black bile, while the most difficult to associate with a concrete matter (except, perhaps, congealed blood), was also most often blamed for health problems and, being cold and dry, associated with the qualities most antagonistic to life.

The prominence of blood and bile may lead us to think of humors as liquids in a literal sense, unless we keep in mind their role as explanatory devices rather than tangible objects of examination. Their definitions, like those of the four elements and four qualities, were to some extent more impressionistic than precise (compare the five elements of Chinese tradition). In a further elaboration of the fourfold construct, the character and movement of each humor responds to a different quadrant of the heavens and to a different purpose of nature's ingenuity. Blood, for example, follows the course of the sun, while it is also moved by nature in the morning so that, produced mostly at night, it may not be tainted by fumes. Phlegm, by contrast, is more in tune with lunar cycles, and nature stirs it in the afternoon so that its superfluities may be purged before night. It is ironic that phlegm, while the least productive humor, was differentiated into four varieties, of which two (the sweet and bitter) were mentioned less often than the thick or "glassy" (*vitreum*) and the "salty" (*salsum*). The latter, which was commonly associated with arthritic miseries, resulted when excessive warmth dried the naturally cold and moist phlegm and left a salty residue, in analogy with seawater.

The prevalence of one or other humor and its respective qualities shaped the emotional bent of one's individual mix or temperament (it is worth noting, at the risk of confusion, that the Latin words *temperamentum* and *complexio* both succeeded the original Greek term for "mixture," namely, *krasis*). Thus, a person with an abundance of blood (*sanguis*), such as an average young man, would by nature have a sanguine or lively and optimistic disposition; the opposite character, with much black bile, would be melancholic or inclined to dark and earthbound depression. Yellow bile made for a choleric or hot-tempered disposition; a polar opposite was the phlegmatic character, which naturally tended toward sluggishness (still reflected in the French expression *j'ai la flemme*)—and which was assigned, stereotypically and with far-reaching implications, to woman.

The combined effects of the humors determined the working of the bodily organs. Each of the organs, in turn, produced one of the humors, in a process that should not be understood too mechanically. The liver produced blood, the gall bladder yellow bile, the spleen black bile, and the brain phlegm—the latter is only mildly surprising if we think of a runny nose. In a less cyclical presentation of the relation between humors and organs, the former were the carriers, and the latter the instruments, of natural forces and faculties that sustained and reproduced life. It is easy to anticipate that these representations required a certain haziness and tolerance of inconsistencies. The spleen, for example, was presented both as the source of melancholy *and* as the agent of laughter. It should be emphasized that the organs were subservient to the humoral complexion. In a wider framework, their role was secondary to the *ingenium Naturae,* that is, the "ingenuity" and "engineering" of nature. Therefore, curiosity in the exact function and anatomy of the organs tended to be blunted by reliance on schematic representations.

In a scheme that grew out of Galen's ideas, the processes of life were understood as forms of slow combustion. In the most basic process, life itself was imagined as the burning of an inborn flame or natural heat. The flame steadily consumed an essential fuel, the radical moisture. The combustion could continue as long as the interaction between heat and moisture remained balanced, avoiding the extremes of burned incineration and drowned suffocation. This interplay was conventionally compared, perhaps even before Galen, with the steady consumption of the oil and lighted wick in a lamp. In this case and others, analogy supplied explanations that made systematic investigation less urgent. Analogies, furthermore, allowed for interpretations that were flexible rather than ironclad and imaginative rather than mechanistic. Nevertheless, even though the interpretations may seem strange—or "bizarre," the favorite adjective of some would-be historians—to another age, the inquiry should be distinguished from unscientific superstition, for it was based on observation and reason. The same caution applies to the realm of more perceivable functions, where life was envisioned as a continued and slow cooking in which the humors were maintained and replenished through three stages of nutrition.

Galen constructed a dynamic image of human life as a digestive process, in which consumed food became bodily substance. The construct was generally adopted by successive authors but modified and cast into an almost dogmatic model by Avicenna. In this physiology, food was digested in the tube between mouth and anus, but primarily in the stomach, which was surrounded and warmed by the lobes of the liver (conventionally five, as Galen had observed in dissections of dogs). Chyle, the product of this first digestion, was sometimes viewed as the initial life-giving moisture and metaphorically characterized as "dew" (*ros*). This moisture proceeded to the liver by way of the portal vein, while useless "windiness" (*ventositas*) and indigestible "dregs" (*faeces*) were expelled—joined, on the way, by impurities of the subsequent digestions. A second digestion took place in the moist and warm liver, which was the center of the nourishment for the entire body. Assisted by the gall bladder and the spleen, the liver produced not only blood, but also choler and black bile, which kept blood from stagnating or inflaming. Venal blood was distributed to the body, but its crucial route was to the right ventricle of the heart, from where it flowed, supposedly through pores, to the left ventricle where it was heated. Part of the venal blood also ran through the pulmonary artery to the lung, which in a dual operation carried off the fumes produced by the heat and drew in new air. From the left ventricle and through the aorta, the now vitalized and arterial blood was distributed through the body and kept from overheating by a contracting and dilating pulsation. This blood, together with the other humors that it carried, nourished the body's parts and periphery by entering all the nooks and crannies, like some paste or loosely woven "tissue" (*cambium*).

The last and most critical stage in the maintenance of life—and one of the theoretical subjects that proved difficult to grasp by authors of manuals and even of specialized treatises—was the third digestion. In this stage, the product of the second digestion became the bond or "glue" (*glutinum*), which held the entire organism together. In a somewhat variant account, the ultimately digested moisture actually changed into the substance of each part of the body (a parallel in natural philosophy to the theological doctrine of transubstantiation, the change of the eucharistic bread and wine into the flesh and blood of Christ). According to yet another scheme, the final product of the digestion was identical to the radical moisture, on which life depended as we have seen. In a puzzling corollary, the by-products of the third digestion reveal the potential for opacity, inconsistency, and misunderstanding. When authors proposed that superfluities were expelled as sweat and skin flakes, they did not clarify the relation with other expulsions. With more intriguing implications, some suggested that sperm was one of the ultimate superfluities, while others taught that seminal material was the residue of the *cambium* after it had nourished the body.

The details on the maintenance of human life may strike the modern reader as esoteric. They are indispensable, however, for understanding the foundation on which all the teaching in the manuals rested. They also help us appreciate the truly revolutionary nature and far-reaching consequences of Harvey's discovery of the circulatory system in the 17th century, after medicine had been locked into a linear vision for more than two millennia. In this vision, which was geared more to conceptual schemes than to precise perception, the heart was both less and more than a pump, let alone, a muscle. The organ received comparatively little attention in medieval physiology and anatomy, even though it was assigned the life-sustaining function of infusing natural warmth. There was much debate, on the other hand, whether the seat of human nature was the heart, as Aristotle proposed, or the brain, as Galen taught. Assigning supremacy to the heart or to the brain was of greater relevance to the philosophers and theologians who wanted to locate the soul, than to the doctors who sought to understand the human body. Physicians circumvented the issue, to some extent by distributing critical roles among factors that were less material, as they attributed organic developments to the design of nature. They incorporated the Greek notions, Arabic elaborations, and Latin interpretations of *physica* on which much of Scholastic philosophy was built. Medical explanations of human life, and of bodily functions and conditions, revolved around invisible agents or faculties.

The most critical faculty was *spiritus*. This Latin term referred, like the Greek *pneuma*, not only to spirit—which was very subtle though not entirely immaterial—but also to the air that surrounds us and that we inhale in respiration for the second digestion as described earlier. Beyond the literal meaning, *pneuma* signifies a wide range of power, of the wind filling the sails of ancient ships, of the Trinity in Orthodox Christianity, and of the compressed air driving the modern pneumatic drill or jackhammer. *Spiritus* propelled the essential actions of the body in three forms, each with a seat in one of the noble organs. The vital spirit, which maintained life itself (*vita*), was derived from the air drawn in by the lungs, refined by the inner heat of the heart and blood, and distributed through the arteries. This spirit also nourished the brain, enabling it to produce the animal spirit, the source of the *anima* or soul, that is, the animation or autonomic movement and the sensation that animals have in common. On the lowest level, the natural spirit, residing in the liver and veins and carried through the body by the venal blood, was the driving force in *natura*, the vegetative operations of nutrition, growth, and reproduction (note the shared root of "nativity" and "nature").

Other sets of faculties controlled more specific operations. Among the latter, nutritional digestion was discussed in the greatest detail. The dynamic agency of a different power or virtue (*virtus, vis, dunamis*) governed each phase of the process, beyond the activity of any digesting organ. An attractive power within the body drew the food inward; the retentive power kept it from escaping, not only down but also up—which is why, as one author explained, people did not regurgitate when they were hung by their feet; the digestive faculty regulated the cooking, while the expulsive faculty assured the disposal of superfluities and waste. In a variation on this Galenic scheme, nutrition involved three more subtle stages and respective faculties, after attraction. The disseminative faculty guided the distribution of the food throughout the body, the unificative the absorption into every part, and the assimilative or mutative the full transformation into the body's substance. In sum, physiology left no doubt that health, while natural, was precarious. It also facilitated an understanding of diseases as contrary to the body's delicate balances, complex processes, and mysterious faculties.

Diseases: Against Nature?

Disease in general was characterized as "against nature" (*contra naturam*) or "outside nature" (*preter naturam*). The understanding of disease and the knowledge of diseases occupied the second branch of *medicina theorica,* playing a role that is remotely analogous to that of today's pathology and nosology. The modern and premodern approaches share an emphasis on precise nomenclature, consistent explanation, and orderly taxonomy. There is a striking contrast, however, between modern reliance on empirical data and the medieval endeavor to anchor knowledge in logical definitions, divisions, and distinctions. Disease was defined and explained as an imbalance of the humors, a bad complexion, or a faulty temperament (*discrasia*) that, in turn, was due to the insufficiency or failure of one or more of the spirits or faculties. It was understood more as a condition than as an event. Unlike the ontological view of scientists who, since the 19th century, have approached every disease as an entity in itself, medieval physicians explained a disease as a quality of the patient.

Qualitative views shaped the criteria for defining each malady, distinguishing different forms or types, and correlating it with other diseases. While the definition of a particular disease might imply various processes and immediate causes, it was ultimately framed in terms of a humoral imbalance. In the framework of rationalist medicine, etiology stood at the center of teaching and of learned medicine. As Chaucer characterized the ideal physician,

> He knew the cause of every maladye,
> Were it of hot or cold, or moist or drye,
> And where engendred and of what humour,
> He was a veray parfit practisour.
> The cause y-know, and of his harm the roote.

Chaucer's focus on the knowledge of causes attests to the victory, not necessarily predictable, of one of several trends among medical authors since antiquity. Three major trends or sects were remembered as Empiricists, Methodists, and Rationalists. Empiricists emphasized observation and prompt intervention, and they professed impatience with attempts to find hidden causes. Methodists devoted themselves to the "technique" of therapeutic procedures, for which they did not consider theory helpful. Rationalists insisted that the Art transcended skillful healing and that all treatment needed to be based on understanding. Their adherence to a set of taught principles (*doctrina* or *dogma*) sometimes accounted for a negative innuendo in their alternate identification as Dogmatists—or in the application of the label "scholastic" to medieval medicine. By late antiquity, medical rationalism emerged as the dominant school. Adherents found their greatest champion in Galen, a receptive audience in the university faculties, and their most eager clientele among patients who admired learned practitioners—and could afford their services. The university-trained doctor was expected to treat most effectively because he was able to justify, whereas treatment by the lay healer was unexplained, erratic, and unreliable. The most solid justification rested on the knowledge of the causes, without which patient care was necessarily superficial—and, literally, casual—since it proceeded case by case.

Doctors differentiated the "roots" of diseases, with great vigor, as primary and secondary causes, extraneous and internal, efficient and final, and a variety of lesser categories. The conceptual and deliberative tendency of this differentiation was overshadowed by the practical and immediate need to identify the disease from distinctive signs and concomitant phenomena or symptoms (*accidencia*). The very first step in the process was taking the patient's history. In the subsequent diagnosis, the practitioner began with a visual and tactile examination and proceeded to taking the pulse and inspecting the urine (uroscopy) and, less routinely, drawn blood. The recognition of a defined disease through clear signs allowed the doctor to foresee the further course and to order the appropriate treatment. In addition, it might allow the doctor to solemnly predict the likely outcome, to the benefit not only of the patients and their family but also of the doctor's credibility and even status.

In the Hippocratic–Galenic tradition, nothing defined the true physician as much as the art and science of prognosticating or, at least, the privilege of foreknowledge or "pro-gnosis." The concern with knowing the past and the future of an illness may be contrasted with the modern doctor's concentration on the moment. Be that as it may, the chronological breadth of vision dovetailed with the holistic belief in correspondence between the course of life and the predictable regularity of the heavens. This belief favored the inclusion of lunar and planetary astronomy in teaching, particularly of prognostication, and in the image of the learned practitioner as astrologer. Chaucer's doctor excelled in his knowledge of medicine *because* "he was grounded in astronomy" and he was able to cast horoscopes by figures of the zodiac:

> Well coud he fortunen the ascendent
> Of his images for his pacient.

This vignette, with the learned doctor attending to the patient, reminds us that diagnosis and prognostication belonged as much to *medicina practica* as to *theorica*. The two branches of teaching overlapped most, however, on the level of dietary medicine or the six nonnaturals. This category, a bridge between knowledge and action, was the part of *theorica* that was closest to everyday life and, at the same time, the part of *practica* that was most ideological.

Diet or Regimen: The Management of the Nonnaturals

The term *res non naturales* should not be misunderstood. Particularly the English translation, as the nonnaturals, may give the impression that the factors in this category were disparaged as not natural or, at least, not essential. Rather, they were called nonnatural only in distinction with the natural components, functions, and faculties; they were viewed as more individual, more circumstantial, and less universal than the naturals. They were, however, emphasized as natural and essential factors in health and disease. The holistic Hippocratic tradition revolved around the physician's duty to take these factors into account for every patient. Their importance in treating disease was surpassed only by their significance in prevention and, most broadly, in the maintenance of health. This significance gave the nonnaturals their own status, as the foundations of a healthy lifestyle and environment. They were the subject of separate compendia, with such titles as "The Governance of Health" (*Regimen sanitatis*) or "The Preservation of Health" (*Conservatio sanitatis*), which might be compared with today's publications on wellness. Regimens were adapted to individual patients or patrons in written consultations (*consilia*). Hippocrates, Galen, and Avicenna each bequeathed a compendium on dietetics. It was natural for compilers of practical manuals to refer the reader to a *Regimen* while abridging the coverage of dietetics in their pages on therapeutics. It is fair to surmise that the abridgment was, at least in part, indicative of an ever-growing shift from conservative to more aggressive medicine.

The inertia of tradition, on the other hand, caused the category of dietetics to become formulaic, with the nonnatural factors standardized as six in number—which included several pairs. The first factor was the air around us, which both sustained and transcended human life. Discussion of this factor naturally entailed considerations of airborne illnesses, seasonal and climatic changes, physical and social environments, and occasionally even of air pollution—for example, with regard to campsites for armies, or the proximity of tanners to towns. Food and drink constituted the second factor but usually, and not surprisingly, drew the greatest attention. The golden rule, hallowed by the Hippocratic tradition, was to maintain moderation, to avoid all excess, and to balance nutritional value with ease of digestion. As a paragon of professional virtue, Chaucer's *parfit practisour* observed the following rule:

Of his diete mesurable was he,
For it was of no superfluitee
But of greet norishing and digestible.

The remaining nonnaturals, which constituted the essence of lifestyle, were sleep and wakefulness; rest and motion or exercise; fullness or retention and evacuation; and "things that happen to the soul" (*accidencia anime*) or emotions. The emotions became as standardized as the nonnaturals, into a limited range of stereotypical responses (anger, sadness, fear), which could readily be linked to a humoral temperament. Except for air and food and drink, the nonnaturals were not always clearly distinct. For example, insomnia overlapped with restlessness and sorrow among the causes of illness. In the most striking manifestation of indistinctness, some authors wondered whether sexual activity ought to be included among the nonnaturals and, if so, under exercise, evacuation, or emotions. In any event, compilers of manuals deemed lifestyle so variable from patient to patient that they usually left the consideration of these nonnaturals to the wit and responsibility of the practitioner, not only in guiding dietetics but also in devising treatment.

In manuals and courses, *practica* was devoted to therapeutics, although it also bore on diagnosis and prognostication as we have seen. The treatment of any disease was supposed to follow the conservative tradition of first addressing the management of the nonnaturals, proceeding to medications, and then adding manual ministrations. Authors, from Hippocrates on, repeatedly emphasized this sequence, but their emphasis risked being overruled by historical developments. An ever-growing interest and trade in drugs—of which quite a few doubled as spices and thus fell under dietetics—easily eclipsed the daily routine of the regimen.

Chaucer's physician, for one, was distinguished by his mutually profitable affiliation with pharmacists and by his readiness to "give the sick man his cure" with medications:

> Anon he yaf the sike man his boote.
> Full redy had he his apothecaries
> To send him drugges and his letuaries
> For ech of hem made other for to winne;
> Hir frendship was not newe to beginne.

Drugges represented simples or ingredients for preparing medicines. Many of these ingredients occurred in culinary recipes as well as in materia medica, as the groundbreaking scholarship of Linda Ehrsam Voigts continues to reveal. *Drugges* were produced by diverse processes, primarily from an immense variety of plants that ranged from the lowly onion (*allium cepa*) to precious ginger (*zinziber*). Simples were also minerals, as base as lead or as precious as gold; others were derived from animals, such as beeswax or chicken fat. *Letuaries* or electuaries (from the Greek word for "licking") were a particularly popular form of compounds, in which various ingredients were mixed, sweetened with sugar or honey, and made into a paste for taking by mouth. The majority of medicines (later called "allopathic") were intended to counteract the antinatural effects of a disease, for example, by cooling an inflammation; a few (later called homeopathic) were supposed to cure like with like, as viper meat for the treatment of poisoning.

Many simples, from ambergris (biliary secretion of the sperm whale) to zedoary (a relative of turmeric), were especially appreciated because they were exotic and expensive. This was true, above all, for gold, which was preferred for any heart medicine (cordial), and which seems to have been an effective placebo for the patient and, even more, a welcome tonic for the physician—as Chaucer observed with a wink:

> For gold in physic is a cordial
> Therefore he loved gold in special.

Physicians and, presumably, patients were most fascinated by substances with one or other "specific" and "occult" virtue that could not be readily explained by their elementary qualities (hot, dry, and so on) or obvious effects (softening, purgative, and so on). Some healing powers were explained by such other qualities as the utter perfection of mother's milk for a host of ailments; some were attributed to the similarity of a plant to an organ, as in the case of liverwort; and others were derived from association, for example, when the brains of apparently frisky sparrows were used in aphrodisiacs.

The growing appeal of pharmaceutics was not the only trend to challenge the long-standing primacy of the regimen. A parallel development was the assertive rise of learned surgery. Much of "surgery" (*chirurgia*) was traditionally limited to manual ministrations, from such mild ones as cupping to the more traumatic application of hot iron or a caustic agent in cautery (somewhat different in meaning from today's procedure), and to the most drastic yet ubiquitous drawing of blood by cutting a vein (venesection, phlebotomy). Until at least the early Middle Ages, the most advanced surgery was not aggressive but restorative, as it lay in the setting of fractures and dislocations and the suturing of wounds. Incisions were by necessity external, primarily to remove growths, with such rare and notable exceptions as the removal of bladder stone (lithotomy). A new confidence in surgery was promoted by various influences. One of these was the renown of physician Abu al-Qasim Khalaf Ibn al-Abbas Al-Zahrawi (936–1013) of Córdoba, who became known in Christendom as Abulcasis or Albucasis. A section of his medical encyclopedia, *Kitab al-Tasrif* ("The Method of Medicine"), circulated separately as *Chirurgia Albucasis* ("The surgery of Albucasis"), and it eclipsed the rest of the 12th-century Latin translation by Gerard of Cremona. At that time, too, several surgeons in Italy argued that their practice was not merely empirical but also rational, and they demonstrated their learning in well-organized textbooks. They opened a trail of impressive surgical writings that reached from Italy into France and England and from the 14th into the 16th century.

Managing Information

A mere inventory of fundamental texts and tenets, as in the survey of the preceding pages, gives an idea of the daunting mass of received information that students and practitioners of medicine faced, already by the beginning of the 12th century. In the course of the same century, the groundbreaking contributions of Constantine and others were followed by a further influx of writings. The study material grew most explosively with the translation of the two monumental Arabic encyclopedias, the *Liber ad Almansorem* of Rhazes and the *Canon* of Avicenna. The growth was spurred, in turn, by emerging schools that, before they became institutionalized, were run by individual teachers among whom the Salernitan Masters were the most famous. The entrance of new texts, teachings, and teachers lent new urgency to the universally human wish to collect all the accumulated information. We have already seen this wish expressed in earlier compilations with such terms as "comprehensive" and "complete" in their titles.

It is worth noting here that, of the 15 authorities whom Chaucer's doctor "well knew," nearly half were remembered for a medical compendium. Three of these were relatively recent authors of manuals known under florid titles. "Gilbertin," that is, Gilbertus Anglicus or Gilbert the Englishman (fl. 1230–1260), wrote a *Compendium medicine* that an early scribe celebrated as "The English Laurel" (*Laurea anglica*). Gilbert retained Salernitan echoes while reflecting vibrant mid-century developments at

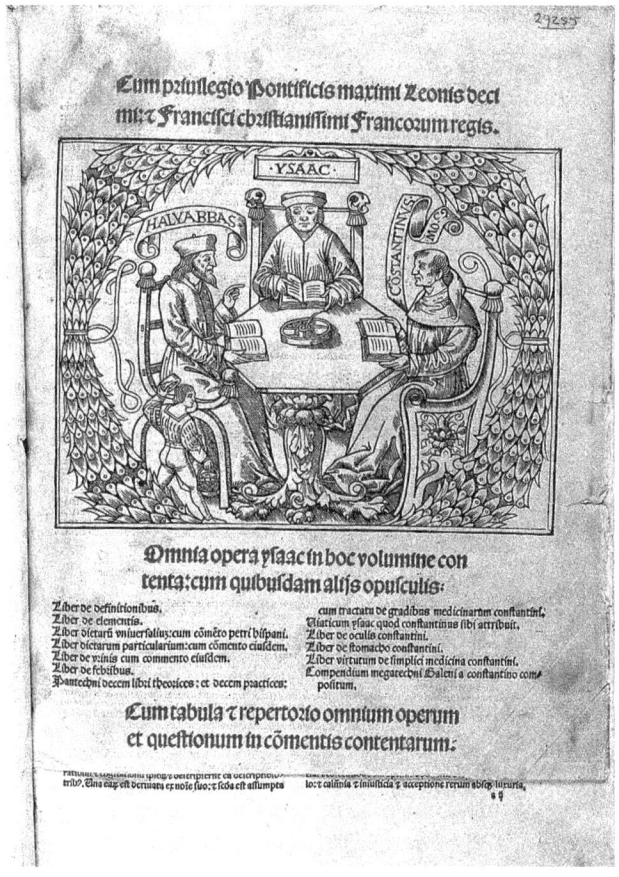

Constantinus Africanus collecting authoritative texts, in conference with Haly Abbas and Isaac Judeus. Title page, *Omnia opera Ysaac,* Lyon, 1515. (Wellcome Library, London. Wellcome Images L0027053)

the University of Montpellier, where he may have written his *Compendium*, as Michael McVaugh argues very cogently. Gilbert's fellow countryman from Oxford, John of Gaddesden (1280–1361) or "Gatesden," compiled a *practica* better known as "The English Rose" (*Rosa anglica*). On the continent, Bernard de Gordon (Montpellier, fl. 1258–1308), completed the "Lily of Medicine" (*Lilium medicine*) in 1305. In these medical compendia, and in the dozens that were produced in the course of a millennium, the compilers evidently faced numerous and mounting challenges in their attempts at completeness. It is worth noting that the challenges, which are also evident in general encyclopedias from Pliny's *Natural History* (ca. 70 CE) to today's Wikipedia, often tend to overrule concerns with reliability. The elementary challenge for any compiler lies in tackling a massive and chaotic amount of information, even within such a circumscribed field as medicine. Authors might circumvent the problem of volume by compressing the data, as Oribasius did in his *Synopsis,* and Constantine the African in *Pantegni*. Another circumvention was, ironically, to disassemble the assembled resource. Thus, parts of the *Liber ad Almansorem* and the *Canon* became quite detached from their encyclopedic context when, as we will see shortly, most teachers began to select the same segments for their courses and commentaries.

Few teachers and students have never been frustrated by individual limitations that hinder the capture of all knowledge. The elusiveness of the target is compounded by the unceasing expansion of information and the unremitting need to integrate new data. This need becomes especially pressing in the wake of historical events, in this case the expansion of Islam into the Hellenized and Persian worlds and, a few centuries later, the influx into Latin Europe of translations from Arabic and Greek. The most ambitious scholars endeavored to collect, assimilate, *and* transmit all the learning that was available in Latin. Medicine, however, presented special challenges that resulted from its ambiguous status between science and craft. For one, a medical compilation might be weighed down by concepts and propositions at the expense of advice and prescriptions, or vice versa. This imbalance was less likely in other fields of advanced learning, whether in a "mirror" (*speculum*) of all nature, a "digest" (*digestum*) of laws, or the "total sum" (*summa*) of theology. On the other hand, a true compendium of the Art of Medicine needed not only to offer more explanation than a collection of recipes but also to provide more practical guidance than a learned treatise. It is understandable that some compilers favored ready remedies at the expense of rationale, while others pursued speculation at the expense of concrete measures.

Accumulated learning is useful to the extent that it lends itself equally to study, consultation, and, for medicine in particular, practical application. This threefold consideration underlay progressive efforts at organizing the subject matter in compendia. The chief objective was to assure that one could promptly find the text applicable to a practical situation, especially when time is short, or in the words of Hippocrates, "opportunity fleeting." However, if the compendium was to be more than a mere compilation of anecdotes and antidotes, the contents needed to be cohesively intelligible and easily accessible. The simplest way to put the subjects in order, by arranging them alphabetically, facilitated a quick search, but it did not contribute to intelligibility. Soon, alphabetical arrangements were applied only to inventories of materia medica—and to indexes that, by the late Middle Ages, were appended to many compendia.

A logical organization of the contents was indispensable for thoughtful consultation, whether by the practitioner or by the professor and student. This requirement could not have found a more receptive milieu than the medieval university, where dialectic was the favorite path of inquiry and where Aristotle and Cicero were revered for the orderliness of their thinking. In addition, in a world where—in sharp contrast with our own—most of learning and life depended on personal memory, logical arrangements facilitated memorization (and so did versification, the adaptation of texts in rhyming, and even metric lines). This is why many textbooks, including the *Articella,* contained outlines and diagrams of the contents. The diagrams probably also served as mnemonic aids to practitioners in the field.

Although the logical structuring of the subject matter was motivated by practical as well as didactic purposes, the danger existed that format might become more important than content. This explains, at least in part, why many students and teachers preferred Avicenna's thoroughly structured and arguably overorganized *Canon* to Galen's brilliant but bewilderingly disorganized opus. While the persuasiveness of Galen's reasoning and the wide range of his writings assured his sovereign stature, the lack of unity in his opus led to efforts, already in Alexandria, to produce a cohesive and manageable Galenism. Avicenna, by contrast, gathered all the information in one integrated and meticulously ordered resource. Even within the *Canon,* however, there was one consistently favored section, namely, Book Four, in which every disease was covered methodically. In a similar fashion, *Liber nonus ad Almansorem* (the "Ninth Book to Almansor") routinely circulated by itself as a convenient tool because it covered therapeutics in an orderly manner. The term "circulated," however, should not be taken too literally here, since it would have been difficult to travel with the entire *Liber nonus:* although only a segment of Rhazes's encyclopedia, this was a hefty tome, even more so when the text became encrusted with commentaries.

A look at any medical encyclopedia, whether in Arabic or in Latin, whether in manuscript or in print, and whether in a premodern or modern edition, leaves no doubt about the physical limitations on their use. Manageable physical size was a prominent concern in the endeavor to make accumulated knowledge fully useful for practice. Today's Medline and, more generally, BlackBerry and Kindle are but the latest (and most rapidly evolving) steps toward this ambitious objective. Early steps included condensing or abbreviating the material into a *breviarium.* The abridgement, unlike a hefty *summa,* would be portable—if hardly a pocket book. It was suitable for accompanying the practitioner, at least in a saddlebag or carried by a page, as a *vade mecum* ("go with me") or a *viaticum* ("provision for the road") and, derivatively, a *viaticus* ("way guide"). Such scholastic volumes, on the other hand, as an encyclopedic *summa* or a specialized treatise (*tractatus*), belonged on a lectern in the classroom or library. There were crossovers, however, though more in one direction than in the other. A formal treatise might not leave the faculty halls or doctor's office, while a manual was readily at hand (*ad manum*) or handy not only for bedside consultation but also for study and even for lectures—especially when it presented practical guidelines with theoretical justifications and in an orderly structure.

Organizing the Manual

While *theorica* naturally tended to be more prominent in a textbook for the classroom than in a manual for the bedside, overlaps and crossovers between both types of books were common. After all, the learned practitioner's *vade mecum* needed to be more grounded in *theorica* than the layperson's how-to book, and the student's textbook was not comprehensive unless it covered the branches of *practica.* The ideal compendium of the Art would be equally useful for didactic instruction and concrete guidance. The *Practica sive Lilium medicine,* which Bernard de Gordon completed in 1305, seems to have filled the dual need. It was assigned to students in the faculty of medicine at the University of Montpellier a century after its completion; it was still required reading at the University of Vienna in 1520. Over time, however, successive copies and adaptations of most *vade mecums* tended to show a shrinking of the theoretical passages and an expansion of recipes. This trend has been viewed both as eroding the advantage of a practitioner's learning and as enhancing the practical value of the doctor's manual.

The ambivalence in the purpose and utilization of a manual is reflected in the organization of the subject matter. For theoretical consistency and didactic effectiveness, each chapter was emphatically (and, on occasion, awkwardly) broken up into sections that followed the Hippocratic sequence of definition, causes, diagnosis, prognosis, and therapeutics. For ease of practical consultation, on the other hand, contents were arranged not only by body part, proceeding from head to toe, but also around diseases, somewhat as in a family health encyclopedia today. Galen was commonly credited with a model for this arrangement, which was called "The Disease Book" (*Passionarius*) and, in fact, compiled by Gariopontus in 11th-century Salerno. In substance, the *Passionarius* was largely copied from premedieval works, most notably from the therapeutics (*De ingenio sanitatis* or *De medendi methodo*) of Galen and the guide to easily obtainable remedies (*Euporiston*) of Theodorus Priscianus (fl. ca. 400 CE). In arranging the contents, however, Gariopontus attested to an interest in improving the immediate usefulness of the sources. The steady growth of this interest is evident when one compares the still fluid format of the *Passionarius* with the stringently logical organization of 14th- and 15th-century manuals that, for example, adhered more consistently to the head-to-toe order and to a uniform structure for the chapters. Logic also played a role in the different place that Gariopontus and later compilers assigned to ailments of the entire body, particularly to the large and weighty category of fevers.

Some writers favored placing fevers and all-body diseases at the beginning of their *summa*, others at the end. We should keep in mind that the arrangement of the subject matter, rather than being purely accidental, often reflected the sources and outlook of the compilers. This is especially true for those who ignored this duality and who either interwove fevers with the other maladies or omitted them altogether from their compendia. A relative indifference to treating fevers by themselves might reveal a preoccupation with practical usefulness and impatience with logical constructions, as exemplified in the *Euporiston* of Theodorus Priscianus. On the other hand, a keen interest in the complexity of fevers might lead an author to treat them separately. Rhazes, for example, reserved them for the tenth and last book of his monumental work for al-Mansur, rather than including them in the "Ninth Book to Almansor," which became a standard encyclopedia of diseases. This may have inspired Michele Savonarola

(1385–1466) to devote a *Practica* to fevers, aside from his comprehensive *Practica medicinae*.

Compilers who did not omit fevers from their compendia but relegated them to the end, and who began with diseases of the head, were avowedly inspired by Aristotelian teleology. They defended the head-to-toe order by arguing that the elevated head was the highest sign of human dignity—with focus on the face since, paradoxically, Aristotle saw the brain as little more than a cooling organ. It would be more logical if they had invoked Galenic teaching on the head as the seat of humanity, which they seem not to have done. Compilers who, to the contrary, placed fevers first were at least indirectly influenced by the importance that Galen attributed to the subject. Bernard de Gordon and others explained that it was proper to begin their compendium with fever because, as Galen wrote, it is "more troublesome than all other diseases."

Some authors, including Gilbert the Englishman and John of Gaddesden and others who placed whole-body diseases after fevers and before their head-to-heel discussion, justified their arrangement more philosophically. They argued, from a somewhat Platonic premise, that one should proceed from the whole to the parts, from the universal to the particular, and from ideas to applications. A few reasoned, in a more defined frame, that it made most sense to begin with fevers because this type of disease was the "most common"; they no doubt understood the term *communis* in the double sense of widespread and affecting the entire body. Aside from justifications, however, these compilers were simply following the most authoritative example. Avicenna opened the fourth and most frequently cited book of his *Canon,* the section devoted to diseases, with a part on fevers (*Canon* IV, *fen* 1). Avicenna's influence is underscored by the fact that this organization gained ground after the translation of his *Canon,* while it was not applied in such earlier Salernitan compilations as the *Passionarius* of Gariopontus and the *Viaticum* of Constantine the African.

Our exploration of the doctor's medieval manual will start with fevers because they most commonly headed the comprehensive coverage of diseases and, more importantly, because they will lead us directly and deeply into the world of medical concepts, observations, and objectives. In addition, they will show, more broadly than the particular diseases, that learned medicine was far less simplistic or two-dimensional than might be expected. The discourse on fevers will reveal numerous paradoxical combinations—of criticism and credulity, common sense and sophistry, logic and imagination, and science and poetry. Poetic license, inspired by the authors' grounding in the humanities and by their wish to attract a broad readership, will allow a free range to literary allusion, wordplay, and metaphor in the understanding of fevers. With the same poetic license, encyclopedias received such fancy titles as "mirror" (*speculum*) or "treasure" (*thesaurus*) of knowledge. Medical manuals were advertised by means of such florid titles as *Rosa, Lilium,* or *Laurea,* as we have seen. One author, Valesco de Tharanta (1382–1417), drew special attention to his manual by naming it *Philonium,* after a compound that was pleasantly aromatic, opium-derived, and, ironically, sleep-inducing. Let us hope that the latter quality does not apply to the following chapters on the physician's manual!

Paradigms of Disease: Fever, Pestilence, and Poison

> Most physicians have erred in distinguishing fevers, by proposing either too many differences or too few. And yet, Hippocrates has given a very good division on the basis of the essence of all fevers, which is unnatural warmth. The differences are taken from the *degree* of the unnatural warmth, from the *manner* in which it comes about, and from the *matter* in which it rages. Hippocrates further differentiated three locations, to wit, the solid parts of the body, the humors, and the dynamic spirits.

This incisive observation is excerpted from Galen's book *On the Differences of Fevers* (Book One, Chapter 1; emphases added for the sake of clarity). The book was central in the faculty syllabus, fundamental in the physician's manual, and instrumental in practical procedures. The excerpt illustrates the tenor of Galen's authority, which shaped all medieval teaching on fevers. It also links the key notions of "fever, pestilence, and poison," which at first sight may seem to form an incongruous trio in the title of this chapter. The common bond is the concept of "miasma," which was crucial in the premodern understanding of epidemics and of disease in general, even though the term did not enter medicine until early modern history. This bond is the reason why poisons are commonly discussed right after fevers in the manuals, and it will lend this chapter a thread of constancy in the flux of definitions and the profusion of differences. The continuum should become clearer when our survey will move from fever to poison, with epidemics as a bridge.

Fever and fevers constituted such a large portion of medical teaching, and they were such a large issue in practice that they will occupy more than half of the present chapter. This first half will adopt the format that was typical of the discourse on each disease in the most logically structured manuals. First, authors methodically defined the disease, spelled out the different forms and distinct features, and identified the causes. This laid the groundwork for the recognition of the specific signs and for the initial—and in many ways most significant—bedside actions of diagnosis and prognostication. The practice-oriented discourse naturally culminated in a section on *cura* or *curatio*, which is more accurately (and more realistically) translated as "treatment" than as "cure." A section, called *clarificatio*, was frequently added for the elucidation of theoretical and practical issues, with echoes of the classroom as well as the bedside: some clarifications were in the dialectical question-and-answer format of scholastic debate, while others concisely resolved a doubt about a particular remedy. Rather than discussing these clarifications separately in this chapter, we will integrate them with the subjects on which they elaborated.

Virtually every discussion opened with a formal definition, which condensed the essence of a disease. Even when a definition was terse and seemingly general, it served as anchor for accurate recognition and appropriate response. A definition was of the utmost importance not only because Hippocratic physicians trusted concepts more than appearances, but also because they were acutely aware that precise terminology was indispensable for the individual and shared understanding of a disease. Paradoxically, efforts to facilitate understanding by recourse to analogy, as in comparisons between human life and the flame of an oil lamp, occasionally diluted precision. The risk of imprecision was more directly compounded by the influx of texts that, after passing through various languages and cultures, required an expansion of the Latin vocabulary. An awareness of these linguistic pitfalls may alert us to the danger of treating several medieval and modern terms as identical. While historical perspective may be enhanced by the recognition of parallels and their implications, it is blurred by the simplistic assumption that history repeats itself. We should resist the temptation to practice what is called a retrospective diagnosis by inferring, for instance, that every medieval mention and even description of *variola* must have referred to what is now known as smallpox.

Forging a new Latin nomenclature, for medicine in general but for fevers in particular, entailed difficulties and dilemmas (which recurred when manuals were translated into vernacular languages from the 14th century on). Quite a number of Greek and Arabic words, for which no exact Latin equivalent was available, made it necessary to choose between linguistic and semantic closeness to the original, with their choice entailing the risk of either not being understood or being misunderstood. A label adopted from Greek nosology might be opaque, as in the case of *epiala,* an intricately complex type of fever. Other borrowed terms might be open to various interpretations: the most important one of these was *paroxysmus,* for a spike or peak in temperature, which some mistook for the *crisis* or turning point in the course of a fever, and a few even confused with the onset or beginning. Translators frequently albeit imperceptibly changed common usage—and, again, risked misunderstanding—when they adapted an existing term, for example, when they applied the adjective *interpolatus,* which meant "altered," to intermittent fever. Moreover, when the wish for intelligibility merged, paradoxically, with the dependence on authoritative tradition, authors occasionally seemed uncertain of their own understanding, lost between the terminology of philosophical abstractions and the concreteness of everyday life, most notably in the allegory of "the innate warmth" (*calidum naturale*) and the oil lamp.

Definitions and Differentiations

Nothing encapsulates *medicina theorica* more comprehensively than the definition of fever; nothing suggests the concrete ramifications more poignantly than the multiple distinctions and divisions; and nothing illuminates *medicina practica* more concisely than the chapters on diagnosing, prognosticating, and treating each variety. Fever was defined in terms that framed the essence of disease, and it was divided into categories that covered every aspect of the physician's art and of the patient's fate. Fever was not seen as a sign or symptom of an underlying condition, but as a malady by itself and with its own symptoms. A long-term consequence of this view is evident in the modern denomination of various infectious diseases, including yellow fever, Rocky Mountain spotted fever, typhus fever, and (the radically different) typhoid fever.

Ancient and medieval medicine defined fever in general as a basic malfunction of the cooking process, in which "the natural warmth turned into fiery heat." *Calor naturalis,* the natural warmth that was life-maintaining when balanced with the *humidum radicale* or quintessential moisture, turned into unnatural and destructive heat. This representation not only matches the universal experience of fever as a kind of burning, but also suggests the imprecision of the alarming perception. The word "fever" comes from the Latin word *febris* and, like "fervor," it is derived from the Sanskrit root for "to be hot"; there is a similar connection between the Greek terms for fever, *pyretos,* and for fire, *pyros* (hence, an arsonist may be a pyromaniac). The perception of elevated temperatures was merely qualitative until the modern thermometer made precise quantification possible. Fevers, more than any other health problems, made the physician's "experience misleading, and judgment difficult," as Hippocrates had warned. Subjective impressions and circumstantial variations were likely to affect the evaluation of the degree to which the patient's warmth deviated from the norm.

Impressions and qualitative judgment shaped the definitions of many types of fever. This is especially striking when it comes to the most feared category of putrid fevers, in which overheating resulted from the putrefaction or decomposition of humors. It is difficult to ignore the analogy with the decay—and, secondarily, foul smell—of juices and other liquids exposed to sustained but less-than-boiling heat. The vivid impressions of putrid rotting, which permeated this understanding, may be contrasted with the more clinical observations that, by way of the notion of tainting, later led to the parallel concept of infection. Impressions further shaped the elaborations of the basic definition, when putrid fever was explained by the excess, thickness, stickiness, blockage, and stagnation of one or more humors. In correspondence with these graphic explanations, manuals prescribed powerful purges of the toxic humoral wastes, and they proscribed such foods that produced foul smells as garlic and onions.

The basic definitions, however, flowed more from analysis and logic than from impression and analogy. These attributed the harmful character of fever to the fact that, ultimately, it was an affliction (*passio*) of the heart. From the overheated heart and through the entire body, blood carried *spiritus,* which inflamed every part. This happened in four stages that, on the authority of Galen, were also recognized in the course of every disease: the onset, increase, hold or siege or duration or "stay" (*status*), and decline or remission. While this internal periodization was critical, for diagnosis and prognosis if less for treatment, it was overshadowed by the elaborate taxonomy in which fevers were divided into kinds, types, and forms. The division generally followed the criteria that Hippocrates and Galen had formulated with logical exactitude, and yet, with ample room for overlap and confusion—as well as for the subtleties and oversights rejected by Galen himself.

The first posted criterion for classifying fevers, namely, "the *degree* of the unnatural warmth," was rarely applied to categories. It was more pertinent to the assessment and outlook of each individual case, which was covered in the manual's section on diagnosis and prognosis; even there, however, it was of limited use for differentiating, as we shall see shortly. Nevertheless, traditional authors taught that the physician's judgment hinged on knowing how much the patient's warmth deviated from the norm *and* drawing the right inference. They emphasized that the extent of deviation depended chiefly on the affected part or organ, and on the nature and amount of inflamed humor or humors. In addition, they recognized that the degree of unnatural warmth varied according to the temperament, constitution, condition, and vigor of the individual, and according to the circumstances, which included the sickroom setting and time of day as well as the weather, season, and climate.

Galen further differentiated a fever by "the *manner* in which it comes about" and runs its course. This criterion yielded several major bifurcations. The oldest and simplest distinction was between chronic and acute fevers. The former lasted 40 days or more, while the latter arose sharply and declined rapidly—if they did not end fatally. Acute fevers drew far more attention than chronic fevers, not only because they presented a greater threat to the physician's abilities but also because, in general (and, arguably, unlike today), sudden affliction and death were dreaded more than prolonged suffering and a slow death. The gravity of acute fever is further evident in the derivation, by way of a French word for "sharp," of the English term "ague" for a severe attack of alternating sweats and chills. It is also worth noting that the label "acute" is reserved today for two specific afflictions, namely, for acute rheumatic fever, which may follow a streptococcal infection and primarily affects children, and for acute Q fever (Query fever), which has been known only since 1935 and is contracted from animals.

A second taxonomy on the basis of *manner* or course differentiated between continuous and interpolated fevers. This was a basic division in the Hippocratic–Galenic tradition and in the manuals. Continuous or continued (not to be confused with chronic) fevers were steady, with little variation in their course. They were subdivided into types with widely varying degrees of urgency. An ephemeral fever, for example, ran only for a day or so, and it rarely brought a patient to the physician. *Causon*, on the contrary, was an urgent type because it was so acutely ardent or burning (compare "caustic") that, if unchecked, it progressed to death in a few days.

Moreover, the burning resulted from red bile or choler, the hottest of the humors; it was concentrated in or around the heart; and it was continuous. *Causon* and the other continuous fevers differed from interpolated fevers, which subsided ("remitted") or ceased ("intermitted") periodically, although these also rose and fell within the time of their recurrence. Commonly labeled "intermittent," they were differentiated further according to the set intervals at which they returned. One singular type, with daily recurrences and peaks (but not to be confused with ephemeral fever) was called "quotidian"—the adjective is now applied most frequently to malaria with daily attacks. There is a greater degree of correspondence between modern malaria and two periodic fevers that were called "tertian," which recurred every third day (with a 48-hour cycle), and "quartan," which returned every fourth day (with a 72-hour cycle). Cases of quartan fever, physicians learned from Hippocrates, increased particularly at the approach of autumn.

A third division according to the *manner* or behavior of a fever drew a line between simple and compound kinds. The group of compound fevers, which was structured more for logic than for therapeutics, eludes sensible discussion in this survey, on account of too many complex differentiations, among "erratic" types, within the single type of "semitertian" fever (*hemitriteus*), between *synochus* and *synocha,* and so on. Among simple fevers, the most notorious was "hectic fever," *febris ethica.* The label "hectic" characterized a chronic, continuous, uniform, deep-seated, and habitual fever. The word was derived from the Greek word *ēthos* for enduring and fixed habit—and hence it means the opposite of what one might expect from the modern usage of "hectic" as rushed and intense (although we have a link in the synonym, "feverish"). There was abundant evidence of bodies succumbing to the steady destructiveness of internal burning. In fact, the discussion of hectic fever regularly spilled over into "*ethica* of old age," which was a slow drying out and wasting of the body *without* fever. Authors noted, with poignant casualness, that this process, while typical of aging, often afflicted children. Allusions to the withering of malnourished children (marasmus) point to another classification, in which the significance of *ethica* became even clearer. In this classification, fever was distinguished by "the matter in which it rages," as Galen taught, and, more specifically, by its location as set out by Hippocrates, "in the solid parts of the body, the humors, and the dynamic spirits."

Hectic fevers, which afflicted the noble organs, flesh, and bones, generated the most intense discussion, with a combination of philosophical wonder and palpable worry about the wasting or consumption that was their essential effect, instead of the putrefaction or corruption caused by other fevers. Compilers identified three types of *febris ethica,* with different degrees of severity, in a division that closely paralleled the Hippocratic set of criteria. They located the first type in the solid parts or, more precisely, in the initial moisture (*ros*) that bedewed the heart and solid members. In this fever, the moisture was consumed in the same way as the oil in a burning lamp is depleted. The moisture of the heart and other principal organs raises a host of questions about physical specifics, as we saw in the first chapter, but the (perhaps unexpected) point of the analogy is that this type of *ethica* was the least fearsome type because—as Galen himself clarified—the moisture, like the oil, can be replenished. The second type was deemed more damaging because it consumed the tissue (*cambium*), that is, the soft flesh throughout the body, in similarity with the flame consuming the oil absorbed by the wick of a lamp. The third type, however, was considered extremely life threatening because it dried up the radical moisture, which is as consubstantial to the entire body as the bond or glue (*glutinum*) is an integral part of the wick itself. This type, together with the third part of the analogy, was universally and ominously applied to the medical notion of consumption or *phthisis* until the discoverers of microbes replaced it with tuberculosis.

In their definition and differentiation of *ethica,* and of fevers in general, the compilers of manuals stayed very close not only to the teachings of Galen and Avicenna, but also to the elucidations and distortions that had accumulated in the many-layered textual transmission. A modern reader may, understandably, find Latin medicine too indebted to tradition, too far removed from tangible reality, and too entangled in subtleties with these distinctions. For a more nuanced appreciation, however, it is helpful to juxtapose the chapters in Bernard's *Lilium* with Galen's treatise *On the Differences of Fevers* and in Avicenna's *Canon*. See Table 2.1. The juxtaposition indicates that Bernard condensed and streamlined the treatises of their sovereign authorities. Other compilers similarly tended to straighten out Galen's discursive rhetoric and to simplify Avicenna's minute categorization. The simplification of traditional doctrines may have not only reinforced some uncritically adopted clichés, but also enhanced the immediate usefulness of the medical manual. Paradoxically, the juxtaposition also helps us realize that logic, when it prevailed over observation, was a tool for understanding a subject that was challenging as well as vital. Prevailing health concerns and conditions often underlay apparent sophistry in the definition and classification of fevers. This is even more the case for etiology, as we shall see.

Table 2.1 Organization of chapters on fevers

Galen *On the Differences of Fevers*	Avicenna *Canon of Medicine,* IV, fen 1	Bernard de Gordon *Lilium,* Part I
Bk 1, ch. 1–2, 4; Bk 2, ch. 1–2; 11–12 Differences	Tract. 1, ch. 1 Definition and types	1. Fevers in general
Bk 1, ch. 3 (Ephemeral fever)	Tract. 1 Ephemeral fever	2. Ephemeral fever
Bk 1, ch. 5–8 (Putrid fevers)	Tract. 2 Putrid fevers [68 chapters]	
	Tract. 2, ch. 42 Causon	3. Causon
Bk 2, ch. 3–4; 10 Tertian	Tract. 2, ch. 37 Tertian	4. Tertian
Bk 2, ch. 12–13 (Synochus)		5. Synochus
Bk 2, ch. 5. Quartan	Tract. 2, ch. 65 Quartan	6. Quartan
Bk 2, ch. 2. Quotidian		7. Quotidian
Bk 2, ch. 6–11 (Composite)		8. Compound fevers
Bk 1, ch. 9–14. (Hectic fevers)	Tract. 3 Ethic fever	9. Hectic
Bk 1, ch. 6. (Pestilential fevers)	Tract. 4 Pestilential fevers	10. Pestilential fevers
Bk 2, ch. 14–18 (*de inflammatione et putrefactione, et accessione febris*)		

Causes

> It is obvious to everyone that some people suffer fever from tiredness, anger, sorrow, heat, cold, sleeplessness, indigestion, drunkenness and satiety. Furthermore, anyone with some intelligence can hardly be unaware that a pestilential quality of the air brings fever . . . It is clear from long experience, moreover, that those who neglect sound habits will be attacked by many illnesses but, above all, by fevers.

With this synopsis, Galen (*On the Differences of Fevers,* Book One, Chapter 3) continued his observation, which we excerpted at the beginning of this chapter. He summarized some causes of fevers that he considered obvious and common. These fall into three broad etiological categories, namely, a physical and emotional condition of the patient, a miasma or "pestilential quality of the air," and an unhealthy lifestyle.

The most obvious causes were indirectly responsible for a fever, through their cumulative effect on a part of the organism, on a phase of the digestive process and, finally, on one or more humor and on the humoral balance. The factors in Galen's first group, which were associated primarily with ephemeral fever, ranged from heat and cold to exhaustion, overindulgence, and emotions. Teachers clarified that excessive heat or cold caused the pores to close and the vapors to be retained. Overheating could result from exposure to the sun or to fire, from a hot bath (stew) or bathing in sulfur springs, from intense physical or emotional movement, or from such hot food and drink as pepper and strong old wine, especially for those not accustomed to it. Many compilers added hunger and sex to the causes of ephemeral fever, as Avicenna had done. In a more intriguing addition, Bernard de Gordon also mentioned swellings (*apostemata*) of the armpits and groin, well before these came to stand out as symptoms of bubonic plague.

When the authors moved from ephemeral to the other fevers, their etiology revolved around the direct role of the humors. They often left the extraneous causes to be inferred from what they called "accompanying particulars." They ascribed causon, for example, to an error in the quantity or quality of yellow bile, with its high inflammability and proximity to the heart and stomach; the only hint at remote factors lies in the observation that causon occurs mostly in youth and is a sign of perdition in old age. For most other fevers, causation was linked to putrefaction. Tertian fever arose when yellow bile putrefied, the vapors accumulated and overheated, and eventually the heat reached the heart and spread through the entire body. Discussions of quotidian and quartan fevers, on the other hand, yield at least a tantalizing glimpse at remote causes. For quotidian, the putrefaction of phlegm was said to result from a range of things that produced phlegmatic chyle: inactivity and overeating. Therefore, quotidian fever readily occurred in winter, in childhood, and in old age, to persons who have what we now call "acid reflux," and to such who are humid and phlegmatic, as fishermen and women (the juxtaposition may seem odd, but it fits in the framework of temperaments). Quartan resulted from a combination between the spoiling of black bile and an autumnal timing, a patient's melancholic constitution, foods that increased black bile or produced too much heat, excessive toil, and intense illness.

Hectic fever induced authors to develop the etiology more fully—so that it affords us the most vivid view of apparently widespread health problems. The indirect causes included all things that steadily dry, heat, and inflame the heart and principal members. Therefore, hectic fever sometimes followed an ephemeral or other fever, when food or cold water was improperly withheld from patients, particularly from those who were dry and emaciated and more likely to suffer from consumption than if they were stout and fleshy. More immediate extrinsic causes of hectic fever were excessive sadness, worry, anger, toil, the exhaustion of the body or mind, and incarceration: briefly, everything that weakens the body. Major internal causes were deficiencies of the liver and the heart. The mention of such deficiencies may seem speculative in the absence of such tools as X-rays or stethoscopes, for viewing internal organs or monitoring their functions. The presence of concrete reality, however, cannot be ignored when the doctors associated hectic fever with conditions that they obviously observed. We have noted earlier their allusions to malnutrition in children and to pulmonary consumption. Hints at tuberculosis are difficult to ignore when they link hectic wasting to deficiency of the lung and chest as well as to empyema, that is, the collection of pus in the pleural space between the lung and the inside of the chest wall. If nothing more, these associations imply a sustained effort to observe the manifestations of disease.

Signs and Symptoms

Unnatural warmth was the essential manifestation as well as the essence of fever; yet, paradoxically (and in ironic contrast with today), it was of limited diagnostic value. Without an objective measure of temperature, the assessment largely depended on the practitioner's subjective perception. Moreover, excessive warmth, as the common denominator of all fevers, did not provide much of a quantitative and divisible scale for indicating one or other type. In most instances, when authors included warmth among the signs for identifying a fever, they did not consider its degree but its quality, location, or time. Aspects of timing normally pertained to prognosis, and it is a poignant exception to see hectic fever recognized in a patient whose temperature rises after being fed. Quality and location were more common criteria. Causon, for example, was evident when an intolerably fiery heat ran through the patient's whole body. Ephemeral fever was indicated, in general, by abnormal warmth that did not feel painful or sharp but more like the overheating from anger or overexertion. A more specific diagnosis could be obtained by palpation: if the ephemeral fever was caused by exposure to the sun, the head would be warm, and the eyes and skin felt warm to the touch; if by contact with styptics, the skin felt intensely and increasingly warm to a prolonged touch; if from consuming hot food and drink, the area of the liver felt hot.

Medieval physicians relied less on touch and palpation than on other methods for the identification of a fever. They favored reading the pulse and urine for a diagnosis, in a ritual that grew out of a centuries-old tradition. There were inherent reasons for cultivating this method. The beat of the pulse and the appearance of urine were observable effects of the inner processes. In addition, both varied over a wide spectrum, which allowed for numerous distinct interpretations. The compilers of manuals usually described signs from the pulse and urine in one sentence, although with more detail on the latter. Pulse reading and uroscopy were also paired in the *Articella* curriculum and, most notably, in the iconography of medical practice. Both methods gave doctors the perfect chance to demonstrate their privileged ability to read signs, in other words, their discriminating knowledge—or *dia-gnosis*—of significances. This opportunity for professional display was greatest in cases of fever, which brought more patients to the doctor than any other complaint, and usually with greater uncertainty about the nature of the ailment and apprehension about its outcome. Numerous contemporary satires of diagnosis by pulse and urine depict an encounter with great potential for a practitioner's vainglory and a patient's gullibility.

Variations in urine and pulse were combined in the differential diagnosis of major kinds of fever. Causon was indicated by a small and rapid pulse together with red and thin urine; tertian by a steady but barely palpable pulse together with reduced and yellow urine; synochus by a heavy and irregular pulse together with livid-red, thick, and fetid urine. Also stages or forms within a fever were differentiated by a combination. Thus, an incipient quotidian manifested itself in a weak pulse and scant urine. Hectic fever again proves particularly fascinating, here in the diagnostic distinction of the three types—more accurately, of two, because Galen and Avicenna taught that the first type was "easy to treat but difficult to recognize." The second type of *febris ethica* is apparent when urination is reduced and the pulse accelerates, in a process that Bernard de Gordon compares with "what happens when water is sprinkled onto quicklime." Using a different analogy for the third type, Bernard describes the telltale pulse as hollow and hard "in the way of a stretched cord"; the patient's urine is oily, and it sounds harsh when it falls onto a stone.

The amazing range of descriptions implies that it required great individual skill to perceive and interpret the fluid and frequently subtle nuances in the pulse. Beyond the obvious indications of a strong/weak and fast/slow pulse, the nuances were so elusive that they needed to be

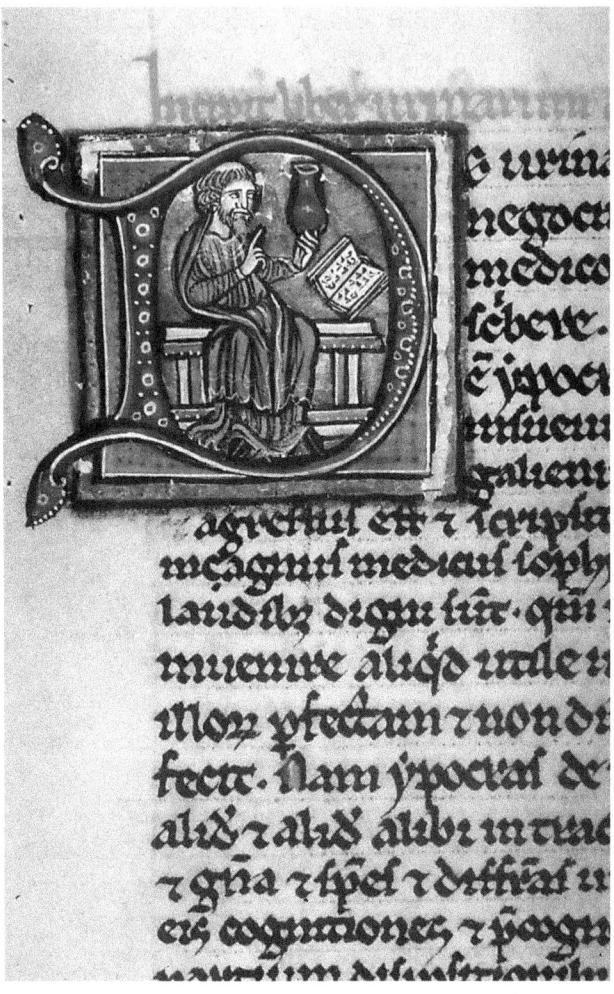

A Master of Medicine, with an open book at hand, teaches about interpreting urine. Initial "D" (for *De urinarum negociis*), under the title "Here begins the book of urines" (*Incipit liber urinarum*). (National Library of Medicine, MS 78, fol.42v. Images from the History of Medicine # A027140)

framed by such analogies as Bernard's. Moreover, it was well known that the heart rhythm was affected by non-morbid factors, particularly the practitioner's haste or the patient's anxiety. The fluctuations did not lend themselves to schematic representation for classroom illustration or bedside consultation. In the end, doctors admitted that it was impossible to teach more than the rudiments of the tactile skill and that no one but Galen ever truly mastered this method. Nevertheless, the silent moment of pulse diagnosis, when the physician held the wrist and began to reveal his verdict, was fraught with suspense, faith, and a tinge of mysticism.

Uroscopy, the visual inspection of the urine, acquired its own mystical cachet, while it was more amenable than the pulse to objective classification and differentiation. The elevation of the urinal vessel or flask (*matula*) containing the patient's urine, which the practitioner held up to the light while pronouncing a diagnosis and prognosis, was celebrated in dozens of images as emblematic of the doctor's privileged knowledge. The examination of a specimen was guided by a considerable number of distinct characteristics that were compared with the norm. The most significant characteristics were the amount, color, consistency or substance, and layers. Aberrations included a reduced output, a lack or excess of coloration, thinness or thickness, turbidity, and unusual sedimentation (*hypostasis*). Extant manuscripts show that various efforts were made to represent the normal and aberrant characteristics in diagrams for teaching and even for quick practical reference.

Since the urine, as the "strained residue" (*colamentum*) of the blood, revealed the internal cooking process, it was an ideal diagnostic marker of fevers. Hence, characteristics were correlated directly—and, of course, often more logically than empirically—to the humoral scheme. Within the scheme, deviations were matched with the definition and subdivision of a specific fever, with a stage in the disease, or with the causes, particularly the offending humor. Thus, abnormally yellow urine pointed to imbalanced bile and the possible presence of a tertian fever. If the urine was reddish, it might indicate causon with inflammation of the blood; if tinted, with dissolution of bile; if ashen and turbid, with advancing putrefaction. If a quartan was due to excess black bile, the urine was thin at first and dark after the paroxysm; however, if it was due to the burning of black bile together with another humor, the urine would vary accordingly: the involvement of phlegm, for example, would make the urine thick. If these diagnostic taxonomies appear simplistic, it is important to keep in mind that uroscopy, while the most visible and celebrated method, was far from the only one.

In addition to the patient's pulse and urine, his or her appearance held vital clues, which the practitioner, guided by the manual, examined and interpreted in a differential diagnosis of fever. These clues ranged from bodily changes to individual perceptions, and to behavioral changes. They might reveal the type of fever, as when a rough tongue, unbearable frontal headache, and insomnia indicated that the entire body was aflame with causon; the degree of malignity, as when a fishy smell of the breath spelled danger in acute fevers; or the stage, as when hollow eyes, tight skin, and a sunken abdomen betrayed the third and most life-threatening form of hectic fever. In several chapters, the signs were distinguished as antecedent, concomitant, and subsequent to the fever. Thus, synochus was announced by redness of the face, heaviness of the head, and pain of the shoulders; it was accompanied by darkened eyes, headache, visions of lighted lamps, and mental disturbance; and it was followed by swelling of the face, weakening of the whole body, and sometimes by measles and pox.

A different offending humor would also account for different signs. Burned blood might be playing a role in a quartan fever if sanguineous diseases preceded and it was springtime; burned bile, if the patient had worked in the sun and eaten bilious things, and it was summer; phlegm, if the paroxysm was prolonged and perspiration limited. Signs could indicate precise causes aside from humoral errors. If an ephemeral fever, for example, was caused by cold, it would manifest itself in a livid appearance; if by toil, in fatigue and aching joints; if by anger, in a red face and protruding eyes; if by sadness, in sunken eyes, and so on. If such precise signs as these proved insufficient, the patient's own communication should supplement the inspection. In fact, while the authors rarely spelled out the details, they certainly assumed that the patient's history and circumstances were indispensable to a reliable examination and interpretation of diagnostic signs.

The complexity of fevers made a reliable diagnosis vitally important to the physician, not only for prescribing the right treatment, but also for obtaining the patient's trust and cooperation. The latter objective was paramount in the reading of predictive signs. In cases of quotidian fever, a particularly elusive kind, Bernard advised that "the physician should say something about what has gone before, something about what is happening, and something about what is to come, so that people will have confidence in him." In another instance, he gave more elaborate advice, in which he combined considerations of treatment and trust with an ulterior motive, the doctor's honor. He warned that tertian fever comes

> with terrible concomitants (*accidencia*), and it tolerates neither ignorance in the physician nor stupidity in the patient; therefore, it is better always to predict future dangers so that they may be anticipated and the physician's

> honor be preserved. Let us suppose, then, that the physician is called after the third paroxysm and it appears to him that a bloodletting should be done and a syrup be administered, and everything is done that ought be done according to reason, but he did not prognosticate anything: then a fourth and strongest paroxysm will come, and the bystanders will say that the patient was killed by the phlebotomy or became much worse after taking the syrup; and thus the physician will have been shamed. On the other hand, if he has predicted such dangers in every disease, the physician will always be praised and he will not be accused of anything.

Bernard concluded with a stern admonition, "Therefore, the general rule should be never to proceed in any disease unless one has first prognosticated. Indeed, prognostication is not to be neglected."

If it was most imperative for doctors to assess the outlook for a patient with fever, it was also more difficult than for almost any other disease. It challenged them to venture far beyond their learning about definitions, causes, and symptoms. In order to anticipate the progress or decline of a fever, they had to take into account the apparent severity of the attack, the estimated vigor of the affected organism, and the established constitution, prior and current lifestyle, and environment of the patient. Each of these factors was complex and variable, whereas predictability hinges on regularity. This truism inspired authors, beginning with Hippocrates, to anchor prognostication in a constant and measurable course. Constancy was provided by the *crisis,* the turning point in the struggle between nature and the contra-natural. This struggle was especially dramatic in acute fevers. Either the patient or the disease gained the upper hand at the critical moment of "judgment" (*crisis*)—often compared with a judge's verdict—in a swift and forceful turn toward recovery or death. Like appeals in court and comebacks in the arena, however, there were resumptions in the contest between nature and disease, and successive crises.

The course of the most serious fevers was marked by "critical days," which occurred at set periods, every other, third, or fourth day. In addition to numerology, the periodicity of cosmic influences secured prognosis, with acute fevers following the lunar cycle and chronic fevers the solar cycle. It cannot fail to strike us that the attempts at forecasting relied more on tradition and faith than on observation and that they left much room for confusion, between major categories of fever, for example, or between such key notions as crisis and paroxysm. Compilers, however, left the finer points to specialized treatises and, occasionally, to the explanatory section that concluded a chapter. With their focus on bedside practice, they drafted instructions for a prognosis by which—as we just saw in Bernard's admonition—the physician could direct his treatment, take a confidence-inspiring stance, and estimate the prospects for recovery or, above all, for death. Thus, a normal ephemeral fever called for little intervention, since it ran its course in little more than 24 hours. While easy to treat, it was difficult to know, according to Avicenna. Therefore, as Bernard assured, once you knew it, you would be able to make the prediction, "This fever will have a swift and good end." On the other hand, it was dangerous to ignore the chance that the ephemeral might cause dryness, which predisposed the patient to hectic fever. In a worse scenario, it might run longer and prove to be the beginning of a putrid fever.

Causon was another fever with a short course, but with far less ambiguous prospects. If all the signs looked good at the onset, recovery could be expected by or before the fourth day; if they were all bad, death would come by or before the fourth day. The patient who happened to survive this decisive day, but then showed signs of jaundice before the seventh day, should be commended to God. Predicting the outcome of fevers, whether swift or prolonged, inevitably linked the likelihood of death with the issue of incurability. There was no hope in treating an acute fever that was known to kill within the first period. The third type of hectic fever, in which the substantial moistures of the heart and organs are slowly consumed, was beyond cure—"unless God wills it," as authors sometimes added. Death was approaching when diarrhea began to deplete the patient's strength, and it was less than three days away when the legs began to swell. Careful attention to the signs made it possible to anticipate the time to recovery or demise. The fast or slow pace of synochus toward death could be gathered from the rate at which the symptoms appeared, including a rumbling sound in the abdomen, difficulty of breathing, and black pustules. Estimating how much time remained—for the practitioner if not for the patient—was an urgent concern in prognostication, not only for deciding how or whether to treat but even for escaping, as some authors advised.

Treatment

> In my youth, when suffering from a quartan fever, I felt the paroxysm come on. I took to my bed, and I had warm cloths, then a warm tile, and then a gourd full of warm water applied to my feet, so that I might avoid the harm of cold. Thus the cold passed, then came warmth, and thereafter perspiration at the end of the paroxysm. Sometimes I also triggered vomiting, at or before the beginning of a paroxysm and after taking food. I should

mention that I did not eat any fresh fruits. By continuing this way, at the end of September I was free of the fever which had begun on the vigil of Saint Lawrence [August 9]. Praise to the living God.

By this personal reminiscence, one of the many that enliven his manual, Valesco de Tharanta intended to confirm the teaching of some authors that quartan fever called for the forcible evacuation of putrid black bile. His story, however, reveals less about treating an intermittent fever than about fighting the chills that torment the patient between recurrent paroxysms. While the anecdote falls short of a case history, it reflects a preponderance of palliation over cure, an experimental or anecdotal slant (suggested by "sometimes") in remediation, and perhaps also a relatively limited confidence in the benefit of writing about remedies.

It does not take extraordinary skepticism to assume that treating fevers was—and to some extent, still is—less effective than defining them, explaining their causes, and interpreting their signs. Indeed, while definitions, etiology, diagnosis, and prognosis merited full attention as fundamental preliminaries to therapeutics, they seem to occupy a disproportionate space in the physician's manual. In addition, the greatest part of the sections with the title of *cura*—which meant "treatment" rather than "cure"—was devoted to prevention and palliation. It is easier to understand these (dis)proportions if we recall the conservatism of medicine before the Hippocratic tradition was progressively eclipsed by the advance of aggressive surgery, the breakthrough of germ theory, and the quest for magic bullets. For a fever in particular, premodern doctors closely followed the standard conservative sequence: they first prescribed dietary measures, then medicinal recipes, and manual intervention only as a last resort. They treated fever on a continuum, one might say, between preserving the natural lifestyle and fighting fevers, which were the preeminent contra-naturals.

The conservative continuum in therapeutics included, paradoxically, a preference for cure by contraries. This was the notion that the most effective treatment of a disease lay in the application of agents with exactly opposite qualities. It is useful here to distinguish the contraries from specifics. Contrary remedies worked by their classified primary qualities— hot or cold, dry or moist—and secondary qualities—purgative or styptic, and so on. Specific remedies worked by their entire substance and unique essence, and they were *experimenta* of which the power, proven by experience, was "occult" or inexplicable by transparent reasons. This power might be attributed to serendipitous discovery by a learned or lay healer, to a resemblance with such a human organ as the liver, or to an association with such animal behavior as the friskiness of sparrows. The power supposedly flowed from "sympathy" with nature's ingeniousness, cosmic influence, or divine intervention. Most of the occult remedies appeared in empirical treatments for topical diseases by similars, rather than in cures of fevers by contraries. The straightforward logic of the latter cures may be illustrated by prescriptions for putrid fever. Putrefaction, to the extent that it was due to occluded pores and passages, was treated with the administration of opening or aperitive remedies that ranged from prunes and spinach to spikenard and laurel oil, and to baths and massages. The preference for contrary remedies over similar substances was not entirely without its critics. Although differences of opinion were far less pronounced than in the later sectarian dichotomy between allopathy and homeopathy, they surfaced in scholastic treatises and even in manuals of *practica*.

Certain authors or practitioners who rejected the application of contraries drew a forceful rebuke from Bernard de Gordon. When he recommended a syrup against the thinning of the blood in causon, he scoffed at "those who are bewitched and possessed enough not to think that thickeners are helpful against thinness." Whether or not his conviction flowed from experience, it evidently harkened to the supreme authority of Galen, who prescribed thickening medicines for tertian fever, and of Avicenna, who admonished, "do not listen to anyone who contradicts this." However, rather than merely copying treatments by opposites from the sources, Bernard devised his own applications of the principle. He asserted, for example, "it is my habit to add syrup of violets," a thinning remedy, when a complicated tertian simultaneously caused a dilution of humors and a blockage in their flow. Such thinning remedies, as vinegar syrup and diluted wine, were the most widely used contraries, chiefly because they counteracted the thickening of putrefied matter while also facilitating its expulsion. Drying agents, including chamomile and sandalwood, reduced the humidity that fed putrefaction; lettuce, rose water, and other cold substances abated the putrefying warmth. These substances were particularly indicated for the acute overheating of certain fevers, when the entire house needed to be cooled by the sprinkling of water and vinegar. In a fascinating vignette, Bernard described a method for cooling as well as soothing, by means of an alembic-like device: water, drawn from a "cantaplora" (surviving in the French word *chantepleur,* "sing-cry") through a siphon, would "flow continuously and, falling into the basin, make the most beautiful melody for the patient."

This fanciful prescription is consistent with the reiterated warning in manuals that the body, however heated by fever, should not be cooled too much or too fast. The recourse to contraries should not be misunderstood as a preference for heroic measures. In addition to cautioning against harsh responses, medieval authors recommended gentle remedies for most fevers and for the longest possible part of their treatment. In fact, they sometimes took a conservative stance in express disagreement with their most authoritative sources. Bernard voiced amazement at Avicenna's recommendation to induce vomiting before and after meals in cases of quartan fever (we may recall that Valesco, on the contrary, applied this method when treating himself). With regard to synochus, Bernard admitted that the treatment revolved almost entirely around phlebotomy, but he expressed reservations about Galen's advice to draw blood fearlessly until a patient of synochus fainted. He mused, "it seems safer to me to let blood several times until the offending matter is knocked out and not the patient: I prefer the disease being prolonged a little rather than death being attributed to me." Moderation was the norm, not only for the drastic yet relatively regular recourse to phlebotomy, but also for the choice of contrary diets at the inception of treatment.

The authors emphasized that the quantity and the quality of nourishment should be carefully adapted to the stage of the fever as well as to the strength of the patient. Quartan fever, for instance, required food that was neither too thin nor too little; and it would be a mistake to withhold all meat and wine in the first 20 days, when the force of the illness surpassed the strength of the patient. The admonition to consider timing in dietary management injects a note of adaptability into the enduring controversy whether one should "feed a cold, starve a fever" or the opposite. While the adage, "starve a fever," is usually traced back only to 1574, at least in English, it was already foreshadowed in the 12th-century teaching of Maurus of Salerno that food should be reduced in a fever's paroxysm, when nature was "in the heat of battle." It is worth emphasizing that starving should be understood here in relative terms, as scaling down rather than suspending nutrition. This measure consisted primarily of limiting the diet to easily digestible oatmeal, diluted wine, and, above all, chicken soup as food and drink. Chicken soup was also prescribed, with some irony, as a reluctant concession to "the men and women who are so picky (*delicati*) these days that they would take none" of the pomegranate, the syrups of julep, violets, and water lily, and the other hardly common ingredients in a medicine for synochus.

The manuals mirror the broad overlaps that existed between materia medica and the household inventory. These overlaps, which have shrunk only in recent history, pervaded not only the management of health and the dietary phase of therapeutics as should be expected, but also medication. Prescriptions drew consistently on common substances of vegetable, animal, and mineral extraction, and ranging from wayside herbs (and weeds) to garden produce and kitchen concoctions. More exquisite preparations contained simples that appeared in everyday life and trade as spices, cosmetics, gems, and precious metals. Recipes with milk, while less ubiquitous than various broths or mixtures with honey, straddled the medical and domestic realms with the most intriguing implications. In view of later controversies about treating tuberculosis, it is interesting to note that milk was recommended particularly for consumptive patients of hectic fever. Bernard de Gordon rated the milk of a woman as the most beneficial, then that of an ass, of a goat, and, last, of a cow (after removal of the butter). For any of these, however, he expressed a caution that was clearly based on experience. If the milk could not be taken directly from the source (*ab ubere*), it was to be prepared in a double boiler and consumed quickly "because milk spoils very fast, like semen." Anticipating the further risk that the milk might spoil in the stomach, Bernard instructed the practitioner to add a little water, salt, and honey, and to boil it by injecting "glowing river pebbles or a piece of hot steel."

The prescription of human milk, in the treatment of fevers and some topical diseases, brings to mind two of the harshest criticisms of premodern therapeutics as polypharmacy and as bizarre. The bewildering profusion of medicines is likely to dominate our first impression of a medieval manual, even if we are duly aware of the modern parallels in pharmaceutical formulas, multidrug therapy, proliferating advertisements, or even the array of pills next to so many breakfast plates. A second look, however, reveals that the multiplicity of medications was expressly linked to rational principles. As the authors acknowledged, numerous factors—above all, the patients' individual condition and disposition—made every case different. The availability of ingredients depended on the place and time, most simples possessed multiple virtues, and the degree of their qualities (hot, moist, and so on) and effects (expulsion, retention, and so on) ranged over a broad scale. Simples, like the colors on a palette, could be mixed into compounds with almost endless variation, which were more than the sum of their parts. Thus, the effect of any electuary or syrup changed with the addition of fennel as a digestive, hydromel as a thinner, or prunes as purgatives. Mixtures also aimed for a balance among the qualities of the compounded simples, and one might be added to temper the quality of another, for example, egg white to temper the cold narcotic and potentially dangerous effect of poppy extract. Aware of all these variables, the compiler of a manual did not intend to present a fully circumscribed treatment but, rather, a collection of possibilities from which, as Bernard advised, the "diligent and solicitous" practitioner should choose.

When Bernard left it "to the conscience of the attending physician" to select from a spread of prescriptions, he pointed out that the Art itself consisted of tailoring the treatment to the particulars, "which pertain to the Art" (*que artis sunt*). This is where experience counted at least as much as book learning, but also where it served every practitioner differently. Some things could be learned only by experience. In a drink for synochus, for example, "five pounds of spring water, one-half pound of white vinegar, and one-half loaf of powdered sugar" should be mixed until it looked "like French white wine, almost greenish," but as the recipe added, the right amount will be "shown by experience." The practitioner needed to be guided by personal experience, beyond the written recipes, because it was not possible—or even seemly, according to Bernard—to enumerate all the variables. At the same time, however, neither the most voluminous manuals nor the longest experience guaranteed satisfactory effectiveness. Bernard admitted that he had never been able to find more than a palliative remedy for a type of quotidian fever, "even though I have tried diligently and frequently."

Helplessness undeniably played a crucial role, not only in spreading a wide medicinal net but also in reaching for exotic remedies. This is still a major incentive for resorting to unusual (if not unaesthetic) remedies, and we are familiar with the power of the plea, "Is there nothing you can do, doctor?" Then as now, many of these remedies transcended rational explanation and reasonable expectation. Mystery, rarity, and preciousness enhanced their promise (and placebo effect). They were worth trying or testing (*experiri*) because they might work where nothing else would or, better, because they were reputedly effective. An *experimentum* resembled the modern experiment to the extent that both involve *experientia,* trial and observation; they were radically different, however, because the former was casual and anecdotal rather than systematic and controlled. *Experimenta,* or empirically proven remedies, were the province of the *experimentator* or empiric, and the boundary that separated them from quackery was thin and shifting. Seemingly far-fetched prescriptions usually coexisted with combination of commonsensical advice. It may be noted that this coexistence continues in every culture and in the response to a wide range of diseases. Moreover, the search for panaceas or wonder drugs is timeless, and the quest for magic bullets became most pronounced and persistent in modern times. Nevertheless, many people spontaneously—and without having to be prompted by *Monty Python*—think of medieval therapeutics as akin to witchcraft, reminiscent of Gothic grotesques, and inherently irrational. Even if we are resigned to the widespread usage of the adjective medieval as synonymous with primitive, we should question the facile application by historians of such dismissive labels as superstitious and bizarre.

The label "bizarre," with meanings that are colored by subjective sensitivities and that run the gamut from strange to esthetically shocking, may not be entirely misplaced for a number of fever treatments. Several of these are undeniably curious. It is entertaining and even instructive to review them, but equally tempting to overlook their context. We should keep in mind that such remedies are most conspicuous where the practitioner deems a conventional cure least promising, and that they account for a small portion of the space devoted to fever therapy. Furthermore, compilers of manuals were generally concerned with gathering information rather than with differentiating between learned medicine and popular lore, mainstream and marginal materials, or conventional and unconventional methods. When compilations were avowedly intended for the public at large, however, they tended to be more indiscriminate. Incantations and talismans, for example, abounded in the 13th-century "Treasure of the Poor" (*Thesaurus pauperum*), a practical manual compiled by Peter of Spain.

Empirical fever remedies normally occur in manuals with a focus on therapeutics at the expense of other aspects. Their significance—and the suggestion of a profit motive—is underscored when the author, ahead of today's advertising ingenuity, not only proclaims the proven efficacy of certain formulas but also intensifies their allure by wrapping them in secrecy. In his manual, called "Sublime Secrets for the Treatment of Various Diseases," Guglielmo da Varignana (ca. 1270–1339) asserted that he did "not need to say much" about the types and causes of fevers because "there is such an abundance of books that treat the matter extensively." He was keenly interested, on the other hand, in "unusual things told by certain authors, and some secret and proven things of ours." Guglielmo's attribution of treatments to his own invention and experience—albeit without obvious preoccupation with secrecy—points to the origin of the English term "nostrum" (Latin for "ours") for a quack remedy. In the most notable instance, he claimed that he had cured many, even of quartan fever, with a medicine of his own, "our nectar" (*nectare nostro*). He professed special "confidence" (*fiduciam*) in the great virtue of this compound of 10 simples, mixed in a thin wine, of which the patient took one spoonful in the morning. The ingredients in this nectar were surprisingly ubiquitous, however: they ranged from borage flowers, dill seed, and other common simples, to more expensive but hardly extraordinary items such as ginger and spikenard.

Before sampling the more curious and colorful fever remedies, a general observation is crucial. The paramount motive for including these remedies was to present a comprehensive manual, rather than to recommend their application. They were consistently presented as hearsay, with the introductory phrase "he said" or "they said" and even regularly differentiated from the compiler's own recommendations. Some were attributed to authors who, while belonging to the scholastic canon, were noted mainly for their practical outlook. Rhazes, for example, according to Guglielmo da Varignana,

> said that, if you take a white spider catching flies, tie it in a linen cloth smeared with a little wax-salve, and apply this to the forehead, it helps a patient who has tertian fever . . . He further said that the spider web, placed on the neck, cures tertian and quartan; and the same when it is drunk with pure wine.

Immediately after this quotation from Rhazes, Guglielmo added, "*I, however, say from my own experience* that the seed of St. John's wort, ground up and given to drink in wine, is very helpful for quartan." It is worth emphasizing Guglielmo's differentiation between the quoted information and his own recommendation, because it was thoroughly typical not only for what he called his "Sublime Secrets" but for most compilations—as a few more instances in the following text will demonstrate. The distance between the compiler and compiled material was expressed so often, indeed, that it gives an indispensable perspective to the most outlandish recipes.

Guglielmo's favorite source of empirical recipes was called *Kyranides* (*Kiranides*) or *Libri Kiranidarum*. This was a collection of hermetic pronouncements, many with roots in Asia, on the secret properties of mineral, herbal, and animal simples; it was drawn up in Greek in the fourth century, translated into Latin in the 12th century. Gulgielmo and other compilers cited and freely adapted *Kiranides* when they listed fever remedies that must have been as extraordinary then as now. It is important, however, to recognize their suggestions of a distance between their compilation and their sources, and even among the sources. Valesco de Tharanta, for example, ranked the marginal *Kiranides* as secondary ("also") to the mainstream authority of Haly Abbas; in addition, he revealed his own cultural context and assigned the cited recipes to a distinct class.

> Haly proposed that long locusts hung around the neck cure quartan fever. It is also written, in the first book of the *Kiranides,* that the heart of the little bird that twists its neck, and that is called 'tortura' [*coturnix,* quail?] in the Béarnais language, cures quartan fever if it is hung around the neck when the moon is waning. These are *experimenta* and even *empirica.*

Guglielmo da Varignana further illustrated the tenor of the citations, distinguished his own position, and underscored the perspective of the manuals when he reported, "*Kyranides* said that a common scorpion, placed in a cup of oil during the waning moon, smeared on the entire back, extremities, and head before an attack, cures quotidian, tertian, and quartan fevers. *We, however,* administer drinks of chamomile root with oxymel in these periodic fevers."

After citing a series of prescriptions for mitigating fever attacks, Guglielmo observed, "we consistently try (*experimur*) the things which we find in books, such as ointments made with oil of spikenard, costus, or castor." In conclusion, he added, "I think that it is safer" to treat by means of "things applied from the outside than things taken internally." The scope of external applications was broader for fevers than for many other internal diseases. At the conservative end, baths spanned the transition not only between dietetics and therapeutics but also between medicinal and manual intervention. When authors recommended bathing, they applied the same humoral and qualitative criteria as in the dietary and pharmaceutical prescriptions. Thus, roses and chamomile would be added to the bath water, as they were to syrups, for their gentle cooling effects. The chief concern was to adjust bathing carefully to the type of fever and other particulars. The general recommendation was that the patient should enter the tub only toward the end of an attack and after the food in the stomach was digested, and should not stay until perspiring. A modern reader who expects that febrile warmth would have been counteracted by barbaric cold baths, may be surprised to find that, on the contrary, frigid baths were shunned as provoking the body's instant reaction of overheating. Ordinarily, the temperature of the water was to be slightly above lukewarm. The patient of hectic fever, however, should be sprayed with cold or near-cold water immediately upon leaving the tub, Bernard de Gordon believed, "because, according to Galen, a bath in warm water is of no use unless cold water follows." In some cases of putrid fever, the noxious fumes could be expelled through the pores, if they were opened sufficiently: this was achieved by a hot bath or "stew" (*stupha*), often accompanied by a massage, the application of a fortifying ointment, or the slow rubbing with such a cooling agent as vinegar.

Massages, rubs, and unctions were only two of several operations that the doctor routinely delegated to a family member, domestic servant, barber, or surgeon. Some ministrations, namely, enemas (clysters) and suppositories, introduced medicinal substances that, for a variety of reasons, could not be delivered orally. The most aggressive manual interventions—short of surgery, which did not enter into fever therapeutics—involved the drawing of blood, in the assumption that it would also drain the putrid part of corrupted humors. There were three methods, but fever treatments seem not to have involved the one that is most often mocked as medieval, namely, the suction by leeches. The next method, by wet cupping (the application of cupping vessels over small scarifications), was far less common for fevers than for other ailments. Phlebotomy or venesection—literally, the cutting of a vein—was the most visible method of eliminating bad vapors while, at the same time, cooling the patient.

Valesco de Tharanta found the cooling effect abundantly proven by experience, humoral rationale, and analogy.

> In my day, I have frequently made this phlebotomy to be performed for tertian fever, in a choleric youth whose urine was fiery, showing a predominance of choler over blood; and I have always been successful. The reason is that phlebotomy induces cooling and ventilation, with a decrease of heat. This is apparent in a pot that is at a high boil: the water jumps out because of great heat, but if a certain amount of this boiling water is removed, the heat decreases markedly and the water will not jump out. This analogy explains how much phlebotomy helps in overheated humors, in tertian and putrid fevers.

Bernard de Gordon, on the contrary, argued against phlebotomy for tertian because it might intensify febrile heat by stirring and thinning the noxious matter. He followed the same logic even for causon, which raged near the heart and was attributed to choler: "by my advice, it should not be done" except in the most urgent cases. Buttressing his position with canonical authority, he added, "let us observe the advice of Avicenna who says that phlebotomy should be delayed as much as possible." The contrast

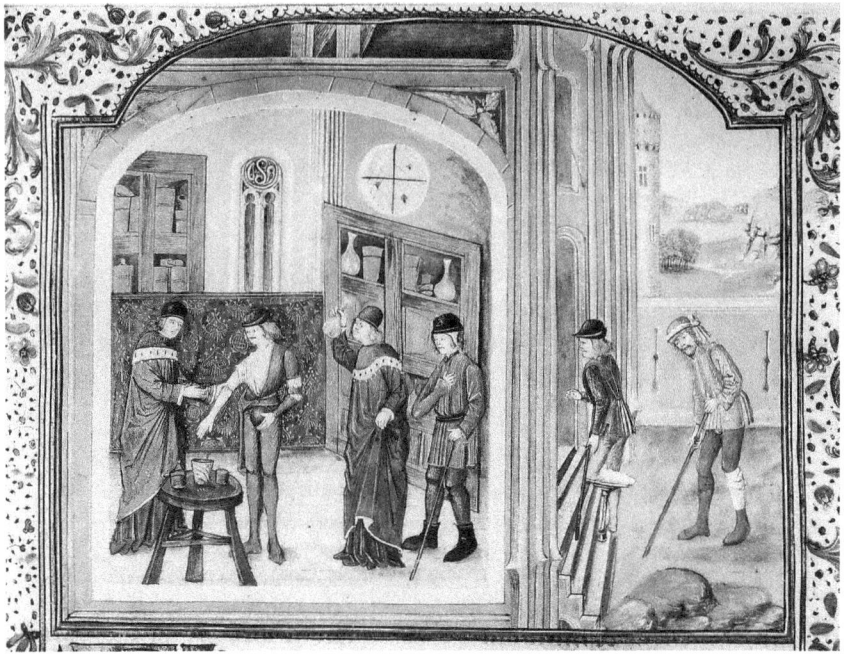

A clinic with a surgeon-physician performing a phlebotomy on one patient and a physician examining the urine of another, and two more patients waiting in line. Illumination from *Livre des proprietes des choses* (*Book on the Properties of Things*) in a 15th-century manuscript. British Library, MS Royal 15 E.11, fol. 165 (Wellcome Library, London. Wellcome Images M0014636)

between Bernard's conservative and Valesco's more confident stance is worth underscoring because it shows that the drawing of blood, while undeniably a staple of medical practice, was the subject of disagreement among medieval physicians. There is much evidence, in fact, that phlebotomy became less controversial and more widespread—in some circles, fashionable—between the 16th and 18th centuries, when it was often recommended without focused rationale, and even applied irrationally to combat pestilential fevers.

Pestilential Fevers

The typical medieval *practica* devoted proportionately little space to pestilential fevers, in comparison with fevers in general and with many other diseases. This may surprise us, because epidemics play a prominent role in the images of Middle Ages as dark ages and, perhaps even more, because our own world is preoccupied with potential pandemics. The limited visibility of epidemics in this context did not mean that they were ignored but that they were not part of the routine practice, that is, the care of one patient at a time, which was the object of the general manual. Beyond sickening individual bodies, epidemics (from Greek *epi*, "upon," and *demos*, "people") attacked entire populations. Their sheer enormity transcended the explanations and prescriptions of the medical vademecum, and it called for separate treatment.

For the compilers, the category of pestilential fevers comprised a vast spectrum of overwhelming diseases while, paradoxically, it might also be subsumed under a broader heading. Thus, epidemics shared a section on fevers with perspiration and poisons in such a well-organized manual as Bernard de Gordon's *Lilium medicine*. This grouping made sense, however, if we consider how much these subjects had in common. In both poisoning and fever, injurious influences spread through the entire body; in pestilence, corrupting influences spread from one body to another—a notion that survived in the name of influenza epidemics. Furthermore, such apparently diverse subjects as pestilence and poisoning overlapped thematically when disease was viewed as ultimately due to influences and emanations rather than to a precise agent (specific etiology), and more as a qualitative condition than as an entity in itself (ontologically).

Aside from the prevailing view of disease, which underlay the structure of most manuals, elementary logic predominated in the organization of the *Lilium*. The first book comprised all the ailments that afflicted the entire body internally. Even when Bernard appended items that fell neither among the all-body diseases nor in the head-to-toe order (and which will be discussed in our next chapter), he aimed for coherence and ease of consultation. His collocation of epidemics with fevers and other internal ailments untangled a complex subject matter for his readers, and by the same token, his logical structure will simplify our summary. First, in an order of ascending gravity (with far-reaching practical implications), he differentiated epidemics from endemic conditions that were widespread in a culture or region but not communicated.

> Some diseases, with various names, are shared by a community as the result of an improper governance of the six non-naturals. Some diseases are regional, such as consumption and empyema in the mountains; diarrhea and dropsy in the valleys; in some regions there are trees with fruits which cause swelling of the neck, while in others the quality of the water causes obstruction of the spleen and liver and hence a bad color [jaundice]. Some

diseases, which are called epidemic or pestilential, arise in corrupt times; these are the worst, and they are deadly because of their radical assault on the principal organs.

It is important to note that, like Bernard, premodern authors conventionally defined epidemics by the circumstance of "corrupt times," rather than by the manner of spreading or the character of impact.

The term "pestilence," which we spontaneously associate with bubonic plague, covered a broad spectrum of epidemics. It circulated, as a generic term, long before the pandemic of 1347–1350, which was called the "Great Mortality" by contemporary witnesses and the "Black Death" by later commentators (and which, according to one early-21st-century historian, was not even bubonic or caused by *Yersinia pestis*). After 1350, the compilers of manuals made fewer references to bubonic plague than one would expect, but the major reason is that they then relegated the subject to a separate literature. It is more surprising that their coverage of epidemics usually did not include such historic scourges as anthrax or ergotism, which they reserved for their section on external ailments (as we will see in chapter 3). At the same time, they retained the traditional focus on other communicable diseases as prototypes of pestilential fever, particularly smallpox and measles. These plagues are tacitly included here, as part of the larger epidemiological panorama, to be revisited later as particular afflictions of the body's surface (in chapter 3) or of a vital function (for example, respiration, in chapter 5).

It is easy to understand that epidemics, with their mysterious onset and massive impact, offered little opportunity for specific identification and classification. On the other hand, they triggered feverish discussions about their general origin and transmission. The faculty of medicine at the University of Paris attempted a learned explanation in a *Compendium about the Epidemic*, which they published in October 1348, as an early response to the Great Mortality. The professors proposed that, "as far as can be understood by the human intellect," the disease was caused, in the macrocosm, by "an unusual conjunction of Saturn, Mars, and Jupiter"; the result in the microcosm was "corrupted air which, breathed in, penetrates to the heart where it corrupts the substance of the spirits." The authors of manuals condensed these elaborate academic speculations. However, they proved to be familiar with the cosmological explanations well before the Great Mortality. In 1305, Bernard echoed long-standing beliefs when he stated that the corruption of certain times ultimately came "from the heavens" (*a superioribus*) and proceeded through "vapors which, released by the powers of the stars, were carried a great distance by the winds, when there is great mortality in some part of the world." He sketched a chain of causation between the cosmos and the body.

> Noxious vapors enter and corrupt the air and water; these, in turn, corrupt other things, crops and fruits, and so on; and then human bodies become infected, because the corrupted air goes to the heart, runs through the whole body, and is fed further by corrupt foods and drinks.

The chain action of vapors caused the unnatural warmth in general, while the condition of each affected individual determined the severity of a particular fever.

The focus on the role of vapors was part of the miasma theory of disease, according to which tainted air, or a polluting atmosphere (Greek μίασμα), was the essential means of transmission in an epidemic. This view (which history books habitually set in contrast with the modern pathogenic or germ theory) originated in antiquity, rather than in the Middle Ages, as some historians assert. The miasma theory persisted, not only because it was an intrinsic part of the holistic Hippocratic legacy, but also because it seemed to fit the observed events. By the same token, it circumvented questions about more specific or tangible causes. Even though "contagion" is derived from the Latin word for touching, in the manuals (as also in the translation of Galen's influential book *On the Differences of Fevers*), the term referred to infection by air rather than to direct physical contact. Valesco de Tharanta conveyed this sense succinctly in the *Libellus de epidemia,* which he composed separately but which soon became integrated into his *Philonium*.

> Since an epidemic is a contagious disease, it can infect not only the weaker and more predisposed but also others, whatever their complexion, because bad, corrupt, and poisonous fumes, and corrupting humors, emanate from the former; the air which they breathe out is already corrupt, it corrupts the surrounding air and those who inhale it.

Such generalizations as this blurred the differentiation between an indiscriminate epidemic and one that targeted the weak. They also muddled the recognition of vernal outbreaks—among populations weakened by winter—while clinging to the authoritative *Aphorism* (3.10), "The most acute and most deadly diseases occur most often in autumn; spring, on the other hand, is the healthiest and least deadly season."

Seasonal criteria and cosmic predictions carried more weight than clinical signs in the diagnosis and prognostication of epidemics. Omens of impending pestilence included the appearance of comets and falling stars, unusual wind and weather patterns, or a profusion of snakes, toads, or mice. Actual symptoms varied from breathing difficulties to, in Bernard's summary, "a foul smell of every discharge from the body, that is, breath, sweat, feces, and urine." This generic summary suggests little interest in precision for individual diagnoses. Moreover, the smell of bodily evacuations was a highly ambiguous phenomenon, as is evident in the case of sweat (which Bernard discussed between pestilential fevers and smallpox, but which we will examine in the following chapter). The author's limited confidence in the ability to assess epidemics was reflected in the observation,

> They all end badly and with terrible and deceptive symptoms. They very often fool the physicians because the urines seem normal and properly layered; and when a turn for the better is expected, death comes. Let us be very careful, therefore, because there are no entirely certain prognostications of life or death for these acute diseases.

Pestilence so utterly confounded diagnostic differentiation and precise prognostication that the authors of manuals presented smallpox and measles not as epidemics in themselves but as *accidentia*—with meanings that ranged from symptoms to side effects.

Grave factors took the epidemic out of the realm of bedside medicine, for which the general manuals were written. Even though the authors recorded various remedies, they seemed to have no illusions about their efficacy. The practitioner could do little to save stricken patients, whether they were about to be claimed by death or would escape inexplicably, "by God's mercy." Often, there was too little time even for alleviating their suffering. As Valesco pointed out, "protecting them is a much more powerful and secure response than treating them once they are actually sick." Most of the preventive prescriptions pertained to the management of the six nonnaturals, which was detailed in a separate class of compendia on the regimen of health. The author of a medical *practica*, then, would concentrate on directly protective measures. Valesco urged that, in the presence of a plague victim, "bystanders should avert their face toward the fire, a window, or a door, in order not to draw in the exhaled corrupt air."

Manuals also itemized aromatics that protected the patient or cleansed the air of the miasma: in cold times, for example, the patient should smell musk, calamint, or amber; on warm days, the air was to be corrected by sprinkling cold water or vinegar and spreading willow leaves.

Aromatic medicines may have made epidemics profitable for a doctor who was in league with an apothecary, "for ech of hem made other for to winne," as Chaucer joked. It makes sense to connect this alleged collusion with Chaucer's cutting remark, a few verses later, that the physician "kept that he won in pestilence." Not much gain would have come either from bedside attendance, which was largely futile, or from preventive advice, which has rarely been a source of profit. A lucrative private practice in pestilence, which is suggested by the famous woodcut in the *Fasciculus medicine,* was probably exceptional. Public service was more likely to be richly compensated because it was both risky and urgent. In fact, public response was indispensable when a disease was corrupting the air, spreading like wildfire, and threatening the fabric of society. Even today, epidemics are the concern of the Center for Disease Control rather than of the National Institutes of Health, the American Medical Association, or any medical college or faculty.

Learned medical practitioners played an important role, however, in the expanding government responses to the recurrent waves of bubonic plague. Even before royal and municipal authorities routinely appointed health officers, they commissioned physicians (and surgeons) to draw up official consultations. The Paris Faculty of Medicine wrote the *Compendium about the Epidemic* at the command of Philip VI of France in 1348. In Florence, the Bologna professor Tommaso del Garbo (ca. 1305–1370) composed an authoritative *Consiglio contro la peste,* which was inspired by the *Consilium contra pestilentiam* of his master, Gentile da Foligno (d. 1348), himself a victim of the Great Mortality. In Montpellier, Jean Jacme (Johannes Jacobi, d. 1384) published a *Regimen contra pestilentiam* "for the benefit of the commonwealth" (*ad utilitatem reipublice*). In the 15th century, health officers in Augsburg, Frankfurt, Nuremberg, and other German cities produced several tracts with the title *Pestregiment.* In England, during the reign of Henry VII (1485–1509), royal instructions guided the preventive and therapeutic response to the plague. A century later, under Elizabeth I, "The best learned in Physicke within this Realme" drew up a manual of preventive and therapeutic measures "upon her Maiesties expresse commandement" (*Orders Thought Meete by Her Maiestie, and Her Priuie Councell, To Be Executed Throughout the Counties of the Realme, in Such Townes, Villages, and Other Places, As Are, Or May Be Hereafter*

Infected with the Plague; see http://historical.hsl.virginia.edu/plague/ for a digital version by the Historical Collections of the Claude Moore Health Sciences Library at the University of Virginia).

The purpose of this quick survey is to point out that, as a growing sense of public interest gave rise to a proliferation of treatises on pestilence, these specialized writings closely paralleled the manuals in their explanations and recommendations. The ultimate causes still lay in the cosmos and the air, on the authority of teachers who ranged from Hippocrates and Avicenna to Gentile da Foligno; the preoccupation with prevention continued, with Tommaso del Garbo advising town denizens to flee to the countryside and as far away as possible; and the materia medica remained largely the same, including vinegar and aromatics. The chief distinction of the *Pestschrifte* lay in the increasing attention for the palliative, curative, and even restorative treatment of actual patients. The far-reaching scientific and societal implications of this increase cannot be pursued here. Suffice it to mention the growing curiosity about the nature of miasma and contagion. This curiosity dovetailed with an intuition of analogies between infection and poisoning, and between the deadly dissemination of an epidemic and the insidious progression of a poison through the body. The association is further suggested by writings with the title "On Pestilence and Poisons" in several manuscripts of the 15th century.

Poisonous Potions and Bites

The authors of medical compendia largely adopted Avicenna's definition and divisions of poison, although a minor modification occasionally affords a glimpse at their own setting. A postclassical fancy for etymology, for example, is reflected in the determination that "venom is so named because it runs through the veins" (*venenum dicitur quia per venas currit*)—although the word actually comes from the Greek for "to kill" (φενω). The more traditional philosophical definitions abstracted the essence of toxicity to an inherent malignity and total hostility to the human body. We are likely to associate these definitions with hemlock (Greek κώνειο, Latin *conium* or *cicuta*), largely because of the death of Socrates. However, few authors of manuals mentioned hemlock. One of these, Antonio Guaineri (d. 1440) of Pavia, reported that birds, when they ate grain soaked in the sap of hemlock, "are stupefied, so that they can be caught by hand"; he proposed, however, that this was different from the compound poison, which the Athenians gave Socrates and which they called hemlock or *cicutam*.

The archetypical poison in medical sources was *napellus,* that is, the monkshood plant (*Aconitum napellus,* also called wolfsbane) and primarily the aconite extracted from the sap. Avicenna suggested a likely application when he asserted that an arrow dipped in monkshood sap killed instantly. Doctor Guaineri also appeared more familiar with monkshood than with hemlock. He documented the actual application of the former in a fascinating aside. When he argued, in his *Practica,* that poisoned cadavers were not toxic themselves, he cited current evidence from the Alpine foothills, "in the region of Saluzzo and Pinerolo," where

> people make poison from the root of a plant which they call *napellus.* They empoison arrows with this for hunting wild goats, which die immediately when they are shot. Yet they eat the goats without harm: in fact, they say that the flesh is tastier when it has been struck by a poisonous arrow.

While wounding with a toxic arrow or iron occasionally appeared in compendia, such as Valesco's *Philonium,* the focus was consistently on "deadly potion"—from which, after all, the word "poison" is derived.

Many potions were both deadly and beneficial, and dosage was recognized as crucial in determining the difference, although their lethality was also mitigated in recipes by the addition of neutralizing ingredients. Most of the ambivalent simples were derived from herbs, among which the poppy was the most conspicuous. Mineral toxins in recipes included arsenic and sulfur, often in combination; and even mercury, as "extinguished quicksilver," with the volatility reduced by "a generous admixture of saliva," according to Gilbert. The fewest but most mysterious dangerous medicines were extracted from such animals as the "sea hare" (*lepus marinus*)," a nudibranch already mentioned by Pliny and Dioscorides, and somewhat similar to the sea slug. The beneficial or noxious effect of each of these simples depended on the amount administered. This criterion was underscored most clearly in comments on saffron. Tradition, as recorded by Constantine the African, held that "saffron has the property of elating so much that too much of it (*nimietas eius*) kills, and the amount for this is three drams." This quantification led Valesco to distinguish two categories when he observed that saffron "kills by making one laugh," but only "when taken in a certain quantity, for otherwise it is not a poison." Valesco's distinction was primarily an expansion of the teaching by Bernard, that saffron was "classified as a poison when the quantity proved lethal." Indeed, Bernard recommended saffron "for fortifying the intestines," while he and other physicians knew that an overdose of the extract (colchicine) caused the facial spasms known as the "sardonic grin"—think of the mien as well as the killing method of The Joker in Batman epics—and led to complete organ failure in less than three days.

The ambiguity between medicine and poison is evident in the Greek word *pharmakon* (for example, in the Hippocratic Oath), and it is connoted in such words as "potions" and "drugs." It is further poignantly exemplified in the categories of narcotic and stimulant remedies. The medieval pharmacopoeia (or, less anachronistically, materia medica) contained many laxative and purgative drugs that were the leading cause of death by accidental overdose, as we learn from caveats as well as anecdotes. Bernard cautioned that, "only very weak laxatives and purgatives should be given" when "diarrhea is what we find most abhorrent." He recommended a safe herbal concoction, so that even "young physicians could administer it, unless prevented by the patient's weakness, loose bowels, or similar circumstances." Accidental overdose did not spare monarchs. The Holy Roman Emperor Otto II died at 28 in 983 after trying to remedy constipation with four drams (one half ounce, or 14 grams) of aloe. King Henry I of France died in 1060 after drinking more of the purging potion—ironically, hoping to prolong life beyond his 58 years—than his court physician, Jean de Chartres, had prescribed.

Purgation and cleansing was the objective of the greatest number of prescriptions in general (*purgativa, mundificativa, evacuativa, expulsiva*). Other indications, however, also called for ingredients that turned toxic when measured imprecisely or administered improperly. Thus, astringent or tightening remedies usually contained lead in various forms: "ceruse" or white lead; "burned lead" or lead sulfite; and "litharge of lead," or oxidated lead; as a poison, lead was said to cause suffocation, presumably if taken internally. Corrosive or caustic recipes for lesions sometimes contained extracts from cantharides, which were known to provoke excruciating urinary burning and kidney shutdown when they exceeded the minute safe dose; the wings of this blister beetle, better known as Spanish fly, allegedly circulated at the court of Emperor Augustus as both aphrodisiac and poison.

The most conspicuous group of ambivalent drugs numbed (*narcotica, stupefacientia, anodina, infrigidativa*) or stimulated (*confortativa, calefacientia*) the body and the mind. It made sense, even beyond the scheme of humors and qualities, to characterize invigorating remedies as warming and inflaming; stimulants, however, represented a relatively small portion of premodern materia medica, in striking contrast with their ubiquity in modern pharmacopoeia. Numbing or stupefying drugs, on the other hand, which were characterized as cooling, appeared in a wide range of prescriptions, though often with a firm warning. Thus, when Bernard prescribed "opium, henbane (Hyoscyamus niger), mandrake, papaver, and the like" for intolerable pain, he admonished that "these narcotics should not be administered except in great necessity and, as it were, out of desperation." It is worth noting here that, contrary to what we might expect, warnings about narcotics did not mention the potential of addiction. They were more insistent because the danger of lethal overdose was so much greater than that for other ambivalent drugs.

Incidents of poisoning, whether primary or by overdose, challenged the diagnostic skills of the practitioner as much as the most acute fever. The authors gave prominence to a set of signs that, especially when they occurred together, unmistakably announced, in Bernard's phrase, "death at the door." The most general omens included, in ascending order, excessive salivation and vomiting, a horrible taste or smell, an ashen color, an odor of the entire body, contortions of the face and throat, and "when the pupil narrows and only the white of the eyes is showing." The diagnosis was further differentiated by means of the hot–cold dichotomy. Hot poisons, such as arsenic or quicksilver, were suspected in burning and pricking sensations, hot and cold sweats, restlessness, and sudden fainting. Cold poisons, most notably *napellus* and opium, were obviously involved if the patient, after showing signs of insensitivity and lethargy, fell into a chill and then into a deep sleep. Symptoms might be specified for particular toxins. Bernard reported, for instance, that the ingestion of ceruse would provoke whitish vomit. He added, however, that the full diversity of symptoms was "something that would be too long to describe."

Bernard devoted proportionately little space to the wide-ranging challenge of toxic substances, which must have been part of medical practice. He appeared less interested in the subject than some other compilers of manuals. Chronology, personal outlooks, and many other factors accounted for the authors' differences in interest. Thus, it is possible that Bernard's avowed aversion to alchemy was a reason why he was reticent on formulas, unlike Gilbert the Englishman who was eager to describe in detail the "artificial production" of litharge, ceruse, verdigris, and so on. It is valid to speculate, however, that in the settings in which Gilbert and Bernard wrote, poisons were less of an everyday issue than in more contentious milieus. This speculation is suggested by a comparative look at the concern with poisoning in a few manuals. While warnings were commonplace in a compendium, some seemed quite abstract and conventional, supported by an ancient literary authority rather than inspired by current circumstances. Gilbert chose to be silent about secret poisons simply because he wished "not to seem teaching something pernicious," and he borrowed Ovid's adage that "we should not add venom to snakes." Similarly, Bernard supported his commonsense recommendation, to be vigilant if someone in the household was suspect, by quoting Sallust, "intimate friendship has the greatest potential for betrayal."

Suffice it to contrast these somewhat detached cautions with the more concrete concerns of two authors who wrote in a different environment. Niccoló Bertruccio (d. 1347), professor at the University of Bologna and physician in the then struggling commune, devoted a separate *tractatus* of his compendium or *Collectorium* to poisons. It may be mentioned in passing that this *tractatus* followed a section on fevers and preceded another on cosmetics. Bertruccio stated, "the first response is that one who fears ingesting something poisonous, as do princes and lords, should not take foods, drinks, or medicines except from a person who is known and trusted, and who has pre-tasted the substance in his presence." Greater tensions, in Pavia a century later, set the stage for more urgent and explicit warnings by Antonio Guaineri. He dedicated the part on poisons of his *Practica* expressly—and, it would seem, without conscious irony—to the notoriously paranoid and murderous Duke Filippo Maria Visconti (1392–1447).

Dispensing with questions that he deemed "of little use except to theoreticians," and aware that "readers of this material wish to get to the practical part immediately," Guaineri turned his attention to preventive measures. He added exact and unusual details to the ordinary warnings of other authors. Thus, someone who was afraid of poison

> should place not only the protection of his body in the hands of faithful servants, but also the things which are necessary for the care of his body. For greater safety, he should have someone enter his bed and warm it by lying in it for at least an hour. He should make one or more persons handle, continuously and thoroughly, his undershirts, cloak, and the like; and make someone else mount his horse an hour before he does.

Most instructions, unlike these, were limited to the danger inherent in food and drink, and to the basic advice of Rhazes and Avicenna "to be wary of anything powerfully sweet, sour, sharp, or salty" and of swallowing "like someone who is starved." Even with regard to safeguarding meals, the manuals seem superficial in comparison with Guaineri's admonition to have the dishes pre-tasted by "a reliable and older person who, after washing the mouth with water, eats the food and drinks the wine to satiety"; he explained that it took time, quantity, and diversity to reveal "if some poison happens to be hidden in any of these."

For a second line of defense against plots, after tests on humans, the literature offered a vast inventory of warning devices. Guaineri collected uncommonly detailed and vivid information on the power of sapphires and other precious stones to signal the presence of poison, although he declared that some talismans "had no virtue other than of emptying the purse, as experience teaches clearly." He was particularly taken with one detecting item, for he stated, "I order that on top of the salt there should always be placed a serpent's horn"; this was a legendary stone (perhaps an erroneous transmission of Arabic mentions of the horned viper, the Latin *cerastes*) that was reputed to sweat in the presence of poison. Guaineri had read, "in some certain little book," about the detective property of a toadstone if it was set in a gold ring. Reading and observation convinced him that a particular gem might possess magical properties while others of the same kind did not, and he argued by analogy: "if not every emerald breaks in the act of sexual intercourse, some do, as I have seen."

Magical properties permeated the recommendations, not only in manuals but also in the authoritative sources, for averting harm preventively or, if needed, after detection had failed. In general, protection lay in "remedies like those with which King Mithridates fortified (*premunivit*) himself," and in "things that break the harmfulness (*malitiam*) of poison," as summarized by Guaineri. He described the twofold defense far more elaborately than other authors; although most also listed antidotes in both categories, they allowed for much overlap. All adopted Avicenna's simple advice that, before a suspect meal, one should fortify the heart and the expulsive faculties by taking almonds, dried figs, or rue. The second method of prophylaxis was more intriguing because it foreshadowed the notion of immunity, as the term *premunivit* in the earlier quotation suggests. Galen observed, and Avicenna confirmed, cases in which tolerance of even the most toxic agents resulted not only from the prolonged use of theriac (about which more later) but even from gradual exposure to the poison itself. It is significant that Valesco extended the observation from poisons to plague: "when taken again and again, such things dispose the body so that the poisonous fury and virulence do not enter so quickly, just as the extended use of theriac before pestilence (*ante mortalitatem*) defends the body from infection by the putrefied air."

A ubiquitous illustration of acquired protection against poison was the evocative ancient tale of the poisonous maiden and her potions. In the

Compendium medicine, for example, Gilbert the Englishman followed Avicenna in crediting Rufus of Ephesus (fl. 100 CE) with the story "that a certain girl was fed poisons so that she would kill kings who lay with her; and she became so strongly poisonous that her saliva would kill animals that came near her." Gilbert and several other authors also cited Avicenna for another case of mithridatism, that is, the acquisition of resistance to a toxin by prolonged exposure to minimal portions. According to an older source, possibly Galen, "a certain old woman began by taking a little bit of aconite, then she continued until she became accustomed to it, and she used it audaciously without being harmed." Galen's authority boosted the reputation of *mithridatum* or mithridate, an antidote to both poison and pestilence, in which dozens of simples were compounded on the basis of a recipe attributed to King Mithridates of Pontus (134–63 BCE).

One antidote that often accompanied mithridate in the manuals but surpassed it in popularity was theriac, a mixture of some 60 ingredients. The antidote received its name from a Greek word for wild and dangerous animals, since it was initially intended as defense against their bites. Over the centuries, however, theriac became a cure-all or panacea, albeit with a distinction between widely variable preparations (the origin of the British word "treacle" for molasses) and "the real thing," *theriaca magna.* Natural philosophers classified it as an intermediate between medicine and poison— so that it was not safe in great quantities or for weak constitutions— because the one essential ingredient was snake flesh (hence, a panacea is sometimes derisively labeled "snake oil"). The reliance on theriac was based on the general assumption that the flesh of venomous snakes was poisonous, on reported observations of victims surviving repeated bites, and on the rationalization that gradual and buffered exposure would provide protection. The appeal of theriac was greatly boosted, however, by the mystique of legend and magic, which were most powerful in the face of the greatest challenges. Valesco advertised one of the most famous legendary antidotes when he claimed, "fame and experience are solid about the horn of the unicorn." Mystique also accounted for the belief in the power of the Asian herb zedoary and of the equally exotic bezoar stone (most commonly a calculus or dried hair ball), to "break the harmfulness of poison," in Guaineri's phrase. It is worth observing that the notion of breaking overlapped with allusions to magic, as in breaking a spell.

Some herbal antidotes were less obviously credited with magical powers, though still trusted empirically without reference to their understood actions. According to Bernard, "the authors whom we have consulted" listed gentian and sage, but they omitted two "that are very helpful against poison, as experience proves." He identified these as tormentil and veronica, but without mentioning the purgative properties of both, namely, laxative for tormentil, and diuretic for the other, veronica—which was then known in Montpellier as *herba tunici* and in French as *l'herbe aux ladres,* "the lepers' herb." In any event, antidotes, whether mundane or magical, usually bridged the preventive and remedial parts of the therapeutic section in a manual's chapter on poisons. Among strictly remedial measures, the most urgently recommended was to make the patient vomit "unabashedly and as much a possible," as Bernard emphasized; he and others also called for administering bloodletting and suppositories, and for keeping the patient awake. As responses to poisoning were naturally accompanied by panic, Bernard urged his readers to "be careful not to accuse someone unjustly." With this admonition, he added a moral tone to Avicenna's mention of an environmental hazard, "when spiders, scorpions, and similar poisonous animals fall into a pot or dish, into the dough, a barrel, or a vessel with wine: this may be due to the uncleanness of some places or because food has been stashed in the woods, in the grass, or in subterranean places."

It may be noted here that fleas (*pulices*), while apparently ubiquitous, hardly drew notice from compilers and that their role in the spread of bubonic plague was not yet known. The more direct threat of spiders, scorpions, and other poisonous animals received extensive coverage in the manuals. At least some of their attention and presentation was due to the influence of their Mediterranean and Near Eastern sources, rather than to the actuality of the European fauna. Although venomous snakes must have been part of Bernard's environment, he associated them primarily with the exotic Levant. He observed that "the inhabitants of Jericho" were familiar with a variety of species, "some of which are called *tyri* [vipers], from which *tyriaca* [theriac] is made; some are called dragons, some asps, and others *basilicus.*" It is difficult to miss the biblical echo of Psalm 91, "On the asp and the basilisk you will tread, you will step on the lion and the dragon" (verse 13 in the Latin Vulgate). Valesco placed greater emphasis on the climatic difference, when he pointed out that the venomous animals mentioned by Avicenna,

> such as big wasps, vipers, asps, are found more in warm than in cold regions. In these parts of Gascony we find only harmless colubers and small green lizards. We could write many things here about reptiles,

but we omit them for the sake of brevity, in order to concentrate on practice.

With remarkable consistency, Valesco showed little interest in the basilisk, a creature that keenly fascinated many authors, including his principal guide, Bernard de Gordon.

The legend of the *basilicus* or basilisk (from βασιλικος, Greek for "royal" or "regal"; and βασιλισκος for "princeling") is surrounded by so much confusion and fantasy that it could easily distract us. Suffice it to touch on the most pertinent points. While, at first sight, compilers simply copied the chapter in Avicenna's *Canon* (IV, *fen* 6, Tractatus 3, Chapter 22), it should be noted that they usually adapted the information to their own context. Niccoló Bertruccio, for instance, dropped several details and added a few others when he reported,

> the basilisk is surnamed "regal" because the head seems to be crowned, or because it dominates all living things by its power. Indeed, it kills not only by spitting or biting but by its mere glance. Because of its burning venom, *the vapors of its body poison the air,* so that no animal can live near its cave. . . . There is absolutely no cure. If you *see a person perish suddenly,* without evident cause, in a suspect deserted place, you should know that this is due to a basilisk.

An addition and a variant phrasing by Bertruccio are italicized in this quotation, because they hint at some of the relevance that physicians found in this seemingly absurd tradition.

The basilisk, no matter how mythical, kindled curiosity about actual puzzles, including death from a sudden and unseen cause, contagion through a medium, the nature of infection, and the role of poisoned air (miasma: see preceding text). Bernard not only expressed this curiosity, but also extended it to other puzzling issues.

> It seems amazing that the basilisk would kill by mere sight, which is a receiving rather than an emitting process; it is even more amazing . . . that the saliva of a fasting person can be poisonous, although it is the residue of the third digestion, which is a continuously rectifying process. I say that, when it comes to images, we receive inward only and emit nothing; otherwise, however, many bad and corrupt things can be emitted: this is how a menstruating woman infects a mirror, a wolf makes a person hoarse. . . . Therefore, it is no wonder that the basilisk corrupts the air and kills over a great distance, since it is a very poisonous animal.

Speculation about the basilisk illuminates the perplexity about infection. More important, it underscores the low expectation of treating—and the urgency of preventing—the effects of poisoned air.

The prescriptions were precise, on the other hand, for bites and stings by most poisonous animals. The manuals offered an interesting mixture of standard therapeutic procedures and folk remedies. For snake bites, Bernard prescribed,

> first tie the extremities with strong and painful ligatures; second catch an old rooster, deplume the anus, and place it on the bite: if the rooster dies it is a good sign because it indicates that the poison has been drawn out; therefore, apply several until you see that the rooster does not die from the extracted venom; third, take a sponge or linen cloth or something similar, place in warm water, squeeze out, and place on the bite, and do this several times.

Further treatment consisted of the repeated scarification and cupping of the bite, the application of plasters, the administration of potions, and

> ninth, have a base person suck the bite forcefully, but he should be careful that his stomach be full, with wine, garlic, rue, and nuts, and that he rinses his mouth repeatedly with wine and oil; and tenth and last, if we have no other way and the involved body part is small, let it be cut off.

Similarly precise though less drastic cures were described for stings by scorpions, which "are found near us in Avignon," Bernard reported. Such simple home remedies as the application of something cold were sufficient for the more common hazards of wasp and beestings.

No home remedy and, for that matter, no learned recipe could do much for the poisoning by rabies, which was named hydrophobia because abhorrence of water is one of its ultimate and most dramatic symptoms. A sense of resignation may have persuaded Bernard to trim the observations and prescriptions of the *Canon,* while adding an occasional rumination. In one, he speculated about hydrophobia as a physical "corruption of the imaginative faculty" in terms that might now be associated with psychophysiology; in another aside, he philosophized about the paradox that dogs, in spite of their classification as cold and dry animals, were so brave and fast. In a more poetic aside, Valesco identified other canine qualities as essential and their absence as a sign of rabies. Dogs proved to have "more sense than other animals," because "they alone recognize their names, love their masters, defend their masters' homes, offer themselves to death for their masters, willingly run with them to the chase, and do not leave the dead body of their master."

This ode to man's best friend, while most likely copied from the writings of Isidore of Seville (*Etymologies*, 12.2, 25–26), may have resonated with Valesco's interest in the quotidian. His down-to-earth interest surfaces in the therapeutic section of his chapter on rabies.

> Let me tell you about the remedies which are used in Béarn. First, someone who has been bitten by a rabid dog immediately goes to the ocean and there drinks salt[y] sea water, bathes in it, thoroughly washes the wound with it, and does nothing else; they say, and it is the common belief (*fama communis*), that no one suffers a recurrence without being protected from hydrophobia. For a second remedy, there is a spring near the place of Morlaàs, in a village called Ousse, and it is said that if someone bitten by a rabid dog drinks from this spring, on an empty stomach before sunrise, for nine days, he or she will be protected by way of prevention. I have seen many who were bitten by rabid dogs and who were saved from hydrophobia by this protection, but the first remedy is more reliable. It is said that those who go to draw the water should not look back, either while going or while returning. I, however, place my trust in the Lord.

A practitioner's trust in divine protection, together with qualified faith in folklore, often made up for helplessness in the face of internal disorders, whether these were caused by bites and poisons or by intangible factors as in the case of fevers. The manuals suggest a greater confidence in treating surface afflictions, in spite of their diversity—which was bewildering, as will become evident in the following chapter.

The Body Surface; Tumors and Trauma

Of the afflictions to the surface of the body, some arise from an internal cause and others from an external cause. Among those from internal causes, some affect the entire body, such as smallpox, leprosy, and morphea; others are limited to a certain part, as alopecia is to the head, and lentigo to the face. External causes include impact, wound, fracture, shock, or submersion: the agents are inanimate objects, as in a cut from a sword, and a fracture from a rock; or animate, as in a mauling, bite, and sting by an animal. Some of the animals are venomous, including a rabid dog and a viper; some are not, including a dog or a man.

Let us begin with external afflictions from an internal cause. The internal cause lies in the excess and corruption of humors and in the predisposition of the receiving parts. The material that produces an aposteme comes either from the essence of one of the four humors or from some inflating air (gaseousness, *ventositate*).

This combined excerpt from the *Pantegni* (Part I, Book 8, Chapter 15) and the *Viaticum* (Book 7, Chapter 15) offers a logical introduction to our chapter on the body surface. Both encyclopedias were among the most influential channels through which Constantine the African brought Galenic teaching to Latin medicine, before being eclipsed by Avicenna's *Canon.* In fact, they surpassed the latter in shaping the contents of the typical manual and the coverage of exterior ailments in particular.

Two characteristics of Latin medicine have far-reaching ramifications for this chapter. First, skin was not recognized as an organ in itself: instead, it was viewed merely as a surface or as exterior and, paradoxically, as integral to each limb or body part. This outlook should provide a perspective not only for the pervasiveness of humoral physiology, but even for some seemingly nonsensical disease categories. A second characteristic of medieval medicine, with direct consequences for the place of surface ailments in practical compendia, was the distinction between two areas of competence. In simple terms, the body exterior was the domain of the manual operator and the objective of the surgeon's *operatio;* the interior was accessible through knowledge of "nature" (*physica*), which was the prerogative of the *physicus,* the learned physician. While the manuals show that this *scientia* included speculations, inconsistencies, and ambiguities, they also document the importance of precise definitions for the accurate assessment, differential diagnosis, and appropriate treatment of the profusely different external ailments and afflictions. The strong link between definitions and therapeutics contradicts the die-hard stereotype of medieval medicine as nothing but scholastic sophistry and shotgun quackery.

Our examination of the medical *practica* will concentrate on the role of knowledge rather than on the application of skill in responses to external health problems. This concentration (and limits of time and space) will result in the omission of trauma and of a host of such fascinating surgical concerns as wounds and hemorrhage, fractures and dislocations, and burns and frostbite. While this imbalance does injustice to the comprehensiveness of medical compendia, it parallels their organization, which was frequently uneven. In general, the compilers found it difficult to maintain the boundaries between competencies, and they drew up open-ended divisions within the external afflictions. One class, directly a surgical concern, included all the external injuries that damaged the victim's anatomy; these overlapped, however, with such injuries as poisonous bites, which, while coming from outside, affected the body's complexion; apostemes constituted the largest group, of external ailments with internal causes, but they also had internal counterparts. The complexity of these divisions, and the ensuing confusion in explanations and prescriptions, was compounded by the ambiguity of one overarching process, namely, ulceration.

Although the demarcation between exterior and interior was far from absolute, the corresponding dichotomy between the hand and the head was indisputably detrimental to medical knowledge and practice in general. Many have overstated the dichotomy, however, from Vesalius in heralding the newness of his *Fabrica* to modern authors simplifying history in their course texts. The alleged chasm was bridged by "the rational surgery of the Middle Ages," in Michael McVaugh's lapidary title, as well as by the surgical details in many medical compendia. Nevertheless, surgical manuals usually presented the external (and the structural) problems of the body more lucidly than their medical counterparts, while physicians readily deferred to surgeons for their knowledge as well as their skill. Bernard de Gordon, for one, ceded the ultimate treatment of difficult external ailments "to the surgical hand" (*ad manum cyrurgicam*)—even though he also admonished surgeons to be more "diligent in knowing the complexion, sense, and nobility of body parts" as well as "the nature of medicinal substances." Valesco de Tharanta, for his part, vowed to keep his chapters on apostemes brief because an eminent authority on surgery, "Guy de Chauliac, of the university of Montpellier, has treated this matter most perfectly and thoroughly."

Guy indeed covered the subject methodically and exhaustively in his *Magna chirurgia* (1363). He suggested, however, that a comprehensive definition of apostemes was not necessary, at least in a surgical manual. "It is sufficient for the surgeon," he declared, "to know that aposteme, tumor, swelling, thickening, ridge, bump, and growth are names which mean pretty much the same thing." In a similar vein, it is sufficient for us to know that an "aposteme" (analogous to what we now call an abscess) was commonly defined as an *unnatural* swelling or tumor. The category included a vast range of localized tumors, most of them external. The umbrella label became deformed in postmedieval English into the word "imposthume." Both the obsolete term "aposteme" and the current "abscess" denote something that has separated from a constituent whole, the former in Greek (*apostēma*, from *apo-*, "away," and *istēmi*, "to stand") and the latter in Latin (*abscessus*, from the prefix *ab[s]-* "away," and *cedere*, "to go"). The primary source of medieval definitions was Galen's book *On Unnatural Tumors*, which built on the basic notion of a swelling, *onkos*—the Greek root of "oncology," for the branch of modern medicine that deals with cancer. Galen introduced this treatise with the blanket characterization of *onkos* as "one of the things that happen to the body." In spite of this generality, he concentrated on tumors due to internal causes—as we will do in this chapter. Apostemes due to external trauma were so predominantly treated by hand, and so closely associated with such injuries as wounds and fractures, that it is logical to leave them to the study of surgical manuals.

Galen discussed a wide variety of tumors, not only when writing *On Unnatural Tumors*, but also in his influential *Method of Healing* (which circulated variably as *Terapeutica, De ingenio sanitatis* and, later, as *De medendi methodo*; and which Constantine adapted in *Megategni*). In addition, he offered numerous definitions, descriptions, and explanations throughout his works. However, he did not draw these together into a conceptual system or even into a unified synopsis. Galen's interpreters, particularly in Arabic medicine, made up for this by constructing elaborate taxonomies. They differentiated apostemes—sometimes to excess—by tying each kind to one of the four humors; they surrendered taxonomic symmetry, however, by incorporating two other factors, namely, "wateriness" (*aquositas*) and "gaseousness" (*ventositas*), which was related to the Galenic notion of *pneuma*.

Tumors and Humors

The *Pantegni* outlined the humoral differentiation of apostemes, but Avicenna developed it systematically in his *Canon,* as may be seen in Table 3.1. Avicenna's categories branched out much further, and the extent of his subdistinctions is reminiscent of scriptural exegesis or legal commentary. The simplified representation in Table 3.1 is useful, however, in various ways. It broadly projects the layout common to most manuals, with the types of tumors (in the right-hand column) that became the principal subjects of dedicated chapters. Paradoxically, Table 3.1 will also indicate on how many points the manuals diverged. Most significantly, it hints at the practical aims of systematic classification. Avicenna aimed at integrating ideas that were scattered through the writings of Galen. This broad objective was matched by his preoccupation with making a very heterogeneous subject matter logically coherent and easy to consult. The synopsis further shows that the scheme of qualities and humors was key to the definition and treatment of tumors, as much as it was for fevers. Since this scheme accounts for the most radical contrast between medieval and modern medicine, it should guide our examination of external medicine in the manuals if we wish to avoid an anachronistic assessment.

The procedure and import of Avicenna's differentiation, while conveniently outlined in Table 3.1, become more evident in a combined excerpt from his *Canon medicine* (IV, *fen* 3, *Tractatus* 1, Chapter 1, and *Tractatus* 2, Chapter 1). The broadest division of apostemes, into "either warm or not warm ones," grows into a veritable tree of unnatural tumors.

> A warm aposteme comes either from blood or from yellow bile. When from blood, it is either from good or bad blood. Good blood is either thick

Table 3.1 Avicenna's humoral scheme of tumors

WARM	BLOOD	GOOD	THICK	PHLEGMON (Flesh and Skin)
			THIN	PHLEGMON (Skin Only)
		BAD	THIN	PHLEGMON (Towards Erysipelas)
			THICK	ERYSIPELAS and PERSIAN FIRE
	YELLOW BILE		THIN	CORROSIVE HERPES
			THINNER	MILIARY HERPES
			THINNEST	ROVING HERPES
COLD	PHLEGM		SOFT	EDEMA
			HARD	SCROFULA
	BLACK BILE			CANCER, LEPROSY
	GASEOUSNESS			SWELLING (*Inflatio*)
	WATERINESS			DROPSY, HYDROCEPHALY

or thin. From thick good blood comes a phlegmon that affects flesh and skin simultaneously, and which is accompanied by pulsation; from thin good blood [comes] a phlegmon that affects the skin only, and which lacks pulsation. From thick bad blood come types of bad swellings: if it is burned and the malignancy becomes violent, it will cause erysipelas or, worse, Persian Fire; from thin bad blood comes a phlegmon that, malignantly and insidiously, tends toward erysipelas.

Differentiations based on the other humors were equally subtle, even though their practical ramifications were often limited, as will become apparent.

From thin bile comes the phlegmon that is called corrosive herpes; from thinner bile, the herpes called miliary herpes, which is less hot and affects the flesh more than the skin; and from the thinnest bile, wandering herpes.

Cold tumors come from phlegm, black bile, ventosity, or a combination of these. Phlegmatic tumors are either simple or composite: simple phlegmatic apostemes, such as edema, are soft; others, such as scrofulas and nodules, are hard. Melancholic apostemes include sclerosis and cancer—you know the difference between both. Gaseous ones ([*apostemata*] *ventosa*) include bumps and blisters.

Avicenna's scheme drew Galen's diffuse teachings into a map of explanations and procedures, for the area of medical learning, which may be called the most chaotic. Even if the scheme was prone to inconsistency and hairsplitting, it not only facilitated the compilation of a manual, but also rationalized the rules of practice.

When science revolved around appearances and deduction, the qualitative-humoral construct of tumors made sense (in a fashion similar to what the Ptolemaic system achieved for the movements of stars and planets). It seems inevitable that the jumble of external afflictions from internal causes would find order and meaning in the fundamental association of each humor with a defined pair of primary qualities (warm/cold and dry/moist: see Chapter 1). The construct allowed for a logical explanation, supported a differential diagnosis, and shaped the specific treatment of each external ailment. It will also guide our survey of manuals, with the caveat that neither our simplified humoral framework nor our selective look at a few typical external afflictions can do justice to the enormous diversity in their discussion.

In line with the most basic level of the qualitative construct, many swellings can be described in terms of temperature or deviation from the normal: some were perceived by the patient as burning, while others felt cold to the practitioner's touch. This initial perception made it logical to link apostemes and humors according to the primary quality that they shared, in other words, to attribute warm tumors to blood or bile (choler) and cold ones to phlegm or black bile (melancholy). Furthermore, tumors often displayed several of the visual characteristics that were associated with a particular humor in the tetragram. They displayed distinct colors and—with some help of preconception and imagination—appeared red as blood, yellowish as bile, pallid as phlegm, or dark as black bile. The physician would also be able to distinguish tumors by touch, according to Gilbert the Englishman, "because softness results from phlegm, hardness from black bile, roughness from bile, and smoothness from blood." In addition, a patient's sensation of pain and pulsation suggested a cause in the blood, while stinging and prickling pointed to bile, moderate pain to black bile, and dull pain to phlegm.

To be sure, the direct and indirect associations between humors and external ailments were treated differently in each manual. Variations in the definitions and divisions of tumors reveal a degree of individuality among the authors and a dynamic dimension of medieval medicine that general historians often overlook. Several compilers ignored the conventional structure of the subject matter, apparently in their haste to provide practical guidance and, to some extent, in relative independence of Avicenna's authority. In 11th-century Salerno, Italy, Gariopontus concluded the

Passionarius, his digest of Galenic therapeutics, with 14 chapters on tumors; in these, he attached little importance to humoral differentiation or, for that matter, to their logical arrangement (the 13th chapter is a synopsis of apostemes). Another Salernitan master, John of Saint Paul (fl. 1200), who wished his "Breviary of Medicine" (*Breviarium medicine*) to be as useful as possible, moved randomly from a single chapter on "The Treatment of Apostemes" to others on wounds and cuts, fistula, smallpox, and warts.

Humoral classifications gained ground after the 12th century, and they tended to frame the organization of manuals. This organization was far from homogeneous, however. While Gilbert stated that "apostemes are distinguished according to the different humors," he scattered related matter across his *Compendium:* he discussed pustules in the face and the entire body, as well as ringworm, impetigo, and anthrax right after the section on the head (Books Two and Three); he addressed apostemes in general in the midst of his chapters on the chest (Book Four); and he placed cancer, lupus, and leprosy among the diseases of the reproductive parts (Book Seven). John of Gaddesden devoted the second book of his *Practica* to "general diseases," with 23 chapters, which began with apostemes but then moved to dropsy, pains in the joints, smallpox, scabies, perspiration, leprosy, rheuma, consumption, and so on, to conclude with poisons. In the *Collectorium,* Niccoló Bertruccio covered scrofula, herpes, and even Persian Fire as well as hair care in the *tractatus* on cosmetic medicine, *de decoratione.*

There were compilers who, on the contrary, followed convention in structuring the subject matter. Even they, however, did not passively or uniformly adopt the humoral organization of the *Pantegni,* the *Viaticum,* and the *Canon.* Rather, these authors adapted the conventional arrangement to their own objectives and inclinations. A penchant for dialectic, for instance, led Bernard de Gordon to observe, "the divisions of apostemes are numerous," and to supplement the standard humoral classification with further categories.

> Some are caused by way of congestion, as when nourishment is excessive for a part that is weak; others when decaying matter is very abundant or very malignant, or both, and flows from a powerful discharging part to a weak receiving part. Some apostemes appear on the outside; others hide inside, such as pleurisy, pneumonia, and the like. Some are in a noble organ, and these are more dangerous; others are in non-noble organs. Some occur in bones and in the soft tissue (*substancia medullari*) of the brain—this is stated because some have denied it.

Here followed the casual but intriguing observation, "some apostemes afflict the poor; others the rich, and these are cured more slowly, because they refuse to do bloodletting or other necessary things, according to Galen." Bernard then added more distinctions, but the ones quoted here suffice for illustrating the contrast between the taxonomies of logical compendia and the almost invisible structure of more narrowly practical manuals.

Guglielmo da Varignana dispensed with explicit categorization, yet his "Sublime Secrets for the Treatment of Various Diseases" followed the traditional order. After a "General Chapter on Warm and Cold Apostemes," he began his detailed exposition with tumors from ignited matter and ended with those from melancholic matter. We, too, will follow this order in our exploration of the manuals. Specifics, however, will occasionally need to be left aside so that we may not lose our way in the tangled underbrush of differences. We will not dwell, for example, on the bewildering differentiations of apostemes that were based on various conditions of a humor (simply excessive, or also overheated, corrupted, and so on), on intermediates between opposite qualities (especially between thickness and thinness), and on combined actions of humors (say, bile with a secondary role of blood). So many diverse types of tumors were distinguished by these criteria that "they could not be spelled out in one day," according to Bernard.

A Double Category by Itself: Smallpox and Measles

Smallpox (*variole*) and measles (*morbilli*) were two types of tumors or, more precisely, pustules that did not fit the hot/cold–dry/moist framework and that different authors classified and explained differently. Avicenna treated them in his *tractatus* on pestilential fevers (*Canon 4, fen* 1, Tract. 4), but several compilers ignored this classification, even though most maintained at least an implicit association with epidemics. We may note in passing that the Salernitan masters devoted comparatively little space to these pustules, as well as to epidemics in general. Subsequent authors varied in their coverage, and they seemed uncertain where in the *practica* this subject belonged, as a quick sampling demonstrates: Gilbert discussed smallpox and measles between leprosy and poisons, Bernard between perspiration and poisons, John of Gaddesden between pain of the joints and scabies, and Valesco after perspiration and ahead of his *tractatus* on epidemics. Bertruccio presented his organization of the subject matter as a return to the earlier tradition:

> It is customary among the ancients to deal with smallpox and measles after
> the discussion of pestilential fever, as seems appropriate because they think

the same way about poisonousness and pestilential fevers. Therefore, we will do likewise.

In keeping with this linkage, he made it clear that the pustules might come from "a certain celestial influence or from the air which is converted into pestilential qualities."

The principal criteria for defining and differentiating smallpox and measles were their immediate causes, blood and bile, respectively. Gilbert implicitly disagreed with a simplistic extension of the differentiation to humoral colors by "*some* according to whom the pustules are called smallpox when they are red and measles when they are yellow." Smallpox and measles supposedly shared a deeper cause in the blood, according to an abstruse theory that the compilers adopted from Avicenna without much elucidation. When a residue of the menstrual blood that had nourished the fetus came to a boiling point, it was expelled and formed blisters; the

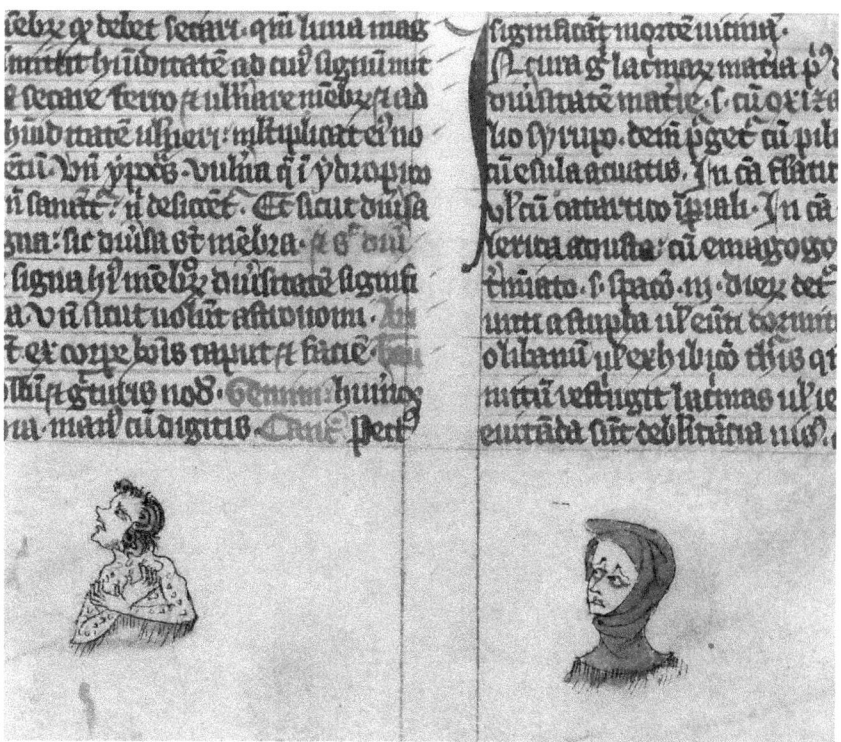

A man covered with spots (likely smallpox or measles), and a woman with inflamed eyes. Small pen drawings in margin of an early 14th-century medical manuscript. *Miscellanea Medica XVIII*. (Wellcome Library, London. Wellcome Images L0037335)

likelihood of this happening depended on how close a person still was to conception and birth. This theory explained why smallpox and measles occurred primarily in infancy and childhood, less often in youth, and rarely in old age. It left much room for speculation, however, about more immediate causes in the diet and environment. In most of these, blood was implicated as an intermediate factor.

The suspected role of blood, particularly in causing smallpox, accounted for some remedies that continue to stir discussion. These remedies, which evidently originated in folklore, appear only in the medical compendia. The descriptions suggest the dynamic evolution and adoption of an empirical tradition. First, Gilbert reported about "old women in Provence"—or in the provinces (*provinciales*)—that they gave "burned purple herb [related to *Echinacea*] in a drink, because it has an occult quality of curing smallpox. The same goes for a cloth dyed with kermes," a red dye. A half-century later, Bernard tersely prescribed, "let the entire body be wrapped in a red piece." A decade or so later, John of Gaddesden added a striking dimension of reality.

> Take a red scarlet and let the smallpox patient be entirely wrapped in it, or in another red cloth, as I did for the son of the most noble king of England when he suffered from the disease; and I made everything around his bed to be red. It is a good cure, and I subsequently cured him without leaving traces of the smallpox.

A century passed before Valesco explained that the remedy was effective because, "by the sight of the red cloth, the blood is moved to the surface, and thus the patient is kept in a warmth that is not excessive."

Valesco, like several others, acknowledged the universal terror of being marked by vestiges of smallpox, especially in the face. Nevertheless, he gave the impression that some of his fellow physicians favored a merciless method that not only may have aggravated pockmarks but also must have entailed serious risk and, most noteworthy, went not only against common opinion but also against the judgment of the learned encyclopedist Bartholomew of England (d. 1272). Some physicians would incise the pustules and apply astringent or even caustic powders in order to prevent them from closing. "This teaching, however," Valesco declared,

> is contrary to the opinion of all the laypeople, who do not wish that [the pustules] be perforated. This lay opinion is shared by the author of the book *On the Properties of Things,* who says, "the nurse or the physician,

whether to a little one or to an adult, should beware that the blisters of such pustules or pox not be broken or opened, on account of itching or for any other reason, especially around the face because, if they are perforated, marks will be visible forever."

Valesco made another memorable allusion to popular opinion in answering the question, "whether smallpox can occur twice or more to the same individual." In contrast with his own position that it could, and foreshadowing the much later discovery of acquired immunity, "the common saying is that an individual is rarely attacked more than once by this disease."

Warm Apostemes from Blood

While the compilers varied in the classification of smallpox and measles, nearly all of them opened the section on unnatural tumors with warm apostemes and, in particular, with those caused by good blood. In other words, these resulted from an excess accumulation of blood and, therefore, of excessive warmth. The role of heat may lead us to associate a warm abscess with the modern word "boil," which, however, has an unrelated origin, in the Indo-European root for "blowing up." In premodern nomenclature, most of the warm tumors received the label of "phlegmons," from the Greek for "to burn" (*phlegein*). The term was eventually succeeded by "inflammation," from the Latin for "setting aflame" (*inflammare*). It is worth noting that the compilers understood *inflammatio* more as a general condition of being on fire than as a localized phenomenon. For centuries, nevertheless, practitioners learned to recognize a local inflammation in the specific signs of "redness and swelling with heat and pain"—and their memory was aided by a rhymed quartet, *rubor et tumor cum calore et dolore.* The terms "phlegmon" and "inflammation" remained largely synonymous in the authoritative tradition, in spite of a few medieval attempts to dismantle the congruence. These attempts foreshadowed the modern differentiations in such labels as "phlegmonous inflammation" and "phlegmonous abscess" (that is, "with acute inflammation of the subcutaneous connective tissue").

The traditional synonymy was exemplified in the 11th century, when Gariopontus introduced his section on tumors by "speaking about phlegmon, that is, about a tumor on fire, or about heat and angry body parts." He further indicated the generic scope of phlegmons by reiterating (*sicut diximus*) that they were "divided into many different, varying, and changeable kinds," which, in turn, called for "just as many variations in treatment."

Some later authors, on the other hand, attempted to assign a more specific domain to the notion of phlegmon. Unlike Gariopontus—and a considerable number of others—who included apostemes from bile, Gilbert the Englishman and Bernard de Gordon restricted the category to swellings caused by blood. Valesco de Tharanta defined phlegmon squarely as "an aposteme generated *from blood* with inflammation, redness, warmth and pain"; he added, with a whiff of impatience, "Galen, however, extends this term to buboes and edemas, quinsies, pleurisy, and many other things."

A phlegmon was the least problematic of swellings if it was due to warm blood by itself, rather than due to a combination with another humor—as seems to have been more common. For a simple condition, the treatment was straightforward and, indeed, predictable. Further distinctions, such as Avicenna had made between the results of thick and thin blood, received limited attention in the descriptive and the prescriptive sections of the Latin manuals. Gariopontus, however, chided physicians who assumed that all phlegmons were identical and should be treated the same way. He claimed, "they make the mistake of ignoring their origin," and in true Hippocratic fashion, he explained,

> First, we inquire what underlies the humoral cause, by looking into the [patient's] age, the physical condition of the body or the affected part, the quality of the place, and the balance of the air: this way, we apply those things which we know to be appropriate.

The patient's condition determined how he or she should be treated and, in particular, whether the excess blood should be drained by phlebotomy or cupping. If so, an almost mythical principle, which was usually credited to Hippocrates, dictated that the bloodletting should be done in the corresponding opposite side, in order not to attract even more blood to the area of the swelling.

The reservations about drawing blood did not extend to the other methods of treating phlegmons. From the onset, the heat should be beaten down by means of "repressive medicines" (*repercussiva*), as long as they did not endanger the vital warmth of a nearby noble organ. These remedies ranged from cold water and vinegar to boiled barley flour in which such cold simples as coriander were mixed. When a warm aposteme advanced (in *augmentum,* which was the conventional designation for the second stage of any disease), its development was to be stimulated by plasters that contained such "ripening" (*maturativa*) agents as mallow or olive oil. Once the tumor reached the third stage of "standing" (*status*) or, in other words, had settled in, the accumulated blood might be loosened by applying such "dissolving things" (*resolutiva*) as compresses with saltwater, white wine, chamomile, or honeysuckle. The overall objective of these measures was to ripen the abscess and to drive out the offending "bloody matter" (*sanies*) in the production of pus.

The warmth, swelling, and hardness of the affected area needed to subside before a ripe phlegmon could receive final treatment. If it did not discharge the pus spontaneously, it "should be opened with a fleam (*flebotomo*) or with a caustic substance (*ruptorio*) which is prepared from quicklime or Jewish soap," according to Bernard. Similarly, it should be "opened with a lancet" in the phrase of Valesco, who added that the wound should be covered with a "tent dressing" for several days. A special procedure, which could either precede or follow the lancing of a boil, was the application of a piece of tow or stupe that had been steeped in a concoction of dry wine and chamomile: this would hasten healing by promoting the formation of pus. The belief in the possibility of a good or, in the standard phrase, laudable pus, was the most notorious and most pernicious legacy of Galen's teaching. The sway of this doctrine, however, has often been overstated because, at least in the medical manuals, pus was characterized primarily as a foul and noxious discharge, *sanies virulenta,* and as an ominous sign.

Warm Apostemes from Yellow Bile

Virulence, while relatively unusual for phlegmons, was the hallmark of the hot apostemes, which resulted from a mixture of blood and yellow bile or, far worse, from the direct burning effect of bile itself (even though bile and boil share an association with heat, they are not etymologically linked). The first aposteme to be associated with inflamed bile in the manuals was erysipelas, from the Greek for "red skin," although it was attributed to blood in the *Canon* (see Table 3.1). Avicenna and the Latin compilers agreed, however, on the distinctive symptoms of this infection: it colored the skin a clearer red than a phlegmon; it spread over the surface with less swelling; it caused a more biting pain; and it was more likely to be accompanied by fever. The further consensus was that typical erysipelas, as a skin affliction due to humoral imbalance or malfunction, differed from various incidences that were due to "manifest" external causes. Such causes, according to Gariopontus, included "wounds, stabbings, cuts by lances, or beatings." Several authors warned, on the authority of Avicenna, that "it is bad when erysipelas results from a fracture below the skin." This warning stirs thoughts of bacterial infection—and the temptation for retrospective diagnosis of streptococcus, which may be strengthened by Gilbert's observation that "sometimes bile becomes heated in a wound that has not been cleaned."

Gilbert continued, "the site becomes black, burned, hard, dry, and difficult to treat: and then we know the site as infected with erysipelas." Inconclusive diagnostic descriptions, such as this one by Gilbert, created a great potential for widespread confusion when they were combined with a fluid nomenclature. This was especially the case for skin diseases when authors used varying names without explanation or correlation. Thus, at one point, Gilbert simply stated, "erysipelas, by another name, is called *Persian* fire," but two centuries earlier, Gariopontus referred to one type of warm tumor as "erysipelas, that is, *sacred* fire"—as Isidore of Seville had done in his seventh-century *Etymologies*. Bernard indicated, at least, that synonymy of the two fires, as well as the distinction between both and erysipelas, was contingent on a developmental stage: "when an erysipelas ulcerates, it corrodes around and makes a scar, *and then* it can be called sacred fire *and* Persian fire." In general, however, these incendiary names and, most notably, "Saint Anthony's Fire" were given to quite different infections by the compilers, and they are often used indiscriminately by historians. In sum, a fluid terminology and facile synonymy designated a wide range of acute biliary or choleric inflammations that, in analogy with flames, consumed and spread at the same time.

Bile caused the greatest devastation when combustion turned it "into a form of burning poison, powerful and pernicious" as Gilbert learned from Johannitius. "A great variety of apostemes," Bernard elaborated,

> come from burned, corrupted, ulcerating, corroding matter that corrupts the flesh, bones, and other parts. Among these are Persian fire—or infernal fire, or fire of Saint Anthony, which is the same thing—and carbuncle, anthrax, touch-me-not, lupus or herpestiomenus, impetigo, serpigo, miliary formication, crawling formication.

The catalog further included a few external diseases from different humoral categories, but the warm apostemes listed so far require some elucidation. First of all, we note not only that Bernard expressly equated three inflammations, but also that here he omitted a fourth, namely, "sacred fire," which, in the same chapter, he presented as synonymous (as we saw earlier). A few paragraphs later he cited, apparently with some reservation, a sovereign authority for an even broader aggregation. "According to the teaching of Avicenna," he observed, "every ulcerating and blackening pustule that makes a scar, as if by cautery, *can be called* Persian fire or coal or carbuncle; this also *seems* to include formication and *some* other [apostemes]."

The definitions and descriptions in the authoritative sources, on which the understanding of warm apostemes depended, were often sketchy or ambiguous. The *Canon,* in particular, presented challenges of interpretation, at least in the Latin translation. As a result, compilers ignored such skin ailments as "burning coal" (*pruna*), when it was unclear whether Avicenna equated or merely juxtaposed them to other categories, Persian fire in this case. John of Gaddesden was one of the few to address the quandary, though not without a degree of doubt, when he wondered, "coal (*carbo*) and Persian fire: these two names *perhaps apply fully* to every pustule that corrodes, raises a blister, burns, and makes a scar." He further revealed his uncertainty by means of a qualifier, "*sometimes* the name 'Persian fire' refers to the fact that it is a pustule, whereas the name *pruna* refers to the fact that it infects and blackens the site in the same fashion as coal first is on fire and then turns black."

The problem of ambiguity in the classification of hot eruptions was compounded by the imprecision of most physicians in their descriptions, and by the flexibility of their analogies and explanations. The comparison with coal, for instance, was applied not only to *carbo* and *pruna,* but also to two kinds of pustule, "carbuncle" (from the Latin diminutive, "little coal") and "anthrax" (from the Greek for coal or, more specifically, for charcoal). Combustion accounted for the blackness of a carbuncle. Anthrax, while less directly tied to the coal analogy, was considered the most choleric, corrosive, and malignant of all external apostemes; it was also highly contagious. It was so named because it causes a "cavity" (*antrum*), as several authors proposed with erroneous if plausible etymology. A penchant for unconventional etymology similarly led some to explain that a related corrosive aposteme was called "touch-me-not" (*noli me tangere*) because it infects one who touches it. The prevailing explanation, however, was that touch was unbearable to the patient of this infection, which primarily struck the area around the nose and eyes.

Lupus and Herpes

The identification of *noli me tangere* as a facial infection is noteworthy, to some extent because it suggests a parallel to the butterfly rash, which is now known as a symptom of cutaneous lupus. More important, it calls for a revision of the persistent claim by historians that lupus has traditionally been associated with the face. It should be emphasized that, except for the generic reference to ulceration, the original category of *lupus* has nothing in common with its namesake in current dermatology and immunology. Another significant point is that no disease was called "the wolf" in Greek, Roman, or Arabic medicine, notwithstanding the primeval and feared presence of the animal in the Mediterranean world. Lacking both an ancient origin and a modern succession, medieval *lupus* typifies medicine of a defined era; in fact, most of its career coincided with the heyday of the *practica*.

The first mention of "a disease called the wolf" was not in a medical document but in an affidavit drawn up in 963 by Eraclius, bishop of Liège in the Holy Roman Empire. Eraclius confirmed that he had been cured miraculously, at the tomb of Saint Martin, of "the ailment that I suffered in the buttocks." Subsequent elaborations of his story demonstrated both the enduring role of popular imagination and the gradual medicalization of the category. A chronicle of the early 13th century related that Eraclius was healed "of a disease *which people call* 'the wolf.'" Adopting the literal interpretation of the vernacular metaphor, the chronicler added that the disease "devoured [the bishop's] flesh in a wolfish fashion." Moreover, he underscored the glory of the miracle by dramatizing the gravity of the ailment. "The only relief was to apply two plucked and eviscerated chickens every morning and evening against this wolfish rage," while the bishop was at death's door "with physicians despairing and with every treatment exhausted to no avail."

The introduction of *medici* and *cura,* in the two centuries between Eraclius's affidavit and the chronicler's amplified version, comes into focus in a passing note by someone who demonstrated familiarity with medicine on more than one occasion. Around 1170, Peter of Blois reported that the archbishop of Palermo had died after "herpes estiomenus, which people call 'the wolf', had severely afflicted his thigh, and all the tools of the medical men had failed." This report was contemporaneous with the appearance of a surgical manual by Roger Frugardi, but there was a clear difference in the designation of lupus. The surgeon Roger and his Lombard commentators presented lupus as a type of cancer, while the medically knowledgeable Peter identified it as herpes estiomenus, which was the classically established term for a slowly advancing corrosion of the skin. Since Peter proposed the identification right after he had spent some time with Romuald of Salerno, archbishop and physician, we may be tempted to assume that it originated in the Salernitan schools. Twelfth- and thirteenth-century masters of Salerno, however, did not mention lupus when they discussed *herpes estiomenus* in their manuals.

Throughout the Middle Ages and beyond, several authors followed the surgeons in classifying lupus as a type of cancer that affected the lower body. The compilers of medical manuals, on the other hand, suggested that lupus underwent a gradual absorption into authoritative tradition and into humoral etiology. In the 1250s, in his *Compendium,* Gilbert the Englishman simply equated the relatively new disease with a category that was as old as the Hippocratic corpus. "Lupus by another name is called '*herpes estiomenus*', that is, 'eating itself'. It results from yellow bile that is burned and thick." In addition to this straight equation, Gilbert proposed qualitative distinctions for a nosological framework.

> If unnatural bile ascends and is burned, the result is erysipelas, that is, holy fire; if it is greatly condensed, the result is lupus . . . Lupus differs from erysipelas because it causes greater blackening and corrosion of the site; it differs from cancer because it corrodes more, deeper, and faster.

The distinction between lupus and cancer, however, lost some of its relevance when Gilbert asserted that "all the things that cure cancer cure lupus and inversely."

The assertion that treatment was interchangeably effective was repeated in therapeutic sections of many a *practica*. This position disregarded the essential difference between apostemes due to bile, including lupus and/or herpes estiomenus, and those due to melancholy, most notably cancer—to which we turn our attention shortly. Among the apostemes due to bile, lupus began to fade in 14th-century pathology and therapeutics; it became largely synonymous with herpes estiomenus; and it would vanish from medical nomenclature, to reemerge in the late 18th century with a vastly changed meaning, and with a complexity that continues to evolve. In medieval nosology, the label *herpes* with a classical pedigree gradually superseded the term *lupus,* which probably originated in Germanic or Gallic metaphor. Where *lupus* lingered on as a disease category, it was occasionally tinged by the popular fears that accounted for the werewolf mythology. The compendia, however, reflected little of this contamination or, more generally, of the literal interpretation of metaphors that characterized vulgar lore. Moreover, literalness became less likely when the stark connotation of lupine or wolfish voracity was replaced by the less patent allusion, to a serpentine or snaky advance, in herpes.

The largest group of hot apostemes was comprised under the label "herpes," which was derived from the classic words for "to creep" (Greek *herpein,* Latin *serpere,* whence "serpent"). Here, too, it is important to keep in mind that modern designations of herpes have little in common with their predecessors. For almost two millennia, classifications fluctuated. Boundaries frequently blurred, for example, between this group and epidemics that ranged from ergotism to anthrax and smallpox. In addition, a variety of criteria governed the distinction of kinds of herpes. The simplest differentiation was according to location: the face was affected by *noli me tangere* and the lower body by *lupus;* the torso was girdled by *herpes zoster* or *cingulus*—the origin of shingles. Other criteria were more ambiguous, and they might support a combined category. Such criteria included not only the subtle humoral variations that we have seen exemplified in the *Canon,* but also the appearance, sensation, course, and effects, all of which were subject to imprecise description and unstable terminology.

In *herpes miliaris,* the skin was covered by small pustules the size of millet seeds; one type, *formica miliaris,* caused the sensation of crawling or biting ants (*formica* is Latin for "ant"). *Impetigo* (from the Latin *impetus,* "attack") erupted abruptly and spread erratically, whereas the infection advanced more slowly and steadily in *serpigo* (from *serpere,* see earlier). Both of these afflictions were accompanied by a burning itch, "an immoderate desire for scratching which induces a false and harmful feeling of pleasure." Either one might be caused "by infection from mouse-eaten bread, because mice have a certain poisonous nature," Bernard noted, admonishing that, "therefore, such bread should not be given even to the poor."

Unequivocal identification eluded even the oldest and most ubiquitous category *herpes estiomenus* (frequently contracted by compilers, into "herpestiomenus"). It may be noted that the meaning of the qualifying adjective (which became the noun "estiomene" in Middle English) is a great distance away from the more specific designation "esthiomene" in modern medicine. Medieval authors expanded the meaning from the original meaning, of "eating" (from the Greek *esthiō*), to "self-consuming," and even "wandering" (*ambulans*): Gariopontus believed that Hippocrates had chosen the name because these apostemes "devour themselves and graze far and wide." Valesco cited Guy de Chauliac for yet another etymology, "as it destroys a body part by deadening and softening it, it is given a name as if it were 'the enemy of man.'" Valesco demonstrated the trust of a physician in the teaching of a surgeon by reporting that, "according to Guy de Chauliac, herpes estiomenus destroys a part by deadening and softening it, and it is called as if it were 'the enemy of man.'"

Valesco made a seamless transition from a semantic point to an actual experience when he recalled,

> I have seen an adolescent of about seventeen who was afflicted by a certain softening and dying of the tissue above his right calf, some four digits from the outside of the leg. The size of a penny at first, it expanded all around, causing necrosis and producing pus. In nine days the flesh was dead and [the lesion] occupied a space of four fingers, soft, with pus and some deepening, but without pain or preceding aposteme. It stayed like this until the twelfth day, when it began to dry without any medication; what was corrupted turned into a crust, which dried and fell off piece by piece.

The anecdote exemplifies the coexistence of precise observation with a lack of specificity in medieval descriptions of skin infections—and, for that matter, of most diseases. This paradox makes it easy to understand the impatience of some compilers. Bertruccio, for one, sighed, "all these diseases are alike in nature and cause, as well as in treatment, so that we can cover them in a single chapter." The confusing subject matter of herpes indeed allowed for streamlined coverage to the extent that it comprised the worst of the hot, choleric, and corrosive external apostemes and, therefore, the most acute threats to external health.

Cold Apostemes from Phlegm and from Black Bile

Cold apostemes, which were attributed essentially to phlegm or black bile, presented a more chronic threat, and they generally occupied fewer pages in a *practica*. The two most remarkable exceptions were the melancholic diseases of cancer and leprosy, with which we will close this chapter. First, however, even a brief glimpse at apostemes from phlegm will reveal that, whatever their ranking in medicine, they reflect a wide spectrum of daily life. Most of the phlegmatic apostemes, which ranged from calluses and blisters to considerable accumulations of fluid, were categorized as edemas (from Greek *oidēma,* "swelling"). These largely belonged to the province of surgeons, and they caused relatively little concern among physicians, except where they overlapped with various forms of dropsy and indicated malnutrition, cardiac insufficiency, or humoral imbalance. Two of the external afflictions from imbalanced phlegm (and a touch of black bile) which stood out in several manuals—probably to the surprise of the modern reader—were fistula and scrofula.

Fistula, from the Latin for a shepherd's reed or a small water pipe, still refers to an abnormal passage into the body surface or between one organ and another. Compilers defined it as "a deep and concave ulcer, narrow on the outside and wide on the inside, caused by corrupt phlegm and alternately closing and opening." Fistulation seems to have been a widespread affliction, and it is puzzling why Valesco wrote, "laypeople say that it is Saint John's disease," which seems to have been the popular name for epilepsy. Fistulas might occur in an injured limb, an infected tearduct, or, most notoriously, a torn anus. Frequent mentions of the latter location hint at problems not only with hygiene, diet, and digestion, but also with horse riding. A fistula might result, as Valesco reported, "when an aposteme has matured and an unlearned barber or surgeon is unwilling to open it," so that the retained sanies corrodes both inward and outward.

The authors unanimously declared that fistula was difficult to cure, especially when it was deep or had been present for some time. The most desperate remedies were *experimenta* from the armamentarium of the empiric, and they ranged from magical pendants to plasters with vile ingredients. When more conventional procedures were still deemed feasible, they consisted of forcefully cleansing and removing the inflamed lining with such caustic agents as orpiment, vitriol, or verdigris. No wonder that, as Bernard observed, "many prefer to remain as they are rather than undergoing such treatments." No wonder, either, that he concluded, "since this disease is extremely difficult to cure, we should leave it to the 'restorers'," or that Valesco considered it "the job of surgeons."

If surgery for fistula was harsh but plausible, it seems utterly torturous and useless for scrofula. Affecting primarily the neck and sometimes the axilla or groin, scrofulas were defined as clusters of hard nodes in soft flesh. In a dual explanation, Valesco and others wrote that the term was derived from the Latin word *scrofa* for "sow" either because scrofula "often affects pigs as a result of their gluttony," or because "it produces many others, just as the sow gives birth to many piglets." It is worth noting that Gilbert the Englishman added that it was "also called the royal disease, because it is cured by kings": his cultural inheritance included the three-centuries-old English tradition of "the royal touch"; inversely, his medical learning apparently did not include knowledge of Celsus, or even of such Salernitan masters as Pietro Clerico, more commonly known as Petrocellus (ca. 1030), who had applied the distinctive name *morbus regius* to jaundice.

Scrofulas occurred mostly in children, Bernard believed, "because they are gluttonous" and careless in their diet. Dietary adjustment, which was the first step toward curing scrofula, entailed refraining not only from repletion but also from "all things that fill the head with fumes, as are garlic and onions, strong wine, shouting, worry, and anger," according to Bernard. When advancing to medicinal treatment, the practitioner should not apply repercussives, which would depress the body's vital heat in an already cold affliction. The nodes might be resolved by an ointment or plaster compounded from lily root, unripe figs, bean flour, nettle seed, or other simples from a wide choice. Beyond this, anyone who was "either timid or delicate" should "go to the kings," Bernard advised, "because they are wont to cure it by mere touch; and particularly the most serene king of the Franks." Only a decade later, John of Gaddesden gave a different color to the cure, by "the touch of the most noble and serene king of the English." The hardy but non-traveling patient might tolerate attempts to rupture the tumors with the help of blister beetles (cantharides) or

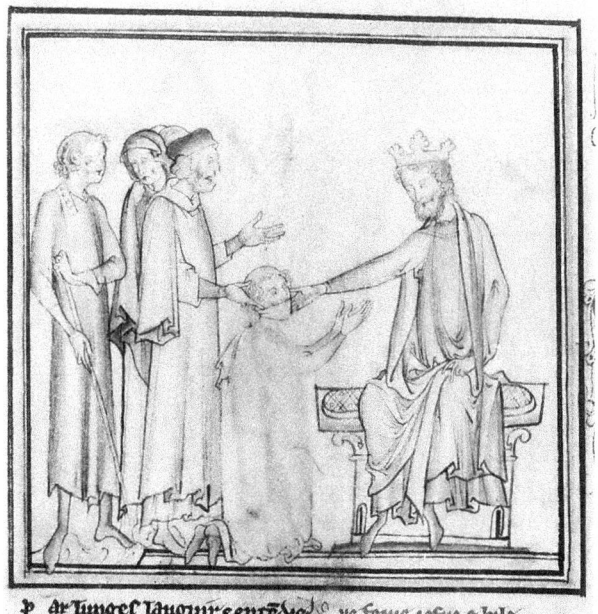

"The Royal Touch": King Edward the Confessor touching for scrofula. Drawing in the 14th-century manuscript of *L'estoire de Saint Edward le Rei* (*The History of Saint Edward the King*). Cambridge University, MS E.E. 3.59, p. 38. (Wellcome Library, London. Wellcome Images M006094)

caustic agents. "However," Bernard admitted, "this treatment is so ugly and difficult that I leave it altogether to the 'restorers.'" Ultimately, it was "necessary to have recourse to the surgeon's hand" for even more drastic methods.

Professional demarcations did not stop some physicians from describing surgical operations in detail. Gilbert instructed,

> when a scrofula is to be incised, it should first be taken into one hand and held firmly. Then the upper membrane should be incised lengthwise, and the flesh be scraped away from it, seized with a clamp, and pulled upward. If another follows, it should also be pulled, and so all of them, as many as are hanging together, together with their membranes. If too much hemorrhaging follows, it should be extracted at intervals, while the wound is filled with a white cloth steeped in oil.

By carrying the instructions into several successive days, Gilbert underscored the extended agony of these procedures. Nevertheless, surgical intervention was hardly uncommon, as may be inferred from Valesco's testimony.

> When the matter is well disposed and not too hard, and it is not resolved, the outside skin may be incised and the scrofula may be extracted with its follicle. Master Guillermus Sagarriga performed this treatment on a beautiful woman in my presence, in Girona, and learned surgeons do it frequently.

It is interesting that Valesco did not mention the royal touch, perhaps in order to maintain neutrality in the Hundred Years' War?

Cancer

The relationship between medical and surgical interventions, as well as differences between the medical and the surgical manual, is most evident in the chapters on cancer. These chapters highlight the general contrast between the surgeon's detailed descriptions and the physician's bent for logical definitions and explanations of tumors. In terms of harsh reality, physicians hinted that recourse to the surgeon's hand may have offered the only ray of hope to the cancer patient. This admission did not preclude an interest in surgical instructions, as we have just seen. However, it also did not negate the principle that humoral treatment, which was the mainstay of medicine, was appropriate for a prototypically cold aposteme from black bile. It was inherent in the competence of the learned physician, moreover, to define and explain diseases, as well as to assess their outlook and curability.

Physicians commonly defined cancer as a cold aposteme from superfluous or, more ominously, burned and corrupt black bile. This definition was derived from Galen's treatise *On Unnatural Tumors* and humoral teaching. However, it was most directly based on formulations in the *Canon* of Avicenna, who assigned a contributing role to yellow bile, in order to explain the eventual corrosiveness of the tumor. The label *karkínos,* "crab" or "crayfish," dated back to the Greeks, who also expanded it into *karkinōma,* for a "crab-like ulcer." The sound of the Greek root seems to have contributed to confusion among authors, and even more among scribes, between *cancer* and *cancrena*. The latter term was actually derived (as is the modern "gangrene") from the Greek word *gángraina* for "gnawing sore." While most compilers demonstrated awareness that this was an entirely different category, and none explicitly confused both words, several left ample room for ambiguity.

Cancrena was normally classified with the hot apostemes from yellow bile and most often correlated with the corrosion of *herpes estiomenus*. However, it lacked clear definition as a disease in itself. Bernard, for example, presented it as "a bad disposition," or what we might call a syndrome, in which the *accidentia* of "a dying color and some loss of sensation" were combined. Gariopontus, too, treated *cancrene* as a condition or a stage rather than a disease, when he clarified, "the name *cancrene* is applied to tissue that is not totally dead but still dying and retaining some life and sense. When tissue or a limb is totally dead and without sensation, it is called necrosis." His clarification, in turn, pointed to another opportunity for confusion, with the melancholic "deadly evil" or *malum mortuum* (English *mormal, mortmal,* or *morrimal*), a type of scabies that most frequently attacked the hips and thighs, turning them blackish, rough, and foul. In the medical lexicon and modern dictionaries, this category is regularly identified as "a bad sore; a gangrene; a cancer."

In an age when words carried enormous weight, semantic connections between crab and cancer, that is, between the animal and the name of the aposteme, burgeoned. They were conveniently drawn together by Bernard, who explained that this unnatural tumor was

> called "crab (*cancer*)" on account of a triple property: first, because it has a round shape, like a crab; second, because it clings forcefully and firmly holds on to its prey, like the crab; and third, because it resembles the crab

with its many long and crooked legs, and with the many different veins all around, which are full of melancholic blood.

Some of the elaborations underscored such sinister analogous characteristics as the hardness (itself the etymological root of *karkínos*) and tenacity that suggested obstinacy; the livid, or blackish-green tint that hinted at malignancy; and the irregular movement that reflected deceptiveness. John of Gaddesden, for example, explained that the tumor, like the crustacean, "gnaws while crawling around erratically, forward and backward."

The manuals varied considerably in the intensity and extent of their coverage of cancer. They generally indicate the degree of Avicenna's growing influence, since the *Canon* was the authoritative source in which the subject was developed most methodically. The earlier Latin compilers, including Copho, Gariopontus, Petrocellus, John of Saint Paul, and other Salernitan masters, evinced limited concern with cancer. Constantine the African covered it in the *Pantegni,* and he mentioned that it had the "appearance resembling that of a crab, because the veins, which are full of melancholic matter, spread out from the side of the aposteme, and they look like the legs of crabs." However, his definition and explanation were sketchy, he did not clarify semiological or therapeutic differences with other apostemes, and he blurred lines by referring to a cancer that "eats and causes a wound." Gariopontus crossed demarcations by mentioning "a herpes which is called 'cancrias,'" and even more by declaring, "I have spoken to you about cancers, *that is,* cancerous wounds." Gilbert still implied that cancers were closer to wounds and trauma than to tumors. This assimilation was explicit in his definition, "a cancer is a wound or lesion left behind by a melancholic aposteme that has not healed properly." For treatment, he indistinctly recommended ingredients "that are good for wounds." A similar lack of distinction was evident around the same time in the title, "On fistulas, cancer, lupus, and the like," for a chapter in a manual that was called *Breviarium* and that was attributed (spuriously, as we will see later) to Arnau de Vilanova.

Later authors showed a growing concern with cancer, and they carefully listed the distinctive signs that they deemed necessary for the diagnosis of the disease itself and of its stages and gravity. They found it particularly important to differentiate incipient cancer from other growths that were also small, hard, and relatively painless in the beginning. Their guidance helped to avoid unnecessary alarm at such less threatening swellings as phlegmons. It was critical for tumors in the category of *sclirosis,* which might be as benign as a callus or as malignant as a scirrhus. Valesco itemized five criteria, of which the first one pertained to etiology rather than semiology, but the other four were readily apparent to any examining practitioner.

> Cancer results from burned melancholy mixed with burned choler, while *sclirosis* results from wasted melancholy, pure or mixed with phlegm; second, cancer is accompanied by some pain and pulsation, which are absent in *sclirosis;* third, a cancer is surrounded by black veins, not red as in phlegmon; fourth, cancer begins on its own, whereas *sclirosis* follows another aposteme; fifth, a cancer is sensitive, *sclirosis* is not.

It was even more crucial to distinguish between an incipient and an advanced cancer, because the former might be curable while the other was not.

The compilers raised the life-and-death implication of careful diagnosis most emphatically in their discussion of breast cancer, a scourge that was known since antiquity. They prescribed topical, humoral, and even surgical treatments for the early stages. Gilbert advised, "if the site is hard around the cancer but the rest is soft and malleable, it may be treated with powder of asphodel (*affodilus*) and a caustic (*ruptorio*) ointment, or even by incision." If hardness, and accompanying pain, resulted from accumulated menstrual blood, which should have been expelled or converted into milk, Gilbert recommended that *maturativa* be applied and, "after softening, that it be incised; and then a tent or wick should be inserted, but with a tail so that it can be pulled out." Once the disease had advanced, physicians faced a heavy dilemma, between the stern reminders that it had become incurable and the proposed options for further treatment. Furthermore, although urged to leave intervention to the surgeon, they were, paradoxically, instructed how to proceed, even with radical mastectomy. The burden of this dilemma loomed large in the admission by Gariopontus that, if the cancer

> has grown too large and come to occupy the entire breast, it is doubtful that the patient can survive, because there is fear of hemorrhage and of extremely acute fevers, which infest the wound, bring danger of death, and make the physician guilty if he has not said beforehand that all these things were going to happen.

Such musings as these must have been on the mind of many a practitioner.

Recourse to surgical intervention was out of the question for most internal tumors, and compilers reminded their readers of the Hippocratic *Aphorism* (6.38), "For those to whom hidden cancers occur, it is better not to treat: indeed, the treated ones perish sooner but the ones not treated last a long time." It is natural here to think about uterine cancer, although diseases of the reproductive organs constitute the subject matter of a later chapter. Few texts are more poignantly illustrative than the section of the *Practica medicinae* that Michele Savonarola devoted to the subject.

> With the veins as its root, when the tumor occurs in a part from which it cannot be extracted with its roots, it becomes incurable. From this we understand that, since this kind of tumor of the uterus cannot be cured, it is untreatable in this location, at least by a real cure.

Refusing to abandon the patient, however, and applying the dual meaning of the term *cura,* Savonarola continued that even this cancer was amenable to treatment. "It can be treated palliatively, that is, medicated; and you can take this on, although in the end you will not gain honor, and you should let the relatives know." His palliative or "soothing" (*blanditiva*) treatment proceeded from dietary adjustments, systemic remedies, and topical applications, to douches and sitz baths with such analgesics as camphor and white poppy.

Leprosy

Avicenna characterized leprosy as "a cancer of the whole body." This was but a small tessera in the complex and cumulative discourse on leprosy by Latin authors until the Late Middle Ages. Furthermore, the compilers were not forced into the same mold by authoritative tradition, notwithstanding the sway of Avicenna's influence. Their chapters on *lepra* serve as a reliable gauge of changes in perceptions and responses, and even in the incidence of leprosy. In the first century of the Roman Empire, authors noted that a new disease was appearing in regions along the eastern Mediterranean. They gave it the Greek name *elephantiasis* or adapted this in Latin to *elephantia,* and they described skin deformities that resembled symptoms of the disease now known as Hansen's disease. Over the course of a millennium, the original name was gradually displaced by another term, from the Greek plural *leprai,* a grouping of various scaly skin conditions that may or may not have included an equivalent for *elephantia.* A decisive turn, with far-reaching consequences that cannot be pursued in these pages, came when the translators of the Bible chose *lepra,* for *zarā'at,* the Hebrew label for a status of ritual impurity and only indirectly for a disease.

The vocabulary change, which appears to have become definitive in or around Salerno, is attested in successive copies of works by Constantine the African and in a sequence of compendia. Gariopontus still called patients "elephantiosos" in the *Passionarius,* but soon thereafter Johannes Platearius called them "leprosos" in his *Practica.* The entrance of the new term into the medical nomenclature may have raised an eyebrow among the learned physicians. Both the transitional stage and the teacher's skepticism are suggested by the casual aside by Bartholomeus of Salerno in the title of a chapter in his *Practica,* "Elefantia, which the common people call 'lepra.'" The unstable nomenclature carried a serious potential for confusion that may be inferred, for example, from Savonarola's chapter "On Elefantia." He was clearly referring to the disorder of the lymphatic system, which is still called elephantiasis, in his definition of "a swelling of the feet," which was akin to varicose veins. He elaborated that it occurred in various parts of the body, including the male genitals, and that therefore it bore different names; "and sometimes it afflicts the entire body, and then it is a second kind of lepra." In the 16th century, Humanists revived the label *elephantia* for leprosy, as part of their return to classical usage. Meanwhile, it should be emphasized that the authors of compendia interpreted *lepra* as a medical category, and they virtually ignored the biblical and ritual connotations, even though they were keenly aware of the social consequences of the disease.

Physicians defined *lepra* in strictly physical terms, as the "breakdown" (*corruptio*) or even as the "rotting" (*putredo*) of the body that resulted from the spread of burned humors. Beginning on the surface, it ultimately ravaged the patient's appearance, limbs, and structure. Black bile was the predominant culprit, but the involvement of another humor accounted for three additional varieties. The result of disordered black bile itself was the prototypical *lepra,* the worst but most slowly advancing form, *elephantia,* in which thickening, cracking, roughness, and knobs made the skin resemble that of an elephant. If yellow bile was involved, it resulted in *leonina,* the second most grave form, which advanced more swiftly, and in which a protuberant forehead, the loss of eyebrows, and the collapse of the nostrils made the face look like that of a lion. The two other types, incidental rather than essential to leprosy, were added in order to accommodate symptoms that were not included in *elephantia* and *leonina* and, arguably even more, in order to maintain symmetry with the fourfold humoral scheme. When burned blood was mixed with the black bile, the chief effect would be the loss of hair in patches, which was named *alopecia* from the Greek for "fox mange" (and which also appeared, on its own terms, among the diseases of the head, as we will see in the next chapter). In the fourth type of *lepra,* the involvement of phlegm caused the cold and moist disposition characteristic of the snake, and it manifested itself in the discoloration and scaliness of the skin: these traits accounted for the name *tyria,* a label with an uncertain pedigree but supposedly derived from a Greek word for "viper."

The compilers mentioned contagion, sex, and heredity among the immediate causes of leprosy. These mentions have stimulated lively debate for more than a century; however, they tend to draw the disproportionate attention of the historian who ignores that they were part of a much larger array. These included such dietary factors as the eating of spoiled meat or too many melancholic foods such bear and boar, or, even more oddly, the consumption of fish and milk in the same meal. Another factor was corrupt or pestilential air, although leprosy was not expressly categorized as an epidemic. This observation is pertinent because the extent of leprosy in medieval Europe tends to be overestimated. The overestimation is due chiefly to one-sided inferences. One of these views the proliferation of shelters (leprosaria) in the 12th and 13th centuries solely as a response to the urgency of a spreading disease, while overlooking the broader surge of charitable foundations. Another slanted inference ignores various reasons for the high profile of leprosy in medieval sermons and in the lay literature as well as in medical writings.

Several compilers, most notably Bernard de Gordon, discussed leprosy in greater detail than several external ailments that were no doubt more common. This was not an indicator of a ubiquitous problem, however, and other considerations underlay this disproportionate attention. In the first place, as Bernard pointed out, "this subject is so sordid that it requires much clarification; therefore, if we prolong the discussion somewhat, no one should think ill of it." Indeed, it was—and remains—difficult to think of a more devastating assault on the human body, a more horrifying vision of slow destruction, or a curse more mysterious in its origin and course. The advancing ravages, especially of the elephantine and leonine forms, dramatically exposed the ineffectiveness of medical treatment. At the same time, the uncertain onset and advance of this disease compounded the challenge to medical understanding. After all, ever since Hippocrates and Galen, the strength of the learned practitioner did not lie in the curing but in the identification, recognition, and explanation of diseases. This strength was a powerful incentive for the physician to demonstrate and contribute his privileged knowledge, if not efficacy, when social responses to *lepra* were at their height.

The most decisive knowledge lay in "dia-gnosis," the ability to differentiate. The identification of the form of the disease determined much of the response. The recognition of the stage, however, had the most specific, urgent, and far-reaching consequences. Social as well as therapeutic ramifications presented the practitioner with daunting challenges. A decision by municipal or other authorities to sequester a patient depended on a formal confirmation that he or she was infected with full-fledged leprosy. Before the rise of medical faculties, and for centuries thereafter in many places, clergy, confirmed patients, or barber-surgeons presented the decisive finding. In the course of the 13th century, an official judgment or *iudicium* increasingly became the responsibility of learned physicians. Their education supposedly enabled them to distinguish not only *lepra* from similar skin ailments but also the acute form from a relatively mild one, and the "confirmed" stage from an incipient one or from a predisposition. These distinctions were deemed vital, protecting society from the spread of a supposedly communicable disease. They were vitally conclusive for the patient as a social being.

John of Gaddesden was one of several authors who listed a broad range of symptoms, including widely scattered spots and inflammations that, though alarming, did not add up to full-blown leprosy. On the basis of these, "a prognosis should be made, declaring that there is inchoate *lepra*, that the patient is disposed, and that he can still mingle with people, but not as safely as someone else." In addition, Gaddesden warned that a person "should not be judged leprous and to be separated from everybody" until the appearance of definitive signs. There was general agreement among the physicians that facial disfigurement and the corrosion of the nasal septum were the conclusive and irreversible *signa confirmationis*. Before these were manifest, however, the tortuous and often slow progress of the disease left much room for uncertainty and even, considering the consequences, agony by the judging practitioner. The sense of hesitation is poignantly evident in the many *iudicia* of which the results have been preserved in archives: a high proportion of verdicts were indecisive and called for a return examination. A corresponding sense of urgency induced compilers to spell out deceptive and ambiguous signs as well as the unequivocal symptoms of confirmed and socially fateful *lepra*.

The diagnosis and prognosis were no less decisive for the patient's fate in directly medical terms. Johannes Platearius summed up the import of this concern.

> To speak the truth, all the types of *lepra* are incurable. When a disposition to *lepra* arises, however, it is possible to protect the patient from future danger. And even when the disease is confirmed, it is possible to palliate, and to protect the patient from greater evil.

After almost two centuries during which the perception of leprosy had grown, Bernard was more emphatic in stating both the decisiveness of the prognosis and the potential for further care.

> We can prognosticate with certainty that *lepra* will never be cured once it comes to the manifest corruption of [the body's] form and shape. However, we can prolong life and, with suitable medications, prevent the poisonous melancholic matter from going to the heart and principal organs.

Paradoxically, Bernard prefaced his therapeutic advice with the caveat that it was intended for the onset of the disease, "when it is treatable; for we do not have to engage in the treatment of the confirmed disease except to prolong [life] and so that, if the physician is asked insistently, he may prescribe something."

Treatments, from preventive to palliative, progressed from dietary adjustments to surgery. An appropriate management of the nonnaturals included avoiding not only many foods that produced black bile but also, most important, all sex—"even though the popular and erroneous opinion is that it not only helps but cures," Bernard noted. Several authors insisted that sex drained the patient's strength, cooled and dried an already imbalanced complexion, spread the poisonous humors through the body, and increased the risk of infection (which they did not state explicitly in this connection, however). Medicines, whether administered topically or to the entire body, internally or externally, aimed for the digestion and elimination of offending matter. There were many methods of purging, but phlebotomy was considered most effective for eliminating corrupt humors, although it was fraught with contradiction. Disregarding the priority of diet in the normally conservative sequence of treatments, Bernard recommended that for *lepra*, "we should begin, first, with phlebotomy." Yet, in the opening rubric of his *clarificatio* he asserted that "phlebotomy is not appropriate per se but only secondarily," when excess blood might entail the danger of blockage or putrefaction in the veins. He further warned sternly,

> I assure you that I every day see people err shamefully in the phlebotomy of leprous patients. I have often seen that physicians aimed for nothing else than drawing all the blood. Therefore, be careful.

Bernard's apparent inconsistency was one more sign of the dilemma which practitioners faced in attending to leprous patients.

John of Gaddesden expressed the greatest willingness to extend the treatment of *lepra* as far as possible. He formulated the prognosis more in degrees of curability than in terms of incurability.

> The disease appears more susceptible to treatment in the beginning, but even then it is difficult to treat in the sense that it will not be cured by the benefit of nature except with the help of the Art. The confirmed stage is more intractable. Once it reaches the manifest breakdown of form and shape, there is no hope of cure, because Avicenna says that then it is not necessary to try phlebotomy or strong medicine.

At this point, however, Gaddesden began to rebut Avicenna on several points, including the proposition that *lepra* and cancer were equally incurable. He followed these rebuttals with a lengthy section on therapeutics, beginning with "preventing and palliating treatments of which, as we should see, some are for the poor and some for the rich." The cheaper remedy called for one spoonful of thyme or thyme dodder with goat's fat per day, in contrast with the expensive "dram of gold shavings, to be given daily with food or drink, in [the] morning or at the beginning of lunch: this is the greatest remedy, and it strengthens the mind and the heart"; even better was "taking a large amount of the gold or silver leaf, which goldsmiths make, if the patient can afford it." Gaddesden then proceeded to the more advanced stages of *lepra*, for which prescriptions ranged from purges to plasters.

Compilers commonly juxtaposed *lepra* with another disfiguring disease, namely, *morphea* ("morphew" is now a largely obsolete term for a scaly skin condition). The same treatment was indicated for both, since they were attributed to the same causes. On the other hand, similarities between identified symptoms heightened the practitioner's anxiety about a precise differentiation. Indeed, the "unsightly spotting" on the body, diagnosed by the practitioner as *morphea*, might have been a sign of incipient leprosy. This was especially the case for white *morphea*, which might correspond to the patches of skin discoloration in Hansen's disease, the modern successor to *lepra*. Efforts to differentiate, between a disease of the skin and one of the flesh, were emphatic but of limited practical benefit. Furthermore, a collation of compendia reveals that, while *lepra* became circumscribed with greater specificity, *morphea* became a catchall for poorly defined skin blemishes. Many Latin authors equated the term with *al baras*, a generic Arabic term for leukoderma ("white skin"). This equation, and their even more than usual reference to Avicenna, Serapion, and Rhazes, gives the impression that the category had not been fully integrated into their lexicon.

The medical taxonomy, as well as the lexicon, remained uncertain for a host of partially similar categories, among which scabies was one of the most troublesome. This skin infection was characterized by an intolerable itch, "delight in scratching, but in the end great pain," in the words of Gaddesden. It attacked the extremities or the entire body, while ringworm (*tinea*) was believed to be a localized form, limited to the head. Scabies was recognized as highly contagious and difficult to cure, particularly in old patients. Most authors believed that only palliative treatment was possible. This did not prevent Gaddesden from offering a recipe as "my own, and satisfactory without any other medication once the body has been cleansed." He recommended the remedy with a personal endorsement that may sound familiar in an age of pharmaceutical testimonials.

> This is a very good ointment with which I have cured many who suffered from every kind of itch and scabies and who looked as if they were leprous: it was so bad that, until this ointment was applied, they needed to have two men scratching them, even during a meal.

Intolerable itching was an essential symptom of scabies, and the pertinent chapter in the *Canon medicine* was titled "De scabie et pruritu." In most of the Latin compendia, however, itch received a separate chapter, as a category by itself.

Another symptom to which Avicenna as well as the subsequent compilers devoted a full chapter was perspiration (*desudatio* or *sudor*). It was viewed as an external affection and, at the same time, as one of the evacuative processes that ranged from urination to menstruation. Deviations from the norm were addressed as a therapeutic concern, but they drew more attention in diagnostics. In Valesco's synopsis, "Constantine, whom [Bernard] Gordon follows, says that one kind of perspiration is natural, the other unnatural, profuse (*diaforeticus*), and symptomatic, as in excessive pain and in the dying." Unlike Constantine, Valesco and Bernard organized their subject matter accordingly. In the *Pantegni,* the chapter on perspiration appeared between one on pustules and another on warts. In the *Philonium* and in the *Lilium,* it preceded the chapters on smallpox and measles. Bernard placed it, most logically, between pestilential fevers and smallpox. His organization reflected the longtime association of fevers with epidemics. This association was most dramatically manifested in the mysterious sweating sickness that swept through England in waves from 1485 to the 1550s.

As a category by itself, sweating often joined the skin afflictions that were treated more for the sake of appearance than for physical health. The relatively minor ones, ranging from liver spots to warts, and sometimes even *lepra* and *morphea,* might be relegated to chapters on cosmetics. The discussion of cosmetics appeared in a separate section at the end of some compendia under the heading "De decoratione." The discussion, which is so rich and complex that full coverage would exceed the boundaries of this survey, demonstrates the significance and the extent of esthetic concerns that contradict the popular assumption that appearance mattered little in the daily life of medieval people. At least some of the cosmetic considerations will become evident in the next chapter when we note the apportionment of aspects in dealing with diseases of the head. By the same token, the chapter will highlight the anthropocentric focus of the compilers on the head as distinctly human, in contrast with the many zoological analogies and derivations (wolf, snake, ants, crab, elephant, fox, lion) that they applied to the body's exterior.

Head Problems, from Hair Loss to Epilepsy

The essential and adjunct parts of the head are as follows: the hair; then the skin, flesh, and tissue; next, the skull; then, the hard membrane, and the thin membrane which is called "secundine"; next, the brain substance, and the cells with their contents; then, two membranes under it, and the rete [mirabile]; and then, the bone at the base of the brain.

This is the anatomy of the brain: it is divided into the cortex; the medulla; and the cells within, filled with spirit . . . The substance of the brain is created cold and moist. Cold, so that it will not be inflamed by the strong movements of the nerves, the imprints on the senses, and the motions of the spirit in changing imaginations, thoughts, and memories; further, so that the spirit will be tempered when, coming from the heart, it enters through two ascending veins. [The substance of the brain] is moist so that it may not be dried out by movement . . .

It should be known that the head suffers all kinds of diseases. Here, however, our focus is on the brain and its membranes, and we are not considering the diseases of the hair. Eight kinds of bad complexion affect the brain.

With these lines, Avicenna introduced 29 chapters on general aspects of the head and brain, opening Book Three of the *Canon medicine,* which covered diseases of the various parts of the body. His introduction, as excerpted here, foreshadowed directions and developments in Latin medical teaching about the head; it will also become useful, further in this chapter, for gauging the extent and limits of his influence on compilers.

It should be noted first that Avicenna addressed the particular diseases before the all-body diseases, which followed in Book Four. The difference between his and our arrangement of the subject matter parallels the diversity among manuals, not only in their organization but also in the degree of their dependence on the *Canon*. As we have seen in the preceding pages, compilers exposed the physiological foundations of medicine in their chapters on fevers and discussed all-body diseases in their chapters on apostemes. This twofold comprehensive treatment left a vast range of particular health issues for the rest of a manual. Before the *Canon* and the *Liber ad Almansorem* became normative, the range was most often covered randomly, as it was in the "Pars Practica" of the *Pantegni,* the influential textbook by Constantine the African, where Book Four, "On diseases in external parts, and their cures," moved from leprosy to diverse skin afflictions, wounds, perspiration, and smallpox, to end with four chapters on hair. There is a contrast, however, between this disarray and the orderly progression of an equally influential main source, the *Viaticum,* which was also edited by Constantine, and in which the first six parts advanced from problems of the head to the "pain of the heel bone" (*calcanei*) known as gout. This order was readily adopted for compendia because, in simple terms, it lent itself best to convenient consultation of the disparate material by the practitioner as well as to the easy review of *medicina practica* by the student.

The head-to-heel arrangement was natural, in fact, because it followed the universal and spontaneous way of looking at the human body. Moreover, the practitioner's concern with health proceeded instinctively "from the care of the hair to the soles of the feet," as formulated in the *Practica,* an early manual that is linked to Salerno and attributed to Petrocellus. A deeper motive for the sequence was suggested in a fourth-century compilation of remedies, when Theodorus Priscianus set out "to descend from the head as if from the summit to the rest of the body": in this wording, the order paralleled the scale of values that philosophers and theologians attributed to body parts, with the raised head and the earthbound feet as emblematic poles of the human condition. The moral subtext was readily enhanced by a pervasive penchant for analogy and metaphor, as we will see. The paradoxical influence of intuitive perception and idealizing contemplation occasionally caused a strange placement in the head-to-toe framework, of issues ranging from sneezing and drunkenness to hunchback. By the same token, the framework itself changed. Most consequentially, intuition and contemplation merged gradually with the rise of anatomical dissection, when the "fabric of the human body" took center stage and the head lost much of its primacy.

The balance between intuition and contemplation—or, more concretely, between an empirical and a reasoning approach—varied from one author to another. This was one of several causes of great diversity, not only in the general range and organization of medieval manuals but also in the chapters on the head, which routinely constituted the first section of the part "on particular diseases." The structure of these chapters was shaped by the objectives of each manual, and it encompassed three or four areas, namely, the hair, the skull and brain, mental function, and motor control. The closely related area of the face, as the location of four of the five senses, involved so much material that authors left it for a separate section, and we will examine it in the next chapter. Still, in their discussion of the head, they allocated substantially more space to the outside than to the contents. The discussion reflected, arguably more directly than other parts, the authority of the main sources. On the other hand, it also reflected the personal outlook of the compilers and their varying concern with practical benefit, taxonomic transparency, and encyclopedic comprehensiveness.

The variations were most striking in the discussion of hair, and they may be reduced to three patterns. Some compilers spent relatively little time on the subject, apparently because their relatively brief compendia concentrated on essential health guidance and on such prevalent problems as headache. In the 11th and 12th centuries, Salernitan masters who shared this pattern included Gariopontus, Copho, Johannes Platearius, Bartholomeus, and Gilles de Corbeil; also Roger Frugardi and other Lombard surgeons adopted it. John of Saint Paul suggested limited personal interest in the subject by asserting that he offered "a few proven remedies (*probata experimenta*), to satisfy those who look for hair grooming." Petrocellus may have made the only exception to the relative inattention at Salerno, by devoting a few chapters of his *practica* to baldness, dandruff, and head lice. The inattention extended, on the other hand, to a few 15th-century authors, such as Antonio Guaineri and Michele Savonarola, who omitted hair from their expansive section on diseases of the head, at a time when it was a standard item in manuals.

Numerous compilers agreed in considering hair worthy of separate attention, but they diverged in their approach, mainly by allocating the subject either to the beginning or to the end of their manual. The distance between these two patterns, together with numerous differences within each group, contradicts the widespread image of medieval medicine as purely derivative. More precisely, the differences belie the assumption that the archetypical and incomparably encyclopedic *Canon of Medicine* established a single and rigid mold. A considerable number of manuals diverged from the *Canon* in their allocation and discussion of hair as a subject. In the first 122 chapters (*fen* 1–2) of Book Three, "on particular diseases from head to feet," Avicenna considered hair in passing, merely as a diagnostic marker rather than as an entity by itself. He left the care and other aspects of hair for a later part, Book Four on cosmetics, where they occupied almost one-third of the chapters. One of the authors who echoed Avicenna most consistently, namely, Niccoló Bertruccio, maintained a similar pattern by relegating hair to the last section of his *Collectorium,* on cosmetics; however, he gave the subject less than one-sixth of this section, whereas he devoted a substantial chapter to leprosy and another to "the fattening and thinning of the whole body." Valesco de Tharanta, too, withheld the consideration of hair until the end of the *Philonium,* where he limited himself to a few chapters and, oddly appended them, as an afterthought, to the extensive Book Seven on apostemes. Guglielmo da Saliceto (1201–1277) reserved hair care for a separate *liber* in his *Summa* or summary "Of Preservation and Treatment."

A third pattern was represented by compilers who not only viewed hair as a medical topic but, with utter literalness, placed it first in the top-to-bottom order—rather than giving the head itself the priority that it held in more reflective yet conventional taxonomies. This pattern had an antecedent in the early-fifth-century *Euporiston* of Theodorus Priscianus. A more direct model, however, lay in an Arabic compendium that, though eclipsed by Avicenna's *Canon,* exerted a pervasive influence on Latin teaching. The *Breviarium* or *Liber aggregationis* (which, like the *Canon,* was also translated by Gerard of Cremona) opened with five chapters on hair; the author, Yaḥyā ibn-Sarāfyūn (870–920), who was known in the West as "Johannes filius Serapionis," gave the subject about one-seventh of his first *tractatus*. This proportion was expanded considerably in a group of manuals that enjoyed a long and wide circulation from the late 13th century on, and that yield the richest material for our survey. Gilbert the Englishman opened the head-to-toe part of his *Compendium* with 10 chapters on hair, and these accounted for one-fifth of his section "de capite." Bernard de Gordon and Guglielmo da Varignana maintained this proportion, even if they also devoted a separate section to cosmetics, usually at the end of their *practica*. It is difficult to gauge to what extent the heightened interest was due to the availability of a certain source, the personal inclination of the author, or social trends of the period. Hair seems too trivial as a medical subject to merit so much attention from learned authors—some of whom have, ironically, been accused of hairsplitting.

Their observations, however, shed so much light on fundamental concepts, proposed and actual practices, and cultural perspectives that here, too, we will give them a seemingly disproportionate amount of attention.

"A Chimney for the Whole Body"

The term *capilli* ("appendages of the head," *caput*) is plural in Latin compendia as well as in today's Romance languages, whereas English and other vernaculars refer to the growth of hair with a singular noun—as Gilbert the Englishman did, in an intriguing exception to Latin usage. The plural is consistent with explanations and prescriptions of learned manuals, which were rooted in Aristotelian philosophy and Galenic physiology. Hairs originated and grew in an exhalation of bodily vapors that were drier than sweat, thinner than the material of fingernails, but thicker than imperceptible evaporations. They emerged through pores that gave them their shape. When pores were too few or tight, as on the palms of the hands and soles of the feet, hairlessness was natural. By contrast, there were places where vapors escaped through wider pores, through "cleansing passages" (*emunctoria*) in the armpits and pubes and other regions. Most vapors, however, rose to the top, as fumes are wont to do. The head, Bernard proposed, "is like a chimney for the whole body." In a maintained analogy with smoke, successive puffs formed lengthening and rounded columns. This cumulative "chainlike process" (*concatenatio*) differed in essence from the intricately managed unfolding in the growth of plants.

The process occurred only when and where the body was balanced in complexion. Thus, men were by nature warmer and therefore hairier than women, but they incurred baldness when they became colder with advancing age. Abnormal cooling also caused some people to lose their hair when they were consumptive, incarcerated, starving, or sexually overactive. By contrast, eunuchs and women did not become bald because their constitution was steadily cold and moist. More elaborate notions added the role of humors to the effects of elemental qualities. For example, a choleric person, with a hot complexion due to the prevalence of bile, tended to be more hirsute yet also to become bald at a younger age—an intuitive sense of the effects of (then unknown) testosterone? One or more humors also gave hair its consistency and other qualities, in explanations that contributed more to speculative excursuses than to practical insights. Without overlooking the compiler's concern with providing information, we may wonder about the therapeutic benefit of some standard humoral schemes. In one, yellow hair was linked to a predominance of bile in a choleric complexion, red hair to a sanguine temperament, pale hair to phlegm, and black to melancholy. In another construct, climate joined complexion to premise the proposition, as quoted by Bernard (undoubtedly from an encyclopedia), that "Indians and Ethiopians have black and curly hair, English and Germans blond and straight, and Southerners in-between."

Hair played an important role, albeit less prominently than the face, in the linking of personal appearance with origin, temperament, and character. The resulting judgments of physiognomy have forever produced stereotypes that simplify life and make things comfortably predictable. In prejudging, physiognomy dovetailed with teleology for answers to profound questions, also in medical theory and even on seemingly superficial matters. Human hair existed for a threefold ultimate reason or *causa finalis,* namely, beauty, usefulness, and necessity. It decorated the head and protected it from heat and cold; hair was further useful by cleansing the body of harmful vapors. For this reason, Bernard objected to the (supposedly modern) practice of those "who prevent the growth of hair on the pudenda of girls, with narcotics or cautery or any other method." The most important rationale, according to Gilbert and others, was the need "to tell the genders apart": this is why "Nature has created beards in men, so that the power of their warm constitution may be recognized on sight, and a partner for reproduction (*ad generationem*) may be chosen decently, without touching." The beard denoted the superiority of male warmth and generative power, and Bernard added a notch to the value scale by noting, "eunuchs do not develop a beard if they have lost their 'pals (*socios*)' before pubescence."

Authors also graded the value of human hair by presenting it as superior to the hairs of other mammals, in the same way as they differentiated almost every body part (without precluding comparisons). They contrasted its dignity in covering the head with the earthiness of the animal coat—and with the shagginess of the wild man. A few hinted at a semantic distinction between human *capilli* and the *pili* of animal fur, wool, or manes. Several authors proposed that graying happened only to humans and not to animals except for horses and that, in the former, it began at the forehead while in the latter—well, they left this to the reader's power of observation. Bernard and others underscored the special dignity of human hair by more solid distinctions. They pointed out a moral dimension by citing the adage, "The grayness of fathers must be honored." Nevertheless, they also drew a line between the natural and moral realms. Physicians alluded to the precept from the Book of Wisdom, "We should honor the graying not of years but of habits," but then they added the paradox that "even if grayness may have moral significance, it represents no natural good." In fact, Valesco argued that it signified a natural ill because it meant that approaching Death had "applied graying to the human head as if it were its flag."

Graying, together with hair loss, fell in an area where core medical theory and practice overlapped with the perennial quest for youth as well as with everyday hygiene and beauty care. Much of this belongs more to the general regimen of health than to the treatment of diseases. Therefore, we will limit ourselves to more narrowly circumscribed health issues, causes, and cures. At the edge of this circumscription was the issue of lice and nits. Most of our compilers included this subject in hair care, but some treated it as part of body hygiene, for example, by addressing crab louse (*pessolata*) infestation of various areas. The declaration, "lice appear not only on the head but, in truth, also on the rest of the body," introduced the chapter that John of St. Paul inserted between scabies and leprosy. Avicenna's discussion of lice followed chapters in the *Canon* on body odors and similar problems. John of Gaddesden digressed in a paragraph on pubic lice, "I touch on many things here because the religious and others who do not care about grooming of the body, like those who frequently use a haircloth shirt, are full of these, and they seek help from medical remedies,"—or, in an intriguingly variant version, "they seek counsel from secret physicians."

Wherever the subject of lice was addressed in manuals or, for that matter, in more comprehensive encyclopedias, it occasioned the most remarkable application of natural philosophy to the understanding of life. The general notion was that lice were produced, invisibly, by spontaneous generation (abiogenesis in modern technical terminology) from nonliving material. Certain putrefying humors, which nature was unable either to manage or to expel cleanly, could become "animated beings" (*animalia*) under precisely favorable circumstances. If the moisture of the exudate was fostered by moderate warmth, it formed flakes that were less dry than mere dandruff. Once they acquired the perfect combination of humidity and heat, the flakes drew "vegetation and vivification from the body's spirits," according to Gilbert; they received "the essence of life," in Bernard's phrase.

The presence of lice was blamed on poor care of the head and body, infrequent change of clothes, and an unhealthy diet, which for several authors included, strangely enough, eating figs. By this presence one could recognize, Bernard claimed, "the poor and the members of religious orders who eat too many phlegmatic and melancholic foods," and "wild (*ferales*) persons" who neglected themselves. The ectoparasites, in turn, caused their hosts to suffer anxiety, sleeplessness, weight loss, and paleness—"to

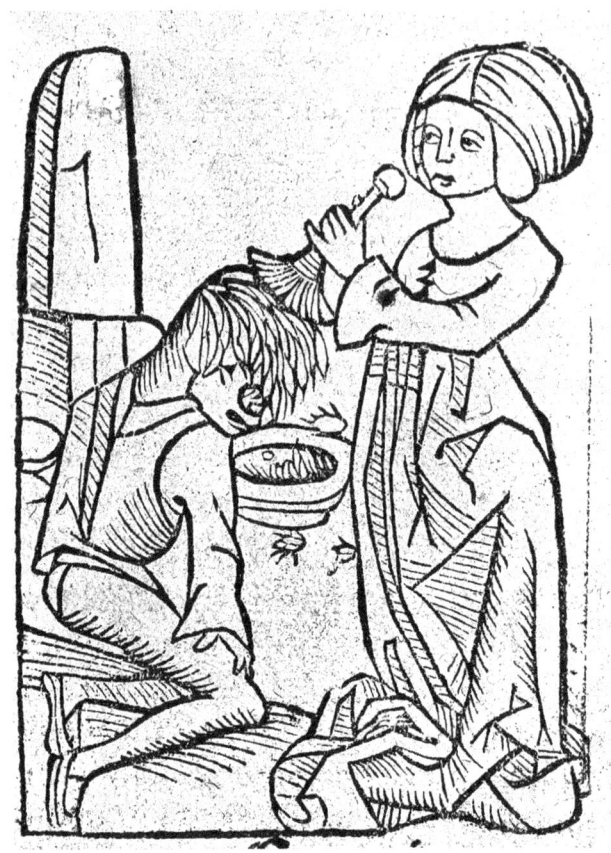

A woman brushes lice out of a boy's hair. Woodcut in an incunabulum of Jacob Meydenbach, *Ortus sanitatis* (*The Garden of Health*), Mainz, 1491, fol. S3v. (Wellcome Library, London. Wellcome Images L0001410)

feel lousy," as we would say. The problem was no laughing matter, but grave enough to call not only for cleanliness and changes in the way of life but also for more drastic prescriptions. One ubiquitous ingredient in these was *staphysagria,* stavesacre, or palmated larkspur, a plant that was also called "lousewort (*herba pedicularis*) because it kills lice by its entire species," that is, by an inherent but occult power. This observation by Bernard directly contradicts the explanation by a recent historian that the plant was believed to *cause* lice infestation in livestock. The name may actually have its root in a resemblance between the seeds of one species and lice. In any event, Bernard extended the benefits of the herb to veterinary medicine when he recommended applying the herb, ground and pulverized, "to birds of prey, for it frees them totally of the pest in their tail."

The powder of lousewort (of which variations are still used to kill parasites) was mildly toxic, but harsher medicines were prescribed for other problems of the hair and scalp. The afflictions that called for the most drastic measures were alopecia, ringworm, and favus. Alopecia or patchy baldness accompanied by ulceration—which also constituted one of the four types of *lepra,* as we have seen in the preceding chapter—was blamed on corrupted humors that blocked the pores. The first treatment, therefore, was to purge those humors by means of bloodletting and laxatives to the extent that the patient was able to tolerate them. Topical remedies began with mild applications to the site after it had been shaven and cleaned. These proved mostly ineffectual, as may be inferred from the crescendo in the recipes for ointments. Increasingly powerful ingredients ranged, since at least Avicenna, from almonds to garlic and mustard, and then from hellebore to pigeon and mouse droppings. We should note, however, that most Latin compilers condensed Avicenna's pharmacopoeia; they omitted his recommendation to apply "leeches, and to prick with several needles," and they eliminated such ingredients as borax, pepper, cantharides or blister beetles ("Spanish Fly"), and bull's gall from their own treatments of lice infestation.

The most extreme remedies were prescribed, in Latin as well as Arabic compendia, for two conditions that were especially troublesome, stubborn, and shameful. Ringworm or *tinea,* and favus or "honeycomb" (now also called *tinea favosa*) were attributed to emanations of putrefied humors, phlegm in particular. Both were considered incurable once they had established themselves. Nevertheless, powerful methods for treating advanced cases were offered in every compendium. The general reliance of therapeutics on polypharmacy, traditional authority, and personal experience betrays a degree of helplessness in spite of claimed success. An instance in the *Philonium* is so illustrative that it merits full citation. Valesco recommended an ointment prescribed by Bernard de Gordon, "which I have found effective in many patients, particularly in a young girl who had suffered ringworm for fourteen years," and which "Bernard arranged from materials proposed by Avicenna."

> Take one half ounce each of white and black hellebore, live sulfur, atrament [a thick black liquid], litharge [lead monoxide], extinguished quicklime, verdigris, cook over a slow fire together with old oil lees and vinegar. Then add the powder of the said substances; finally add one ounce of pine tar and fresh wax as needed, and make into an ointment.

Continuing to quote verbatim, Valesco added, "this ointment is, without a doubt, of such great power that, in a purged body, it cures every kind of infection that is curable by human science, whether it be ringworm, scabies, dead flesh, or morphew. This is why it should be honored and revered, as Bernard says in the *Lilium*."

In this and many other matters, however, authors cautioned that the administration of strong prescriptions depended on the patient's ability to tolerate them. In a warning about the possible dangers and ill-advised interventions, Valesco reminisced about

> a certain knight whose nephew for a long time could not be cured of ringworm. The knight applied a poultice of arsenic, sulfur, verdigris, and mustard seed. The boy, who was twelve, was found dead in bed the next morning. The knight had found this remedy in his book. Thus was borne out the *Aphorism* of John of Damascus [Mesue], "Although the depth of medicine is immense, the use of books without intelligent understanding is risky."

The temptation to resort to rough treatment for resistant diseases was intensified when these diseases were also known as contagious, disfiguring, and stigmatizing. *Tineosi* (see the French *teigneux*) were called names and shunned; "even if they might be cured, the disgrace would be forever," Bernard claimed. He observed that ringworm could be caused "by the nurse of an infant, or by the presence of an infected man or woman." The fear of contagiousness, however, may have been second to revulsion in causing social rejection. Favus was graphically distinguished by its honeylike discharge, and ringworm was described as "scabies of the head with flakes and crusts, the falling out of hair, itch, ashen color, foul odor, and loathsome appearance."

Headache

At first sight, concern with appearance seems to explain why there were three or four times as many chapters on hair as there were on headache in compendia. The apparent slant, however, was due to several factors. Most important among these was the contrast between a simple object with discrete facets, which lent themselves to separate discussion, and a complex subject with overlapping aspects that defied neat categorization and that presented the compilers with a dilemma. For ready consultation, headaches belonged in one chapter as if they constituted a single syndrome; for comprehensive discussion, headache was an elusively multiform notion. An additional challenge was to integrate, in a format appropriate for a *practica,* a bewildering mass of observations, rationalizations, and recommendations from the sources. The oracular terseness of Hippocrates, the diffuse demonstrations of Galen, and the intricate classifications of Avicenna made it especially difficult to collate and condense the information on the types, causes, and cures of headache.

Definitions and differentiations of the various types were cast, firmly but not uniformly, by an accumulated tradition. As Valesco introduced his chapter, "note that there are many names for referring to headache, due to the diversity of authors and of usage, and to the particular locations of the ache." While honoring Hippocrates as "the first of the masters of things natural" (*primus naturalium magistrorum*), he began with seven divisions that were proposed by Galen, and then he adopted eight others from Avicenna; he further added several more, for a total of 21. This exceeded the number listed by any single predecessor, even though Valesco concluded his enumeration by crediting Bernard de Gordon who "has ably and adequately tracked down the said divisions: and this is where I have run for them." When Antonio Guaineri noted that "the numerous names for headache" were accompanied by different interpretations, he called upon a common refrain to claim, "I care little about the distinctions of names, since this knowledge of practice (*sciencia praxis*) deals with things rather than terms"; nevertheless, he proceeded to enumerate several terms.

The nomenclature and taxonomy of headaches defy synthesis, and a selection is more likely to give an idea of the compilers' preoccupation with precise definitions and with the implications for etiology, diagnosis, and therapeutics. A sampling will also illustrate, more colorfully than a summary, the connection between the manual and the bedside. Physicians largely assumed that headaches were part of daily life and that only the severe ones merited their attention or discussion. The worst kind, and apparently a widespread bane, rated a separate chapter: this was migraine or (*h*)*emicranea,* which affected one side of the head (from Greek *hemi,* "half" and *kranion,* "skull"). The severity of the suffering brought many authors back to questions about the essence of pain—with the stock definition, "the feeling of something contrary"—and about the extent to which it was "a disease, a symptom, and a cause of disease." Other philosophical questions or *dubia,* for instance, whether the brain is sentient and subject to pain, pertained more directly to the subject at hand. As an object of learned practice, general headache acquired an appropriately technical label, either *soda* from Arabic sources or, more commonly, *cephalea* or *cephalicus* from the classical tradition. Characterizing *cephalicus* as a "difficult and horrible illness," Copho proposed, "the name should not be applied unless the pain lasts for one or more months." Gariopontus, too, emphasized that the term was appropriate only for "a headache that persists a long time."

Specific terms and graphic descriptions underscored the ordeal of *cephalea*. Such names as *galea* or "helmet," and *ovalis*, which was derived from "egg," reflected the all-surrounding and tight oppressiveness of the total headache. The patient might perceive the agony as being struck with a hammer, jabbed with keys, or pricked with needles. Subjective perceptions overlapped seamlessly with slightly more objective symptoms, which ranged from tinnitus and dimmed vision to oversensitivity to noise and light. The transition from a descriptive sketch to differential diagnosis was almost imperceptible, although it was accompanied by an increase in complexity. Signs and symptoms, moreover, easily became omens for a dire prognosis. According to Guaineri, for example, "a headache that depresses the appetite and causes sleeplessness and insensibility is mortal, for it indicates great harm" to the vital and mental faculties. This observation, like many others, shows headache in the ambiguous position between symptom and cause.

The detailed discussion of symptomatic headaches was normally left for chapters on the problems that they revealed, while the section *de capite* concentrated on the diagnostic signs that indicated the nature and therefore the causes of the ache itself. Visual inspection, palpation, and information from the patient and bystanders were normally sufficient for recognizing such external causes as insomnia, exposure to the sun, or sulfur baths. Blows and wounds were mostly left to the surgeon's examination, assessment, and skill, while the holistic consideration of the patient's body, behavior, and circumstances fell to the physician. Habits might be responsible for headaches, as in the case of women who, Gariopontus observed, "oil their head repeatedly while working on their hair: if they are not careful with the ointment, nasty aches ensue." Other external causes were more incidental, and these suggest an inconsistency between their momentary effect and the definition of a true headache as persistent. Bernard and others were probably not thinking of a long-lasting impact when they mentioned "the terrible sound of thunder or big wheels," vapors inhaled while "peering into old pits or deep mine shafts," and "excessive coitus." Bernard was silent on the alternative, proposed by Guaineri, of "excessive abstinence" causing headache by "rising fumes when the retained sperm turns into poison."

Internal causes, which were more likely to have chronic consequences, could be identified only by means of a more sustained inquiry and, particularly, by the examination of external signs. When Guaineri proposed, "a pain in the meninges inside the skull extends to the roots of the eyes," he buttressed his insight with personal observation, "for, as I have seen, most frequently it makes the eyes protrude from their sockets." Symptoms of a qualitative or humoral imbalance were also apparent to the senses, with predictably standardized criteria. An unusually warm forehead and red face pointed to excess warmth or blood as the cause of a headache; sour breath and a yellow face, with pain on the right side, to bile as the offending humor; a cold and pale face, with occipital pain in the back of the skull, to phlegm; a cold left side, a livid face, and nightmares, to black bile or melancholy.

A headache might result indirectly from a disorder elsewhere in the body, especially in the stomach, liver, or spleen. If so, it was likely to be intermittent. Most of these cases were covered in the chapters on the organ in question. One case, which Saliceto mentioned in his chapters on the head, is worth quoting because it exemplifies the link between diagnosis and etiology as well as the overlap between physiological and physical explanations, but it also poignantly illuminates a social subtext of the headache.

> Children, gluttons, and those who have sticky humors in their intestines sometimes, indeed often, incur headache from worms produced in the bowels. Signs of this are an itch in the nose, hollowness of the eyes, paleness of the face; the stench of the worms is perceptible, the patient's breath smells, and involuntary movement is felt in the intestines.

Humors played the dominant role in disorders that were communicated to the head by other organs. Since this role called for applying the principal diagnostic techniques, compilers regularly referred the reader to the abundant literature on urines and on the pulse for further information on the signs and causes of headaches.

Once the immediate and underlying causes were identified, they became the exact targets of therapeutics based on the principle that contraries cure. Treatment proceeded from general to topical remedies, and from dietary adjustment to medication and manual intervention. For headaches as for all diseases, the first phase of therapeutics aimed at restoring the patient's humoral balance by regulating the six nonnaturals. This phase consisted mainly of such obvious measures as switching to lighter foods when indigestion was the basic problem. Authors unanimously banned leeks, onions, garlic, cabbage, and nuts as smoky foods and therefore responsible for headaches. When excessive sex was to blame, Bernard prescribed a fortifying diet of "broths, meat juices, and egg yolks"; with a mixture of leniency and censure, he added that if the patient, "by misfortune, was unable to abstain, he should not engage in sex after eating his fill, or when he is hungry."

A broad and gray area between diet and medication contained a variety of diuretics, laxatives, and emetics. These were supposed to assist nature in the elimination of the superfluous humors that were directly or indirectly responsible for the headache. The spectrum of purgative remedies recurred in nearly every chapter of the manual. At the milder end, and close to the kitchen cupboard, were the prunes, marjoram, and lavender in one of Guaineri's recipes. He thoughtfully recommended the prescription for a headache from black bile "in case your patient should prefer a gentle potion, which you may offer at dawn without any further care." On the more drastic end of the spectrum was the ubiquitous laxative *Hiera picra*, which had aloe as the main ingredient and became known as "the bitter pill." Nevertheless, patients probably preferred this pill to the emetics that were prescribed for treating headaches from an upset stomach. Guaineri was thoughtful on this matter, too, for he advised to "purge by vomiting as long as your patient can do this with ease," and he prescribed an alternative digestive.

Once the superfluities were evacuated, the patient's complexion could be returned to balance by means of pills, potions, and inhalants. The superabundance of materia medica is readily disparaged as polypharmacy and ascribed to the cumulative tradition, particularly to Arabic influences. It was also a response, however, to the challenges presented by the disease and even by the public. Gaddesden admitted,

> I am writing a diversity of things here, because headache is a common problem and difficult to cure on account of the hidden causes. Sometimes it is necessary to satisfy people and to tell them different things: tell one to use sage in any manner he or she may wish; tell another to use betony; another, to use lavender; some, to use peony; others, mountain siler; and still others, to use mace, nutmeg, cinnamon, or tragacanth seed.

Beyond these panaceas—and, literally, placebos—simples and compounds aimed for more precise benefits. Thus, cholagogues targeted the excess yellow bile or choler that was blamed for many a headache. Their place in everyday practice may be inferred from Bernard's recipe for making a syrup from borage, violets, and six other relatively ordinary ingredients: he added a persuasive yet qualified recommendation, this concoction is not dangerous in itself, so that young physicians may securely administer it when they need it for purging choler, unless it is contraindicated by the patient's weak condition, diarrhea or constipation, indigestion, aposteme, pregnancy, and the like.

With a broader target, allopathic drugs counteracted a qualitative imbalance: balsam oil by warming a shivering patient, purslane by cooling an overheated patient, and so on.

A group of cooling substances, ranging from lettuce to poppies, affected the mind as well as the body. They followed the correction of the patient's complexion and humors, in two stages of "the sedation of pain," as outlined by Gaddesden: first, "by inebriating, that is, gently inducing sleep"; and then, "by stupefying." Latin compilers included these drugs in oral and external headache remedies, but with more caveats than we find in their Arabic sources. Bernard, for example, voiced reservations so insistently and repeatedly that they suggest an intense fear of overdose. He urged to administer only "moderate refrigerants" to patients "with weak heads, such as the elderly, women, eunuchs, and children." A more emphatic warning followed his advice to "add opium, henbane, mandrake, white poppy, and the like" for cooling the head more forcefully: he added, "we should be careful, however, that these narcotics are not administered except in great need, as if in desperation." The administration of narcotics was primarily external or by mouth, but it also included inhalation, as we may infer from Guaineri's casual remark, "many authors add opium in odoriferous preparations, as you may do if you wish, especially if the patient has suffered prolonged insomnia. In any kind of case, however, avoid opium as much as you can."

Guaineri reported having used narcotics in his own practice, but with implicit reservations even about topical applications. For analgesic compresses, he recommended to "add a little opium if the pain should be persistent or, as often happens, unbearable: I have done this frequently and, by the grace of God, successfully." Guaineri's pharmacopoeia was one of the most extensive in the manuals, so that it may not be surprising to find willow leaves in several of his preparations. For one of his lotions, he clarified, "if the patient should wash the head with this concoction, he would not commit a mortal sin"; and "even washing the legs and feet with this concoction is helpful for a headache." Anyone who is familiar with salicin as the core ingredient of aspirin may be intrigued to find willow derivatives used only in external applications and, even more, to learn that the mention of willow in the *Canon* drew virtually no comment from compilers. Even when they closely followed Avicenna, they simply and silently included it in generic cooling compounds. One exception was Saliceto, who placed willow in relief and treated headaches with *oleum salicis*.

Saliceto cited the *Canon* with book and chapter, but he introduced two noteworthy differences. He added a willow oil ointment for the forehead to Avicenna's prescribed vaporizers for counteracting the "drying effect" of bad odors. More significant, while Avicenna stated that willow oil had "a greater moderating and moisturizing property" than other fragrances, Saliceto expanded the praise by claiming that, "by its property, it cures headache caused by a fetid substance." The phrase, *de proprietate curat*, conventionally characterized a medicine that worked by an occult virtue beyond mere complexion, and whose effectiveness was known empirically from experience rather than deduction. The presence of such medicines, called *empirica* or *experimenta*, usually indicated special challenges to treatment. Guaineri characteristically collected the most extravagant remedies "for any kind of headache." The collection included "rubbing the blood of a water turtle onto the forehead and temples . . . ; wearing a ring in which is enclosed a little of the umbilical cord of a newborn infant . . . ; hanging plantain from the neck, according to Gilbert; and combing the head with an ivory comb." It is easy to see how these treatments, like some others, earned the translation of *empirica* as quack remedies, but it is also facile to ignore the desperation by which they were motivated.

Whether or not they adopted *empirica* for stubborn headaches, the authors viewed the most aggressive treatment, by manual intervention, as the last phase of therapeutics. Drawing blood or, with it, another offending humor, was the predominant procedure, especially when the suspected cause was a humoral imbalance or excessive warmth. Venesection was presented as commonplace and as normally performed on the cephalic vein (perhaps not only because it was easily accessible but also because the name was derived from the Greek for head, *kephalē*). The application of leeches and cupping was a somewhat gentler—if, to us, no less disagreeable—method of drawing blood. Guaineri, who was in the habit of citing numerous sources, preferred a method that, judging from the compendia in general, seems to have been uncommon. He distanced himself from traditional doctrine as well as current practice when writing that, after purging the body,

> as a rule, you may proceed to drawing blood . . . Galen commands to cut a vein in the temples or forehead or nose. Avicenna and Rhazes agreed, in accordance with the [Hippocratic] *Aphorism* [5.68], "Cutting a vein in the

forehead helps for a posterior headache." Some apply leeches to the said veins, and you may do this if you like. I, however, in that case induce bleeding from the nose by means of a bristle or something else, which is safer and more convenient.

Guaineri's conservative stance, which may have been sufficient for relatively mild headaches, stands in contrast with the aggressiveness of some practitioners in tackling tougher problems. Bertruccio declared, for instance,

> For every chronic and persistent headache, it is most helpful to perform cautery with a hot iron on the top of the head, penetrating down to the skull where the right commissure runs together with the coronal suture toward the forehead and with the lambdoid suture toward the occiput: this dissolves the material and redresses the balance of the brain's complexion.

In addition to suggesting a determination born of despair, Bertruccio's declaration was in character for the teacher of the famous medieval surgeon, Guy de Chauliac. More important, it highlights an aspect of the medical manuals that is largely invisible in the previous pages, namely, the localization of diseases, their symptoms and causes, and their treatments.

Thus far, we have encountered only scattered glimpses of localization, in the spatial definition of migraine, the diagnosis of internal pains, the distinction between immediate and remote causes, and the topical application of medicines. A very slow and long imperceptible shift in perspective on disease, from an all-body condition to a process in one or more parts, was a counterpart to—and, arguably, a powerful stimulus in—the development of anatomy since antiquity. Galen interwove structural anatomy and qualitative physiology throughout his authoritative writings. Avicenna combined "parts" and "complexion" in the foundation of his teaching on the head, as illustrated in the opening excerpt of this chapter. The same excerpt also shows how Avicenna projected this combination onto two areas, namely, the "movements of the nerves," and "imaginations, thoughts, and memories."

This duality paralleled, albeit very superficially, the division between psychiatry and neurology. Shifting the division somewhat, compilers assembled problems with mental functions into one group of chapters and problems with mobility into another. We will adopt their arrangement, even though it will soon become evident that their demarcations were less than precise, their taxonomies not always logical, and their coverage rather spotty—especially from a modern viewpoint. Thus, Bertruccio

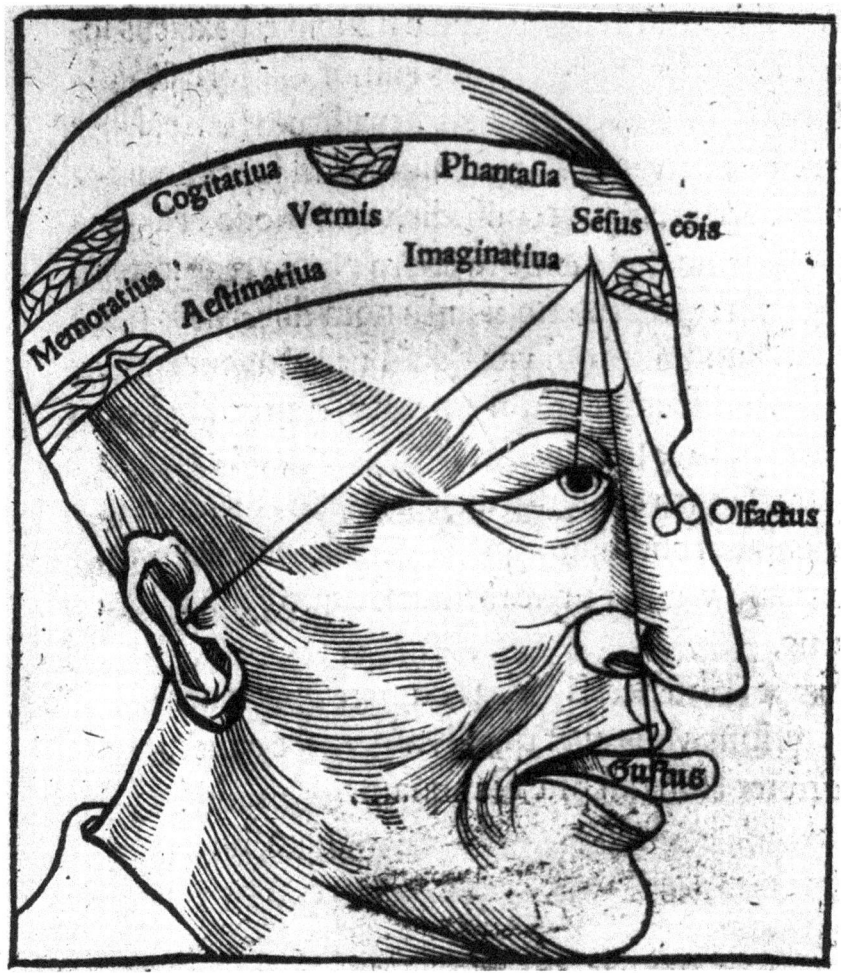

Map of the brain, faculties, and senses. Woodcut in Guillaume Le Lièvre, *Ars memorativa* (*The Art of Memory*), Paris, 1523, fol. 5. (National Library of Medicine, Images from the History of Medicine # A016194)

discussed *stupor* among the diseases "of the head," and he then included it again in a distinctly separate part on diseases "of the nerves." Other forms of catalepsy, such as *rigor* and *congelatio*, proved equally difficult to classify exclusively either as mental or as neural disorders. Compounding such difficulties, there were several overlaps and gray areas between problems of motion and of sense. A basic ambiguity is suggested by the fact that, whereas Avicenna treated paralysis as a disorder of the nerves, Latin compilers presented it less distinctly as a disruption of motion.

The compilers were keenly aware of the taxonomic difficulty, which was compounded by the need to forge a fixed nomenclature from fluid terms in at least three languages. One small example of the terminological challenge was the confusion about *stupor*. Some applied the term to the narcosis that Avicenna called *subeth*. Others understood it as a "total loss of sense and motion" due to a brain failure, according to Bernard, who objected that this was "not *stupor* but apoplexy or epilepsy." Still others, he claimed, equated it with *mollificatio,* an extreme softening of the nerves, "while this is not precisely *stupor* but paralysis." He concluded, "by stupor I understand a lessening of sensation and motion in a part of the body, which is popularly called the 'sleeping' of a limb, as when someone, after keeping the legs crossed, has little feeling and is unable to move easily until he has stood for a while." Such quandaries had implications for diagnosis and treatment, and they should not be dismissed as sophistry. On the level of teaching, they underscored the need for precision in defining, describing, and explaining brain malfunctions. Even when the compilers placed a disorder in one class of diseases, they warned that it might span the entire spectrum by causing "multiple harm to the mental, sensory, and motor faculties."

The Brain and Mental Malfunction

Sensory and mental disorders were defined and explained as a combined result of complexional imbalances and anatomical abnormalities. Latin authors seemed primarily interested in the role of humors and vapors, in contrast with Avicenna, who gave priority to anatomy. Nevertheless, the compilers also considered localization when classifying mental disorders. The prevailing map divided the brain into three cells (which correspond, roughly, to the ventricles of modern anatomy) and allocated one or two faculties to each. In the first cell, the *sensus communis* brought together what was perceived by the five senses, and the imaginative faculty or *fantasia* produced these perceptions into images, figments, and notions. In the second cell, the rational faculty processed the products into concepts, by the *cogitativa* power, and into judgments, by the *estimativa* power. In the third and softest or most impressionable cell, imprints were stored by the faculty of memory, *memorativa,* and, according to more elaborate maps, commands for the body's movements originated. As the center of the nerves—and of animation by the soul, *anima*—the brain was not only protected by the skull but also cushioned by membranes, of which the pia mater and dura mater were mentioned most often. This is a simplified outline, and variations included the five-cell system of Avicenna that may allow us to gauge his influence on one or other compiler.

Temporary Brain Malfunctions

Anatomical allocations were most evident for transitory disorders, which chiefly affected the front and back of the brain and, respectively, the perception and storage of information. Explanations relied on a combination of anatomy and humors, and mental malfunctions often merged with disorders of the senses (which properly constituted the subject matter of a separate section, and of our next chapter). This was the case for vertigo, and also for clouded vision, or "the seeing of flies," in *scotomia* (which covered more than the current medical term "scotoma" for a blind spot or an isolated area of diminished vision). Both of these, while due to a faulty transmission by the optic nerves to the *sensus communis*, were glitches in the receiving imaginative faculty, which produced phantom images. Further causes were fumes or moisture that distorted not only the optical perception but also the reception of sensory input in the frontal brain.

When vapors accumulated in the back of the head, they were likely to cause amnesia and *litargia*—which was more distinctively pathological than "lethargy" in current usage. The vapors interfered with memory, because perceived impressions were stored in the soft and moist posterior brain, as imprints on wet clay. The front and back of the brain could be affected simultaneously, by an excessively cold complexion, for instance. The disruption of both perception and recall caused unnatural sleep and shock or "freezing" (*congelatio*)—today's term "congelation" designates the very different category of frostbite. The unconsciousness of *congelatio* was so deep that, "when common people see someone like this, they believe that he is in rapture and speaking with God and his angels."

Transitory problems of perception and memory called for allopathic treatment, whether they were profound or not. The inability to shut off mental activity, in insomnia or "watchfulness" (*vigilie*), which could become a chronic condition, was treated with psychological as well as medicinal contraries. If sleeplessness was due to sadness, worry, or other *accidencia anime,* it should be remedied with "joy, the performance of music and songs, and the contrary of the responsible emotion." Medicaments for insomnia ascended from such mild soporifics as willow leaves to narcotics that triggered the same caveats as we have encountered with regard to headaches. Quite a few physicians apparently preferred nonmedicinal remedies for sleeplessness, including "the rustling of tree leaves, running water through the house and on the roof, a gentle rubdown, and soft sounds." Bernard added, "if everything fails, let the patient begin to say the Divine Hours, and he will go to sleep right away." He believed, however, that "there is no good remedy for insomnia in the elderly."

Except for the secondary condition of insomnia, passing mental problems resulted from brain deficiency, which was to be corrected by stimulation. Stimulating remedies, again, ranged from non-medicinal correctives and mild medications to stronger stimulants and forceful manipulations. In some cases, prevention was more likely to be effective than treatment. Someone prone to vertigo should not look "at such fast moving things as big wheels, rushing waters, and clouds that seem to fly; also avoid looking down from the tops of high mountains, towers, bridges, or ships." For other disorders, on the contrary, the most forceful intervention was necessary. Bernard passionately, one might say melodramatically, stressed this necessity for a *litargicus* patient,

> as I have seen many. Pull the hairs of his beard and chest, and also his nose; tightly tie his fingers, folded double, and bind his extremities. Forcefully, and without any mercy rub the extremities with salt and vinegar. Place sows with piglets in front of his face and make them squeal loudly; let there be trumpets, big bells, a drum, and many big irons that are beaten with a hammer all day; bronze vases that emit terrible noises; and very loud shouting. Otherwise they die sleeping.

This concern was no doubt based on an experience of many fatal outcomes.

Bernard's concern was intensified by his indignation, as a physician, at the stubborn ignorance of laypeople.

> Many die because the bystanders do not allow such things to be done, believing that it would be disgraceful malice. Do not give in, however, once the danger is predicted, for I have seen many escape by means of such violence; I have often accused bystanders of murder because they did not let me proceed and they scornfully dismissed me. These and other methods have cured many. On the other hand, many also have died when we were unable to attend to them because of obstinate bystanders.

A dual bias, one professional and the other sexual, tainted Bernard's bitter memory of a fatal case.

> Our master, who was sixty and suffered from burnt bile, died from *litargia*. A group of masters was present, and they all agreed that his hemorrhoids should be opened. This is what a surgeon did by himself, with no master present, and he is said to have drawn an excessive amount of blood, so that the patient kept getting weaker, until he died. In my opinion, it had done

him great harm to be filled with ground chickens by the women, for one is hardly able to observe a proper diet where women wield power.

If this master seems to have succumbed to a heart attack or stroke as a result of an unhealthy diet, it is worth noting that Bernard differentiated his *litargia*, at least implicitly, from *apoplexia*, which he discussed among the disorders of motion, as we will see at the end of this chapter.

Dietary excess was most notoriously responsible for drunkenness, in which disordered motion was compounded by mental malfunction. The process of inebriation was described as the rise of thick and sticky fumes by the drinking of wine, when the amount or strength exceeded the digestive capacity of the stomach and liver. Ascending to the brain, these fumes weakened the nerves and darkened the senses, like clouds do to the sun. Bernard drew a puzzling distinction, between wine as a genuine inebriant and "many things which have an effect *similar to drunkenness*, such as ales, meads, and the seasoning in bread." Real intoxication varied widely in degree and character, according to complexion and temperament: a drinker with a cold stomach was more likely to get a headache; the sanguine tended to become childish, the choleric furious, the phlegmatic sleepy, and the melancholic sad. The effects appeared first in the highly innervated tongue, with "stuttering and the mangling of words," before other faculties begin to fail.

Physicians viewed inebriation as an occasional condition, and they did not extend the purview of medicine to what is now called alcoholism. Nevertheless, those who classified it as a separate disease tended to inject a censorious if not moral tone. Bernard roundly rejected Avicenna's recommendation of a monthly purge by getting drunk, because "there are many other methods, and this one is disgraceful and not even entirely safe." The dire prognosis for constant drunkenness was "death in apoplexy, paralysis, epilepsy, tremors, or gout." Valesco elaborated bluntly, "I have often seen gluttons and drunks sleep on the table, and I expected that they would die a sudden death: and this is what happened, praise be to God." He believed, in fact, that in his day drunks were "so many that they could not be counted, and they are so habitual that they believe not to need a doctor." Doctors may have limited their practical concern to occasional drunks or to side effects, if we may judge from the compilers' relative terseness or complete silence on habitual inebriation.

Some relegated the habit to a secondary tier, together with "the ancient practitioners" who, according to Valesco, "did not devote a chapter to drunkenness but to headache from inebriation." Other compilers subsumed it in the etiology of more unusual disorders, as Gariopontus did when he stated, "*scotomia* arises in people *given to* drinking wine." An extract from his symptomatology indicates that his focus was not on the perception problem of *scotomia* but on a phenomenon closer to intoxication.

> Persons who suffer from *scotomia* have these signs: they see circles or wheels fly before their eyes, and every time they incline or lean toward the ground, they fall and their head becomes heavy. They fall as weighed down by sleep, they lose their mind, thinking that they are turned around and fall with everyone. They vomit, are sad all the time, and become emaciated. Unless they are cured quickly, they become either insane or epileptic.

In another indication that drunkenness fell short of a full-fledged disease category, Saliceto began a chapter with "the smell of wine and things which make one drink much"; he ended it with "the treatment of inebriation"; and, most tellingly, he placed it in his section on cosmetics, right after presenting "things that cover the smell of garlic, onions, and leeks"!

Chronic Mental Disorders

Drunkenness and other transitory afflictions of the brain were attributed primarily to lifestyle or certain actions, in contrast with permanent mental disorders, which were blamed chiefly on a humoral imbalance. However, the dichotomy between transitory and permanent conditions did not correspond invariably with the causal distinction between conduct and complexion. Constantine crossed the divide in the *Pantegni* by declaring that a temporary impairment could be due to an excess cooling of the humors, "as is proven when the mind becomes alienated by the drinking of opium and mandrake" (cold narcotics). Nightmare (*incubus*)—somewhat akin to intoxication but even farther away from modern nosology—also bridged behavioral and humoral causations. "A bad diet in quantity and in quality" caused thick vapors that blocked the brain passages, according to medical teaching as summarized by Valesco. This made patients feel "as if someone were sitting on them like a hen incubates chicks or eggs." The populace believed that the cause "might be a demon or a phantom, but it is nothing of the sort."

The distinction between transitory and chronic disorders was blurred in the category of brain infection, called *phrenesis* or, in the medieval spelling, *frenesis,* which is the origin of the nonmedical modern terms "frenzy" and "frenetic." A further element of confusion was added by the occasional application of a similar label, "phrenitis," to hypochondria as a brain condition caused by vapors rising from the diaphragm or "the abdominal area beneath the ribs." The label is now obsolete and replaced by two distinct ones, namely, "encephalitis" and "delirium." Be that as it may, *frenesis* was defined in the compendia as a hot aposteme in the brain membrane, which was caused by putrefied yellow bile or boiling blood. Some of the described symptoms suggest nonfatal amentia rather than modern meningitis. *Frenesis* might be life-threatening, however, when it lingered with escalating signs until the patient had "death in the feet, and the physician should flee hastily," as Bernard warned. Before mortal signs appeared, cooling remedies could prevent "impending shipwreck." Nevertheless, permanent dementia might set in, which was accompanied by excessive coldness, and which called for desperate measures.

For Bernard and several other compilers, extreme measures included the application of a still warm animal organ to the patient's head. For Constantine, the organ was simply "the warm lung of a sheep, wrapped around the head." Gilbert's instructions, more graphic, were to "let suckling kittens be cut in the middle of the back, or chicks, and be applied warm." Gilbert explained that such applications dissolved the offensive matter and that, if they did not work, "the last treatment or counsel is the application of narcotics, and this in desperation, for inducing sleep." Bernard also mentioned the kittens and "the lung of a goat, pulled out through the back of the animal while it is still alive"; unlike Gilbert, he viewed this remedy, rather than narcotics, as "the last resort." Valesco cited Bernard, but he altered some details in the treatment, and he explained that it worked by inducing sweating. He apparently had greater confidence in his own concoction of a dozen more such ordinary ingredients as cucumber, plantain, and almonds, compounded into "a marvelous medicament that I made for Austerus de Lucca, suffering from *frenesis*."

Valesco's claim reliably documents the actual treatment of brain disease with medication, but it does not allow us to estimate the extent of such treatments—let alone, of the more exotic ones—or even the extent of practitioners' attendance to patients with mental illness. John of Gaddesden made a remark that might cause some skepticism. He characterized the major mental disorders as "diseases which are particular not only because they affect one part of the body, but because the physician seldom earns money with them: these are *litargia,* mania, madness, and melancholy" (Gaddesden included *frenesis* in the latter). His characterization, however, warrants neither the inference that these diseases were rare, nor the conclusion that they were left utterly unattended by the physician. It reflects, rather, their stubbornly chronic nature, the uncertainty of their remissions and recurrences, and the sobering fact that their treatment was less lucrative than that of bodily illness.

The two principal chronic mental diseases were mania and melancholy, in each of which the naturally balanced cold and moist complexion of the brain was disturbed. Both diseases overlapped substantially, in the generic area of madness (*alienatio* or *desipientia*), yet they were also sharply differentiated. Mania was defined as a disorder of the imaginative faculty in the frontal cell of the brain and characterized by fury and explosive energy. It was attributed to an imbalance or inflammation of the hot and dry yellow bile that, in turn, might be due to dietary errors or such emotional triggers as anger. Mania was most likely to occur in spring and summer, and in youth. Melancholy was understood as a malfunction of the *estimativa* and *cogitativa* faculties of reason in the central cell, which was manifested by suspicion and gloom. Predictably, it was most common in fall and winter. It was blamed on superfluous or burned-out black bile, which might be caused by vapors arising from some foods or from incomplete digestion, not only in the stomach but also in the liver and other parts of the nether regions. Foods that produced too much black bile included various meats, "such as those of fox, bear, mule, and the like, which are eaten in some regions, or because of bad custom or of hunger," as Bernard claimed to have read in Galen. In a third and less grave form of *alienatio,* memory was lost when the storage of impressions in the rear cell of the brain was disturbed by excess phlegm or another cause.

Gariopontus pointed out that there were "many kinds of manics: some laugh suddenly, others become angry, tearful, or frightened; some sing, others talk a lot, and others rave irrationally." He suggested—perhaps with a wink—that people struck with mania included "philosophers, orators, and those who read or think too much." Patients, as he and many authors pointed out, might be aggressive and so dangerous to themselves and others that they should be tied. Valesco differentiated between a "wolfish" (*lupina*) and a "doglike" (*canina*) or less furious and more obedient rage, of which he remembered a case.

> I have seen someone in Paris who was like this, when his brother and I were near a well: there was a maid with a bunch of pewter vessels which stood on the edge of the well, and with one strike he threw those vessels to the bottom of the well; when he was scolded, he became a little ashamed.

This case resembled one cited, more famously, by Galen to demonstrate that in mania, the imaginative but not the rational faculty failed, so that the man had lost the sense of reality but retained a sense of right and wrong.

Manic behavior was so perplexing that explanations seemed to call for causes beyond humoral imbalance. As Gariopontus reported, "mania is allegedly named from possession by deities, for 'divine' is called 'manes' in Greek." Several compilers echoed the effort, rooted in the Hippocratic tradition, to distance natural etiology from the popular explanation of mania and also of melancholy. Several compilers summarized the distancing, as did Valesco.

> It is the opinion of laypeople, and of some physicians, that mania and melancholy are demonic, but Avicenna says that, in so far as we teach *physica*, we do not care whether this happens from a demon or nature, for their immediate cause is black bile. If a demon is able to produce black bile and to turn a complexion into this, then it is the antecedent cause. The demon, however, is not the concern of the physician, except for fleeing his works.

For greater emphasis, Valesco added, "and we do not find Hippocrates saying anywhere in his books that God would cause any disease. Nevertheless, some of the Ancients called mania demonic on account of the harshness of the disease."

The harshness of mania was matched by the heaviness of melancholy, a bane that seems to have been the more prevalent. This disorder, too, was said to encompass a broad variety of derangements, "and the whole day would not suffice to describe all of them," as Bernard assured. All patients tended to be sad, fearful, and withdrawn. Individual manifestations, however, ran the gamut of delusions—which we might associate with imagination rather than with reason, unless we keep in mind that they were failures of the rational ability to recognize reality by thinking and judging, with the *vis cogitativa* and the *vis estimativa*. Galen sketched the most stereotypical melancholic behaviors, and Gaddesden was but one of several authors who proved particularly impressed by the image of patients who "think that they are roosters and, raising their arms as if they were wings, try to crow." Compilers wove their own vignettes of melancholic conduct around Galen's sketch, bringing the diagnostic model up to date and adding their own experience.

One of the most vivid expansions of the original sketch was Bernard's portrayal of patients with a variety of delusions.

> To some it seems that God is getting old; to others that the angel who moves the earth is getting tired, and they keep fleeing so that the sky cannot fall on them; to others that they are being swallowed; and to still others that they are glass or clay vessels, and they fear being broken when touched.

Here Bernard moved to examples that were clearly closer to his own milieu.

> To others it seems that they are masters in everything knowable, and they begin to lecture and teach, but they say nothing reasonable; others that they are prophets inspired by the Holy Spirit, and they begin to prophesy and to predict much about the future, such as the state of the world and of the Antichrist.

It has been suggested that this depiction may have been an allusion to one of Bernard's own colleagues. Valesco offered a glimpse of his social environment in his assertion—putting the cart before the horse, perhaps—that "jealous women often are melancholic, and I have seen many of those."

A contemporary setting was also echoed in Gaddesden's remark that some melancholics think "that they are bishops, and they want to confer prebends," that is, ecclesiastical stipends. Gaddesden added a personal experience about patients "who are seized by terror when they hear talk about the devil": one of these was

> a woman whom I had in my care. I saw that she did not dare to speak of the devil, or even to look out the window in case she might see the devil; she was even afraid of every man dressed in black because he might be the one.

Valesco cited similar cases that had exemplified some of the innumerable forms of delusion in his practice. He reminisced, "I have seen those who believed to be kings. I had a woman in my care who claimed that the devil had copulated with her every night, but in the end she was cured with God's help."

Regardless of the specified differences, mania and melancholy were paired in one chapter by most of the compilers—in a pairing paralleled by such modern denominations as manic depressive and bipolar. The interaction of yellow and black bile might be complicated by the involvement of a third humor. In addition, both imbalances played a combined role in intermediate categories. The most notable of these was "heroic love" (*amor hereos*), the melancholic–manic infatuation of "those men and women who love inordinately," in Gaddesden's words. Savonarola explained that this affliction "most often befalls heroes or aristocrats because these, more than anyone else, press themselves on others unimpeded." He added, more pointedly, "the passion commonly affects those who live in pleasure or solitude, the celibate religious, and those who lead a life of ease." Even though *amor hereos* affords a prismatic view of medical thought—and it has been the subject of fascinating literary studies—a detailed examination would greatly exceed the confines of this survey. Nevertheless, it will be indispensable in a glance at psychotherapy *avant la lettre*.

If *amor hereos* may be seen as an intermediate category between mania and melancholy, there were also mixed conditions, in which incessant restlessness coincided with misanthropic wretchedness. For one of these, the compilers adopted the intriguing Arabic term *cutubuth* (or *cucubuth*) from Avicenna. They agreed on Avicenna's definition of the disorder, and on his assertion that "it occurs most often in February," but they embroidered variously on his etymology. His "little creature on the surface of the water" was identified by Bernard as an erratically moving long-legged aquatic spider, which

> is called 'water goat' in the vernacular. Thus, when people see someone who acts or speaks foolishly or childishly, they say 'that one is a water goat'. Indeed, when reason is completely lost, the movements of feet, hands, tongue, and eyes are irregular, never keeping one way or order.

One may wonder whether the phrase "water goat" (*capra aque*), as Bernard took it from the vernacular, did not rest on a faulty Latin deconstruction of the French "chevreau" to *chèvre* and *eau* (oddly, a medieval translator of Aristotle interpreted "capricorn" as "chèvre d'eau"). In any event, Bernard's excursus was mild in comparison with Avicenna's portrayal of the *cutubuth* patient as one who "flees the living, likes to be near corpses and graves," and runs to and fro at night. Avicenna similarly dramatized the description of a manic patient as "not looking like a human but, rather, like a wolf." These two characterizations in the *Canon*, together with elaborations in the compendia, produced an interpretation of *cutubuth* that merged with myths of the werewolf until at least the 17th-century *Anatomy of Melancholy* by Robert Burton.

The most general treatment of chronic mental disorders was by remedies that directly counteracted the emotional and humoral causes. For example, if "the loss of money" was the cause of despair, Johannes Platearius advised, "you should pretend that it has been recovered." He recalled,

> I saw someone who, while recovering from a fever, became melancholic upon the news that his treasure chest had been broken into and his money had been stolen. Brooding incessantly about his debtors and their debts, he set out for them in insane melancholy, and he argued about debt even with those who owed nothing.

The professional prescription may have raised some eyebrows. "On the advice of the physicians, several of his friends were brought to him with money: they began to pay him as if they were debtors, and thus he was freed" of his madness.

Joy, the principal antidote to any kind of depression, was to be procured by means of bright rooms and pictures, flowers and perfumes, and music and pleasant company. The latter included "beautiful women" with whom, Johannes Platearius declared rather bluntly, the patient "should do it (*utantur*) occasionally, because moderate sex cleanses the spirit and removes bad suspicions." Sex played a more ambivalent role in the psychological treatment of *amor hereos*. On one hand, the principle of *cure by contraries* was applied in the nearly universal prescription to denigrate not only the object of infatuation but also women and even lovemaking itself. On the other hand, sex could be remedial. Philandering was prescribed for defusing single-minded love. Valesco, expanding on Ovid's *Remedies for Love,* suggested that it was "helpful to love several, to kiss them, and to talk with them frequently." A hardly more ethical suggestion was to resolve the lover's insane passion by "handing him the one whom he loves heroically." Valesco ascribed the latter idea to Rhazes, but he left no doubt about his own opinion. "The prognosis is that these are in danger of becoming fatuous, losing their honor and spending their entire substance unless they are helped immediately. And among those I have seen some rich folks who became impoverished down to their breeches."

Valesco observed, however, that at the time "few if any become 'heroic' lovers, for they so dissolutely do it with different women that their love is unable to settle on one, and that one is loved with words and not with the heart." Promiscuity was "most evident in the powerful and noble, for they neither fear any woman nor feel any shame in abusing this business." He also agreed with Savonarola in claiming that aristocrats were most prone to lovesickness and that, as he added, "gravediggers and laborers, who spend life in toil, hardly suffer from this." Valesco outdid other compilers with his 13 therapeutic recommendations that, he claimed, cured any form of depression and helped "those who may be forced to act well and manly as if nothing were the matter." On the premise that "the entire treatment consists in distracting the imagination," he recommended hunting and fishing, fencing and jousting, and playing dice, chess, and cards. After waxing poetic on "walking, with friends, through green pastures, woods, and flowering gardens, where birds sing," he added an epicurean note on "well prepared meals with three or four kinds of wine and exquisite dishes and fruits."

With diet as the first phase, the entire humoral treatment targeted the imbalance that was suspected of causing the particular chronic disorder. For prevention, Bernard taught, one should avoid such things that "are melancholic or burn the humors," as moldy bread, old cheese, and beans or lentils. A dangerously dry complexion was corrected by sleep and baths and by "humidifying" food and drink; these ranged widely, from chicken, lamb, and soft boiled eggs, to clear wine. Oil of roses or willows, vinegar of sea onion, lotion of chamomile, and similar ingredients were applied to counteract choleric heat. Valesco's pharmacotherapy culminated in a relatively simple powder

> that I have tried very frequently and which has restored the health of mind and body for all who have used it. It is a medicine of Haly [Abbas]. In cases where other remedies do not work, this one works by the will of God. It is a noble medicine that should be treasured and kept very secret.

His praise concluded with the boast, "I have gained great profit and honor from this blessed powder."

If even marvelous but mild medications were ineffectual, more forceful intervention began with a series of purges. A sanguine imbalance, revealed by uncontrolled and persistent laughter, was to be remedied by bloodletting "from the cephalic vein, which is in the curve of the arm," or from another vein, "assuming that it is necessary and that the patient is strong enough to tolerate it," Bernard proposed. As last resort, he called for a radical method.

> In the end, when all else fails, shave the head, make a cut in the form of a cross, and then administer one cautery or many: this will work, beyond doubt, for the evacuation of the humors. I once saw a melancholic patient who, by accident, had been wounded by a sword and suffered a skull fracture: he was perfectly cured as long as the wound was open, but the mania returned as soon as the wound was healed. I think that, if the wound had remained open longer, he would have been treated appropriately and would have been cured.

Already Gariopontus (and possibly earlier authors) had described a similar method, in more graphic terms: first, "the head should be shaved and the artery of the head incised"; and further, "both parts of the occiput should be cauterized down to the bone, so that next you also shave the bone until you feel drawing flesh out of the bone."

The Nerves and Disorders of Motion

The etiology and therapeutics of mental disease, however complex, were straightforward when compared with the responses to neural malfunction.

The treatment of mania and melancholy culminated in severe and almost punishing methods, which stand in marked contrast to the methods of treating diseased nerves. This contrast becomes already apparent in the discussion of epilepsy, which lay at the intersection of brain and nerve disorders. The compilers recorded virtually no heroic treatments for this disease, although it was one of the most baffling diseases since antiquity, and the subject occupied disproportionately long chapters in their compendia. On the other hand, these chapters contain the greatest amount and range of magical remedies, as well as of anecdotes from practice, which was probably not sheer coincidence. Most of the extraordinary cures recurred from *practica* to *practica*, which attested to the continuity of a core tradition. Numerous variations, however, serve as more evidence that compilers were not mere copyists. Traditional prescriptions were usually presented as "proven by experience" (*experimenta*), while the personal ones were distinguished by such claims as "I have used this"; both kinds were sometimes presented as "secrets" (*secreta*), which made them more mysterious and therefore more enticing. The extraordinary remedies, which have too often been lumped together under the facile label of "superstition," ranged from the use of substances with occult powers to religious rituals and charms, categories that were not always distinct.

The most intensely ritualized prescription dated back at least to Constantine the African, who promoted "this very powerful medicament" for a patient with full-fledged epilepsy.

> His father or mother, if he has one, should bring him to church during the Ember Days, and hear mass on Friday and Saturday. When Sunday arrives, let a priest or a religious man write the Gospel where it says, "This kind is not cast out except by prayer and fasting" [Mark 9:29, Matthew 17:21]. Without a doubt he will be cured, whether he be epileptic, lunatic, or demonic. It should be noted that this does not work for those born from incestuous unions.

It is interesting that compilers omitted the concluding restriction, while they added various details. Bernard, for example, narrowed the designation of "a priest *or* a religious man" to "a faithful priest"; we are left to guess whether this change had any implications. Gaddesden placed the remedy not only in a historical but also in a personal context. He declared, "since epilepsy afflicts many children and others who are unable to use medicines, we should use the *experimentum* which Constantine gives in the fifth book of his *Practica*, and Gualterus [Agulinus] in his *Practica*, and Bernard, Gilbert, and everyone." Then, endorsing the remedy, he claimed, "and I have found it true."

As if to underscore his endorsement, Gaddesden spelled out some ecclesiastical aspects as well as the instruction (also mentioned by Bernard) for the Gospel to be read by the priest "over the head of the patient," and for the written text to be worn "around the neck." Sacred texts were indeed both read as incantations and written down for amulets. Such dual use was also illustrated in the widespread prescription to recite three times, directly into the ear of a patient in paroxysm, the verses, "Gaspar bears myrrh, Melchior frankincense, and Balthasar gold: whoever carries with him the names of these three kings will, by the grace of the Lord, be freed of the falling sickness." This belief most likely rested on the portrayal of the Magi in Matthew 2.11, "and falling down they adored him: and opening their treasures, they offered him gifts; gold, frankincense, and myrrh." Savonarola assured that the prescription "is also praised by our masters, who were Christians." Religious ritual and magic were also combined in a specific claim, cited by Petrocellus, that antimony cured "if taken together with the holy water which Greeks bless on Epiphany, and with Our Lord's Prayer sung three times in name of the patient."

If these rituals are reminiscent of priestly exorcisms, they also overlapped with popular charms to ward off evil (apotropaic). Guaineri, for one, expressed awareness that the adoption of charms and rituals by learned medicine might be called into question. He scoffed, "some, who think of themselves as philosophers, I say, wonder that this disease should be removed by those methods" and why anyone would add rituals. To the second question, he argued,

> you should answer that this is done so that greater faith will be had in a medicine, for the patient will take medications more avidly if he likes them, and they will work much better. And this is why we perform so many ceremonies in medicine. For example, we prescribe an uneven number of pills because the common folk think that this is far more perfect than an even number.

He concluded, "therefore, if I will describe some things in the manner of old wives, keep in mind that I did not write these as based on reality. Even though they may look to you like incantations, none of them lacks a rationale based on natural principles."

Guaineri formulated the fundamental rationale in his answer to the first question, about the treatment of epilepsy by magical methods. Because a poisonous character, "venenosity," cannot be repelled by such a simple quality as heat or moisture, an effective agent must have "a certain hidden (*occulta*) quality," which is contrary to the poison.

Now, since epilepsy happens on account of venenosity, the repelling remedy must have a hidden opposite contrary, which may exist in a toad's liver, a dog's blood, or something else. Things possess so many properties that are still unknown to us.

So many of these specific substances with hidden powers were prescribed for epilepsy (and, often jointly, for mental illness) that only a brief selection is feasible here. Mineral simples included such gems as jet, coral, and lapis lazuli as well as, most curiously,

the little red stones found in the gizzards of swallows, which are forever helpful if they are hung on the patient's neck. After catching the swallows on the nest and cutting their gizzards, remove the stones in the middle of the day: they are useful, for they cure epileptic, insane, and lunatic patients.

It is worth pointing out that Gaddesden adopted this prescription from Constantine, as did several other compilers.

Two celebrated plants with occult power to cure epilepsy—and a host of other diseases—were mistletoe and peony. The latter was mentioned as a remedy for possession in the fourth-century *Medicine of Pliny*, which was based on the *Natural History* of Pliny the Elder (23–79 CE). Johannes Platearius recommended the use of peony for epilepsy, either in a concoction or in an amulet. He invoked the sovereign authority of Galen and, we may note, so did his brother, Mattheus Platearius. This author of the "Book on Simples," a catalog of materia medica better known and widely circulated as *Circa instans*, reported that peony "has occult virtue" in an amulet, "as Galen testifies about a child who did not suffer as long as it was hung around his neck but was afflicted as soon as it was removed." Mattheus added a qualification: "right now, however, this effect is not seen, so that some say that it is true only for a certain species." This may be why Bernard specified "Roman peony." Peony root also appeared in natural remedies for epilepsy without the mention of occult qualities, for example, in Savonarola's formula for suppositories. He cautioned that these should be administered, inferentially to children, only "in so far as it is possible, for sometimes they cry and toss so much that greater harm might follow."

Animal ingredients in special remedies for epilepsy ran the gamut, from sparrow brains to bear testicles. Two enjoyed exceptional status. The rennet from a hare's stomach, which Aristotle and Pliny praised as a panacea, bore the highest stamp of approval since Galen "said that he had tried it for epilepsy." A second animal with specific power against epilepsy was

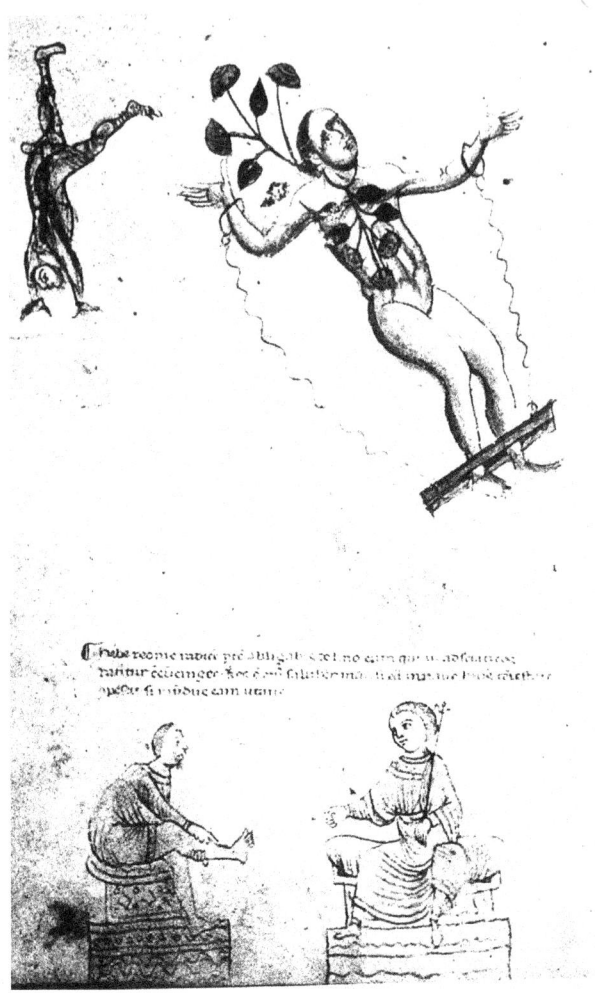

A manic patient does cartwheels and, restrained, is treated with sprigs of peony (at the bottom, a physician prescribes peony root to a patient with "sciatica" [*sic*]). Drawing in a 13th-century manuscript of Pseudo-Apuleius, *Herbarium*. Vienna, Oesterreichische Nationalibibliothek MS 93, fol. 72v, in Loren MacKinney, *Medical Illustrations in Medieval Manuscripts*, London, 1965, Fig. 39. (Wellcome Library, London. Wellcome Images L0001410)

the cuckoo. After a cuckoo was carefully incinerated in an oven, the ashes were to be served in a drink. In addition, as Gaddesden explained,

> some carry a cuckoo's head around the neck. It is preventive and, at least, it alleviates the illness greatly and slows it down, as I have experienced with many children who cannot take medicine. The reason of its value is because the cuckoo has epilepsy every month, so that some say that it has the prop-

erty of curing this disease by drawing the matter to itself, just as rhubarb draws yellow bile.

This brief statement is remarkable for a double and intertwined paradox. Gaddesden deferred to hearsay while also claiming personal experience, and he endeavored to give a reason for a hidden property.

The compilers shared some significant characteristics in their presentation of extraordinary epilepsy remedies. They persistently distanced themselves from exotic recipes by underscoring their hearsay source, "it is said." Even Guaineri introduced incantations with a similar and oft repeated expression, "*some say* that the patient will rise immediately," in this case upon hearing the sentence about the Three Kings and their gifts. Secular authors, from Dioscorides and Galen to Avicenna and Constantine, were regularly identified in order to lend credence to prescriptions. Johannes Platearius cited a domestic authority to inspire confidence in an arguably peculiar remedy,

> an *experimentum* of my father regarding epilepsy, to give three drams of blood, drawn from the shoulder blades by scarification, together with a raven's egg, at the end of the onset when the patient is still dazed, because right then he would drink even poison.

When sources were not identified, they belonged mostly to Greco-Latin learning, but such sources as prescriptions of camel's brain and similar Levantine simples were more likely of Arabic origin. Vernacular lore probably accounted for Constantine's report that "Some say that, if a goat's brain be drawn through a gold ring and given to swallow by infant before he/she sucks milk, the infant cannot become epileptic (*caducus*) or deluded (*fantasticus*)."

A second constant in the compendia is the secondary status of extraordinary remedies in most therapeutics. They were intended as supplements to the conventional methods of adjusting the diet, digesting and expelling the offending matter, and counteracting the humoral imbalance with contraries. Moreover, they complemented the most advanced attempts—when surgery was out of the question—with the administration of such universal antidotes as Constantine's "greater theriac or the mithridate of emperors." Petrocellus, who limited himself to ordinary remedies, claimed, "God is my witness that I have cured someone with nothing else than white violet." Even in routine therapy, discretion was required. Johannes Platearius warned that, except in case of prolonged stupefaction, "sneezing should not be provoked in epileptics, because many have choked on the excess production of liquids, through the fault of undiscerning physicians."

There was a general, though rarely voiced, understanding among the compilers that extraordinary methods were reserved for paroxysms while routine methods addressed the quiet stages in between. This understanding had more explicit parallels, in the distinction between curable and incurable epilepsy, and in the fluctuation between confidence and despair. Before spelling out the therapeutic triad of diet, contraries, and specifics, Valesco asserted confidently, "I say that we ought not to despair about a cure of epilepsy but to hope for improvement, because many have been found cured, children as well as others who have been attended to promptly, before the disease became fixed." He highlighted this view with a case from his own career. A 65-year-old patient who, in addition to having suffered a mild stroke and being paralyzed,

> had fifteen or more attacks of epilepsy, which lasted as long as it takes a person to say the Lord's Prayer five times. With God's help and great diligence and effort, I cured him so that within a month from the beginning of his illness he was healed of the stroke and of epilepsy, and he was even able to walk on his feet, with a slight trace of the paralysis remaining in his hand and tongue.

Guaineri claimed more bluntly, "I have cured many, among whom a sexagenarian who had suffered from the disease for many years." These boasts were enhanced by the patient's age, which defied the odds. Petrocellus, together with many other authors, categorically stated, "from infancy to early youth, epilepsy merits treatment; but if it attacks later, it is incurable."

The differentiation between ages, as well as between ordinary and extraordinary remedies, may explain an apparent inconsistency in Bernard's outlook. He seemed optimistic in offering ample recipes; at least one, for a concoction with shrimps, was so elaborate and redolent of alchemy that it may have been his own. He pledged that "long use" of the universal antidote mithridate "cures all epilepsy"; and he prefaced a catalog of specifics with the rather sweeping statement, "there are many things which cure epilepsy." These passages contrasted sharply with Bernard's admission, in one of the most poignant expressions of helplessness,

> I assure you that I have had many in my care, young and old, poor and rich, men and women, with nearly every kind of epilepsy, yet I have not seen anyone being cured, either by myself or by someone else, even though I was most diligent and the patients were most obedient. I do not know the reason, God knows.

Combining realism and ethics, Bernard added, "I am saying this so that, when patients come to you, you will not disgrace yourselves with vain and false promises in the treatment of epilepsy, because almost every form is eradicated with great difficulty, provided that it can be eradicated."

It is important to emphasize three aspects about the elaborate therapeutic sections in the manuals, for a mostly incurable disease. First, numerous supernatural remedies were included but, as Guaineri insisted, even these were "based on natural principles." Second, it is remarkable that this inclusion was not matched by recourse to supernatural etiologies of the disease. Third, and most significant, the profusion of prescriptions was motivated by a determination to cover any and all possibilities for fighting this "horrible kind of disease," in Savonarola's words. The same determination inspired the compilers to reach beyond rationalized treatments into the realm of ultrarational remedies. Their inclusion of *experimenta* and *secreta* did not necessarily mean personal confidence or experience. Hearsay was the source of the standard refrain, "it is proven" (*probatum est*), which should be viewed as closer to today's drug advertisements than to scientific proof. In fact, there were tensions between the observation and the understanding of epilepsy that corresponded to the fluctuation between pretended confidence and admitted despair. The compendia richly illustrate the challenges of defining and explaining this disease, of differentiating it from partially similar conditions, and even of fitting it into a physiological framework.

The Salernitan masters endeavored to correlate the various names by which epilepsy was known, beyond the close translations from the Greek as *morbus caducus* or "falling sickness," and especially to match the popular and medical terms. Both nomenclatures coincided where epileptic seizures, perceived as periodic occurrences, were associated with lunar phases and hence with lunacy. This association found a rationale in Galen's teaching that epilepsy was very moist during the waxing moon and cold during the waning moon. It was echoed, in turn, in prescriptions for remedies that were to be collected during the corresponding phases of the moon. A more sinister association emerged in the reference to "epilepsy as it is called in Greek, but which the Latins commonly (*vulgo*) call 'possessed by demons (*demoniacos*).'" This distinction was drawn by Petrocellus, an author who was exceptionally conscious of the transition from the classical vocabulary to the newer medical terms with vernacular origins. Three centuries later, Guaineri added context to the continued difference between medical and popular appellations. First, he opened the broad perspective that "this disease dwells among all nations, and it is far more familiar than they would wish, so that it is called by various names." Then, addressing the popular association with possession, he explained that epilepsy, by blocking the senses, banned distractions from the rational faculty and thus sometimes enabled it

> to apprehend future events; hence, once the seizure is over, patients often predict many future things. The common folk (*vulgares*), ignorant of the cause, think that this happens by the power of demons. This is also the reason why several ancients called this disease "divinatio."

Bridging semantics and practice, Guaineri recollected, "I have seen a choleric youth who said that he always saw marvelous things during seizures; he very much wanted to commit these to writing: no doubt he hoped that these were things to come."

The compilers did not cite the Hippocratic work *On the Sacred Disease*, but the references to antiquity reflected indirect knowledge of the seminal treatise, and they exemplified the Hippocratic legacy of natural explanation. Johannes Platearius stated that epilepsy "was called *ieranoxon*, that is, the sacred disease, by the ancients because it afflicts the sacred parts of the body, namely, the brain which is the seat of the soul." Guaineri underscored this explanation with somewhat verbose embroidery: "the ancients saw the contemplations of the soul primarily in the brain, which they called the temple of the soul, from 'contemplating'; and as temples are commonly sacred, they called the brain a sacred place, and hence they spoke of a 'sacred disease.'" He applied a similar historical perspective to yet another name for epilepsy. "This disease is called *comitialis*, from the *comitiae* or assemblies of the Roman people, which were held in the Field of Mars on the first of January for electing the magistrates. If at that time the disease happened to attack someone, they postponed the assemblies to another day." Valesco cited the lexicographer John of Genoa (died ca. 1298), for a slight but interesting variant, that the disease was called *convivialis* "among the gentiles because, when it happened to one of them on the day of the assembly, they dismissed the assembly"; and, as an alternative explanation, because fear or shame brought on seizures in assemblies.

The subjective consequence of the disease, as well as a mental aspect, also emerged in Bernard's description of different patients: "there are some who after the seizure remember neither the fall nor the affliction, and some who remember and are ashamed." Bernard further distinguished, with perceptive precision, two forms.

> Sometimes the seizure is very strong and long, and sometimes brief. I have quite often seen one so short that the patient needed only to lean against the wall or something like that, and to rub his face and it ceased. Sometimes he did not need support but a disturbance came to his head and a cloud to his eyes and, with presentiment, he said a Hail Mary and before he completed it the seizure had passed; and he spat once and it was totally gone. This happened repeatedly during the day.

These descriptions of momentary episodes may make us think of what is now called "petit mal." Earlier, Petrocellus made a less incisive distinction when he noted "two kinds: one in which patients fall suddenly without knowing it; the other, in which they spit and snore, do not fall readily, and the limbs do not contract."

The different manifestations of epilepsy, together with the intermingling of psychological and neurological aspects, caused not only conceptual problems, for defining and classifying the disease, but also diagnostic difficulties, for precision and differentiation, and hence therapeutic quandaries. Definitions presented the disease as essentially an obstruction in the brain, but they were ambiguous about the primary cause and about the role of the nerves. For Petrocellus, patients "suffer a tremor in the brain, and all the innervation that descends from the brain labors under a melancholic humor and cold phlegm." Guaineri captured the elasticity of the definitions in his summary of medical doctrine. In the first place, "Galen, Avicenna, and most of the other authors agree that this disease is located chiefly in the back of the head, otherwise all patients would remember the seizure." In the process itself, "the brain contracts, and this causes the contraction of the nerves near their origins." The spasm of the nerves, in turn, "occludes the paths of the spirits, prevents them from reaching the members, and deprives the latter of movement and sense, so that the patient falls." Guaineri concluded, however, that "the immediate cause of epilepsy is a vapor, windiness, or humor" according to Galen, Rhazes, and Avicenna. They had proved the thesis by dissecting epileptic sheep: "if these are anatomized at the time of a seizure, a poisonous moisture is always found in their heads." In the end, ironically, the dissection served to confirm qualitative explanations rather than to broaden anatomical knowledge.

The combined reliance on humoral constructs and on reported inquiry rather than direct observation compounded the inherent difficulty of understanding the nervous system (to use an anachronistic term). It is even striking how little attention compilers paid to Avicenna's detailed descriptions of the origins, branches, and paths of the nerves—and how much they might have benefited from adopting his dual division of the subject matter, between diseases of the brain and of the nerves, and between sense and motion. The compilers largely limited their purview to a general image of channels through which the *spiritus* traveled from and to the brain, and which were susceptible to blockage, softening, and hardening. This framework was of little use for differentiating disorders of transmissions through the sensory and motor nerves from malfunctions of faculties in the brain (the *virtus motiva* and *virtus sensitiva*). The compendia give the impression that differential definitions and diagnoses depended chiefly on semantics and speculation. This was evident, for instance, in efforts, from Johannes Platearius to Guaineri, to contrast the incomplete loss of sense and motion in epilepsy with the total loss in *apoplexia*. Platearius added a largely speculative anatomical contrast between, respectively, an obstruction "in the principal ventricles" and "in all the ventricles" of the brain.

Transient and peripheral episodes presented the greatest challenge for differentiating, classifying, and explaining neural malfunctions. Some distinctions, between tremor and spasm, for example, were readily indicated by mere observation but less easily correlated with physiology. Bernard and others distinctly attributed tremor to weakness, but their definition as "a lessening of the motive faculty" left room for conceptual confusion with the "loss of motion" in spasm, notwithstanding further clarifications that the latter was a "contraction of the nerve toward its root" and that, in the vernacular, it was called *grampa* (the origin of the modern word "cramp"). Facial spasm (*tortura*), on the other hand, was treated as a separate category and attributed to paralysis of the nerves. The authors, however, assured that medications were largely identical for most of the categories, whether separate or not. All this leaves us with the impression of a certain nominalism, which was most pronounced with regard to an uncontrolled movement that the Greeks called *palmos* and the Arabs *ikhtilāj*. Constantine translated the name as *iectigatio* but Gerard of Cremona as *saltus*. Except for common associations of this "jerking" (which may be derived from *iectigatio*) with internal "windiness" and exterior cold, the accounts of the compilers were too semantic, speculative, and varied to be summarized here.

Diseases of the mind and disorders of movement dominated the part of compendia on which we have concentrated in this chapter. Sense perception will play a larger role in the next chapter. A continuing theme, however, will be the difficulty of transcending the construct of humoral physiology that supported broad explanations and purposeful therapeutics. This difficulty was more apparent in compendia than in thematic treatises. In addition, it was most predictable in discussions of mental and motional health, because cerebral and neural functions eluded dissection, both in the literal and in the figurative sense. The senses, on the other hand, lent themselves more to close observation, and their organs were more amenable to dissection. Even here, however, greater anatomical interest and knowledge proved of limited practical benefit to concrete explanations and applications. This will become apparent in the following pages, where we will see the limitations, as it were, eye to eye.

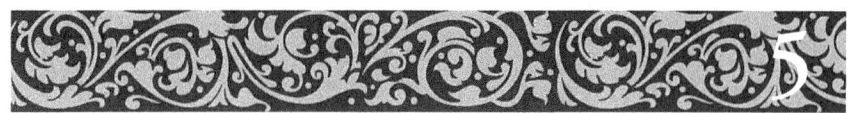

The Face and the Senses

Among the faculties of sense, sight is subtler than the others, because it has the nature of fire, which is subtler than all the other elements. As proof of this subtleness, sight perceives the most distant objects, but the other senses only nearby ones. Hearing is next in subtleness, because it is of the nature of air: sound is the striking of the air, and the voice is nothing but the air being touched. Next is the sense of smell, with the nature of smoke, which is between earthy and watery. Taste is next, watery in nature and related to all the fluids. Touch is coarser than all, because it is earthy in nature. They each fulfill their task, that is, to adapt and change into the natures of the things which they sense and which the mind, when it senses in turn, prepares for the intellect . . .

Constantine the African appropriately makes a second appearance here, introducing the second of our two chapters on the head with (greatly condensed) excerpts from the *Pantegni,* his avowed summary of Galenic teaching and his most comprehensive compendium. He seems to have exerted greater influence than Avicenna on the compilers with his philosophical outlook on the instruments of the senses, which is exemplified in the quotations. The medical discourse on normal and defective sense perception was anchored more in the nature of things than in methodical observation; it relied more on elemental and humoral qualities than on mechanical interactions; and it focused more on the purpose than on the structure and function of organs. The philosopher's preoccupation with concepts and definitions competed with the practitioner's concern with concrete conditions and bodies. The competition was compounded by the learned physician's reliance on written sources and logical cogency over firsthand observation. Moreover, the correlation of concepts, observation, and patient care is a perennial and inherent challenge of rational medicine. Nevertheless, as this chapter will show, the compendia richly document the dynamic coexistence if not complete integration of thought, care, and experience.

The lines from the *Pantegni* illustrate the teleology and value scales, and the underlying anthropocentrism, which structured the medieval discourse on the senses. Teleology, which was at the heart of the Galenic legacy and at the core of human superiority, gave the eyes not only immeasurably more value than the other sensory organs but even priority over the brain and the head. Avicenna's authority reinforced this preeminence and its far-reaching implications, and it promoted the teleological order to a virtual dogma.

> Galen says, the purpose of creating a head is neither the brain, nor the instruments of hearing, smell, taste, or touch, for these parts and faculties are found in animals that lack a head. The purpose is the right position of the eye, elevated above all the parts of the body.

Bernard de Gordon and other compilers reverently invoked Galen for the formal declaration, "the brain is caused for the sake of the eyes, so that they may be in the highest part of the body, like the watchman in the tower." Value judgment colored such statements as this, by Valesco, "the eyes are more noble organs than all the parts of the face, because their action is one of the two most powerful actions of the intellect."

The Eyes

The preeminence of sight, which characterized most of the compendia—and, for that matter, the medical literature of any age—led Constantine to compose a separate *Book of the Eyes,* based on a work by Hunayn ibn Ishaq. The *Pantegni,* too, devoted special attention to the eye, in the theoretical first half as well as in the practical second half. The first of the two following excerpts gives an idea of the basic eye anatomy that the compilers adopted, with varying degrees of adherence, adaptation, and revision. They shared one characteristic, namely, that they offered more anatomical details here than in most other parts of their manuals. As the second vignette shows, however, a focus on anatomy did not preclude the preponderance of humoral constructs in the area where they would seem least applicable. In a similar paradox, it will become apparent that even informed and elaborate accounts on optics were of limited relevance to the treatment of eye diseases.

The Instrument of Sight

The instrument of sight is a crystalline humor [the lens]. It is covered, in the back, by a humor that is clear as glass [vitreous]; and, in front, by another [i.e. aqueous or albugineous] that resembles egg white. Three tunics lie in front, three in the rear, and the seventh [surrounding the retina] is called the spider web. A network of veins and arteries surrounds two hollow nerves that come from the brain. This network brings the *spiritus* to the lens. One of the three front tunics is called grapelike (*uvea*); the cornea is hard and white like horn (*cornu*); the conjunctiva connects the eye to the surrounding bones.

Things That Happen to Sight

Sight may be removed entirely, diminished, or faulty. The possible causes are a defect of the lens, or the *spiritus* not reaching the eyes, or a defective auxiliary part. The lens may suffer from a bad complexion, too cold, warm, wet, or dry; or from a wrong position: when it is moved forward, the eyes acquire a bluish grayness (*glaucitatem*). The *spiritus* may be blocked in an anterior brain ventricle or in a hollow nerve, or it may be deficient. Defects of the auxiliary parts include: excess aqueous humor, called cataract, which reduces vision; a dry complexion of the cornea which weakens sight, especially in old age . . .

These sketches of eye anatomy and nosology from the *Pantegni* encapsulate the Greek legacy as transmitted in Arabic writings, interpreted by Constantine, and integrated into many of the Latin compendia. They are also useful for recognizing the diversity among compilers. Bernard de Gordon, for example, seems to have relied directly on Galen rather than on Constantine for his synopsis of eye anatomy. He described each humor and tunic or layer methodically, and he even claimed to introduce a new observation, that the uvea—which encompasses the iris—determines eye color whereas "the *Tegni* makes no mention of this coloration." His precise description of the optic nerves included an explanation why they "join in the form of a cross" (the optic chiasma). He also faithfully summarized Galenic teaching on the course of the "animal visible spirit" through these nerves. Bernard was more interested, however, in proceeding to the real objective of the *Lilium*. "We have given the anatomy as concisely as possible so that we may have a better understanding of the diseases of the eyes, because the eye suffers every kind of disease." Even so, he admitted that, "with the grace of God," he would treat the subject matter "briefly and plainly, because the diseases of the eyes are very difficult to know and to cure." This difficulty led many compilers to gloss over the details of ocular anatomy and, even more, over the complexities of optical physiology.

Medieval medicine inherited competing or, worse, hybrid theories of vision from two philosophical mainstreams. Plato explained vision by an extramission from the eye itself: this emanation combined with external light to hit an object, from which sparks ("particles") then traveled to the eyes. Aristotle rejected this theory on the grounds of observation combined with logic: he gave the eye the more passive role of receiving light reflected by an object through changes in the medium, that is, the air. The lens played an active part, however, in processing the colors from the incoming rays. Galen adapted some aspects of Plato's teaching, and he interpreted the emanation as the *pneuma psychikon* or *pneuma optikon,* an "animal" or "visual spirit," power, or faculty. This *pneuma,* in this case a form of light rather than air, resided in the lens. It interacted with surrounding reality and conveyed resulting images to the brain by way of the optic nerves.

The compendia offer ample evidence that the concept of "visual spirit" (*spiritus visibilis*) or "spirit of sight" (*spiritus visus*) eluded clear definition. Furthermore, the paramount authority of Galen did not completely overrule the fundamental natural philosophy of Aristotle—and the result was an ambiguity that paralleled those on more vital issues, such as whether the seat of humanity was in the brain or in the heart, or whether a woman really contributes to conception. Compounding the confusion, the *Canon* and other Arabic treatises fused Aristotle's principle that objects emit rays, with the Neoplatonic concept that objects radiate a power (*species*) that can be received. The Salernitan masters who preceded the expansion of Arabic influences largely ignored this complexity. Indeed, Gariopontus, Petrocellus, Bartholomeus, and Johannes Platearius in their compendia bypassed eye anatomy and vision physiology in order to concentrate on taxonomy and therapeutics. Their omissions are somewhat surprising in view of the geographical and chronological proximity to Constantine's contributions.

There is even greater irony in the failure of the later Latin compilers to benefit from the careful thinking of such 13th-century natural scientists as Robert Grosseteste (ca. 1168–1253), Roger Bacon (ca. 1214–1294), and John Pecham (ca. 1230–1292). The English provenance of these three makes it intriguing that the most elaborate examination of optics appeared in Gilbert the Englishman's *Compendium,* where it complemented a careful synopsis of the anatomy and physiology of vision, as well as one of the most lucid summaries of eye medicine. This seems to have been a rare medical *practica* in which traditional and current optical theories were addressed methodically.

Gilbert collated authoritative teachings in a dozen *dubia,* or topics for debate that strongly suggest not only an academic setting but also a facile familiarity with Aristotle and Avicenna. Gilbert cited Avicenna but concentrated on parsing Aristotle directly. He focused on a central question of natural philosophy, namely "whether vision happens by inward reception." The elaborate answer consisted primarily of a close and animated gloss on the Aristotelian proposition, "to which some are objecting." One argument for dissent was that receiving an object in the eye would invalidate the role of rays and thus, "the book on mirrors would perish." Even though Gilbert left us guessing who, of several possible authors, had written this particular *Liber de speculis*—historians consider it unlikely that it was Roger Bacon—he was evidently familiar with the literature and the controversies on optics. Gilbert declared, "others are of the opinion that sight happens by 'extramission' only, but Aristotle refutes them." While largely adopting the Aristotelian arguments and underscoring the role of rays, Gilbert may have had a somewhat divided loyalty. This is suggested not only by the wording of his conclusion but also, as we will see shortly, by the premise in one of his prescriptions. He concluded his *dubium,* "Therefore, some concede that sight happens only by receiving inward and not by sending anything outward, if their words be taken accurately."

The most striking dichotomy in Gilbert's chapters and in most compendia, including the *Pantegni,* was between *theoria* and *practica* or, even, between theory and practice with regard to the eyes. Teaching on anatomy and optics seemed to stand by itself, with limited bearing on the rules of diagnosis, etiology, and therapeutics. Descriptions of the eye were more detailed than for any other part of the body, but they proved almost entirely copied from the accumulated translations from Greek and Arabic. In fact, many details from the sources were omitted in the Latin compendia. Also largely absent are references to empirical inquiries that might have emulated the dissection of monkey eyes by Galen or, from at least 1300 on, would have drawn on human dissection. Nevertheless, a keen sense of observation shines through in various discussions, of which we will see some examples shortly. The medical manuals described surgical interventions in breathtaking detail while their physician-authors, paradoxically, deferred the majority of eye treatments to surgeons. Gaddesden allocated the entire treatment of eye ailments, including pain and even blindness, to the third and, as it was titled, "most useful and primarily surgical" book of his *Rosa medicine.*

Savonarola left no doubt that for such problems as apostemes, growths on the cornea, wounds, and injuries, "it is necessary to run to surgery," but he also suggested that this contributed to a neglect of eye care by physicians. He diagnosed the general quandary of medicine in a characteristically astute analysis.

> Physicians should devote intense consideration in treating eye diseases, because sight is most highly prized. However, because most of its care lies in the hands of the surgeons, they superficially pass over the treatment, unwilling to enter it with their hands as they feel that manual work does not become them.

The other side of the problem was linked to social responses and responsibility.

> There is another reason, for those who suffer in the eyes are so often disobedient that most treatments do not succeed. When this happens to the eyes, the outcome is always brought into the open, and thus it becomes a public testimony of a bad operation, from which loss of reputation and profit is expected. It takes someone with knowledge to prevent all this, unlike quacks (*trufatores*) who do not care for reputation but aim only for profit.

This is what motivated Savonarola "to write, right now, about treatments only, in order to satisfy the physician. Nevertheless, on occasion I will insert some things that are useful to the purpose, for I rank the health of the eyes above the other senses."

The determined focus on treatment, which was a consistent characteristic of the medical *practica*, entailed the risk of leaving natural anatomy and physiology to peripheral attention. It also allowed the compilers to be less concerned with structuring the theoretical material than with covering every practical aspect. Their preoccupation with widely varying attempts at comprehensiveness and rather haphazard arrangements make it particularly difficult to summarize their sections on the eyes. A concise survey becomes more manageable by dividing the subject matter into two panels, one encompassing diseases of the eye and the other disorders of vision. This division is somewhat arbitrary and porous, but it is inspired by a quandary in Bernard's *Lilium*. He noted an apparent inconsistency in Galen's book *On Disease,* and he wondered, "for love's sake," whether an infection of the conjunctiva was to be labeled simply as a disease of the eye or also as an affliction of vision. After shrugging, "I do not know what to say about this, if the statement is true as it stands," Bernard bridged the dilemma by reasoning that the infection could affect vision by spreading to the pupil or lens.

Eye Diseases

Infection of the conjunctiva—now known as conjunctivitis or, popularly, pink eye—was subsumed under the broader category of ophthalmia or inflammation of the eye (Greek *ophthalmos*). Some compilers introduced the discussion of ophthalmia with a general chapter on "pain of the eye," which resulted from another health issue or directly from such an outside factor as extreme cold. Most, however, began their "ophthalmology" (a modern term) with afflictions of the conjunctiva. These eye problems, which may have been the most prevalent, ran the gamut from itch, swelling, and growths to ulceration, bloody discharge, and fistula. Internal causes were blamed for some of them, and these were identified by such stereotypical humoral symptoms as redness for a sanguine imbalance in the body. If the physician determined that this imbalance was the cause, he would address it systemically, by ordering phlebotomy from the cephalic vein, for example, before prescribing topical remediation, by ointments and the like. Among the external causes, wind, dust, and smoke were noted as common irritants. Savonarola (or his source) believed that conjunctivitis occurred more "in southern regions, on account of the abundance of humors and vapors."

One insidious external cause of conjunctivitis, namely, contagion, seems to have been recognized at least dimly. Without engaging in retrospective diagnosis, we may suggest—possibly for the first time—the presence of a bane that was more severe than ordinary conjunctivitis. Scattered clues in the compendia point in the direction of a highly contagious bacterial infection that, through the centuries, has spread most rapidly in milieus with poor hygiene and that is now known as trachoma. A related condition was implied in several descriptions of *ophthalmia*. It was probably disguised, more particularly, in such terms as *lippa* and *lippitudo,* which referred to runny eyes and a crusty accumulation of discharge. This symptom, which was underscored in juxtapositions with earwax, indicated a particularly acute infection. Compilers wrote separately, sometimes in dedicated chapters, about a film on the cornea (*pannus*) and the inversion of eyelashes, which are also symptoms of trachoma. The most persuasive clue, however, may lie in the classification of *lippa* among the contagious diseases. The versified *Flower of Medicine* ("Flos medicine"), which has traditionally been attributed to the School of Salerno, included *lippa*, together with scabies and anthrax, in a mnemonic list of *contagia*. Bernard quoted the verse in support of his differentiation between some growths on the eye, such as "web" (*tela*), which "are not infectious because they shed little or nothing," and other growths, including *lippa*, which are infectious "because they shed something."

Aggressively advancing conjunctivitis was identified as one of the causes of lacrimal fistula, that is, an abnormal opening in the tear sac. This must have been a widespread problem if we may judge from its relatively high profile in the compendia. In extrapolating, however, we may draw some caution from the realization that compilers also devoted a separate chapter to the excessive shedding of tears, which were supposed sometimes to flow from the brain. Be that as it may, there is little reassurance in Gilbert's observation that "sometimes, worms are produced in the corners of the eyes and in fistula." There is even less comfort in his prescription to "take fresh cow dung, right as it comes out of the animal; press it so that the liquid runs onto the worms; and plaster the cake onto the site for three days, and then the worms will be found dead and as if cooked." Bernard prescribed, more agreeably, a drink of white wine in which agrimony and olive leaves were steeped, and he claimed, "doubtless, if the body is cleansed and the patient has a good regimen, this potion cures all fistula." Savonarola cited the prescription and added some dosage details, but then he expressed reservations: "we should have recourse to other weapons or, I assume, there is no peace with the disease, whatever [Bernard] Gordon says. Some say that the concoction should be placed in the fistula, and that this is how the text should read, and this seems more reasonable."

Savonarola urged to do everything possible to forestall surgical intervention for lacrimal fistula. Bertruccio, on the contrary, proceeded early in the treatment to "cautery of the spot with a heated blunt silver needle." This more aggressive stance may have been related to Bertruccio's closeness to surgeons as well as to his worry that "unless cured, fistula threatens the eye with corrosion and the consumption of its seven tunics, as well as with the melting of the crystalline humor, all followed by blindness, which is the dregs and mire of bodily miseries." Other conjunctiva problems that presented a threat of blindness, albeit less urgently, included *ungula* or "little hoof," that is, the growth of a dense nail-like raised white tissue (now called pterygium). It may be mentioned in passing that authors commonly also associated *panniculus* with the conjunctiva, whereas this was actually opacity on the cornea (now called leukoma). In either case, such abnormal growths were known to affect the entire eye, even though they tended to advance unnoticed, in contrast with problems with the eyelids, which received seemingly disproportionate attention in the manuals.

Savonarola noted that authors counted up to 26 diseases of the eyelids, but he argued that many of these coincided, "such as itching, burning, redness, and heaviness." Nevertheless, he still distinguished 12, ranging from swelling to the loss of eyelashes, which he (and most other compilers) adopted from Avicenna. "Because we love this sense too much, I have decided to speak of these diseases more in particular and as briefly a possible, always following the leader whom I have chosen." Suffice it to mention one affliction that appeared in almost every *practica,* probably attesting both to Avicenna's influence and to widespread occurrence. When Valesco began his chapter on the "many diseases of the eyelids," he believed that, "first, we should talk about their lice." According to Savonarola, this was a place where "we sometimes find *platones,* called *piattole* in our vernacular, which adhere strongly, and which are normally found in the pubic area; they are a species of lice." Gilbert stated that "they are called *plactili,*" the term for flat lice which appears to have been used in Salerno. As for remedies, a constant ingredient was the boiled sap of peat and stavesacre (*staphysagria*). Valesco concluded his section on treatment with the simplest method: "it also helps when a girl with good vision pulls them gently from the site where they are attached."

Compilers naturally associated eyelid infections and infestations with hygiene, and lice in general with lifestyle, as we saw in the preceding chapter. Only one, it would seem, broached a more far-reaching association in these chapters. Whereas most authors reserved physiognomy for the section on appearance and "De decoratione," Gilbert inserted a lengthy inventory of characterizations or "significances" into his section on the eyes. After enumerating diagnostic interpretations of various shapes and colors, he strayed into a more marginal albeit integral area of medical learning. A few nuggets, while amusing, may give pause and afford a glimpse of a less rational yet powerful strand of perception.

> Someone with deep-seated eyes we call crafty and deceiving . . . If the eyes are small and protruding, like those of a crab, they signify stupidity and

dullness . . . Big eyes which are directed upward, like the eyes of cattle, and which also seem to laugh, signify a very bad, dull, dumb, a drunk person . . . Long eyelashes prove arrogance and shamelessness.

Physicians addressed various abnormal appearances as medical issues, including strabismus, sunken and protruding eyes, and dark circles. Their coverage was largely pro forma, however, because it was of limited relevance for diagnosis and, particularly, for their interventions.

Injuries, by contrast, ranked high among the extraneous eye problems that called for accurate assessment and prompt treatment. Most of these fell to the surgeon's competence, but Gilbert reported his successful intervention as physician, probably in the late 1240s during practice in the Holy Land (which would no doubt have sharpened his interest in vision and eye diseases). He presented an eyewash of his own design,

> a salve that I made for little Bertranno, the son of Lord Hugo de Iubileto. As the result of a hit to his eye, his entire pupil was covered inside and outside by a white liquid, and he lost sight so that he barely saw the daylight. Distinguished Saracens as well as Christian Syrians despaired about a cure.

A compound was prepared laboriously, with numerous ingredients that ranged from gold shavings and amber to tutty (zinc oxide) and vulture's gall. Then, "I applied it twice every day. With God's mercy, the whiteness receded, exposed the center of the pupil, and cleared away from the uvea." Thanks to the daily administration of a further refined powder, Gilbert achieved the child's complete recovery. Nevertheless, he admitted that "the Saracens and Syrians" knew a remedy which, "according to the authority of their books, was more helpful in eye injuries"; he further reported that they "made a salve with the bile of eagle, vulture, partridge, and crane." Savonarola also intervened in a case for which the surgeon would normally have been called, but which presumably resulted from an injury: "for a two-year-old child who had a large extrusion of the right eye, I applied a plaster from burned date pits, together with clove and rose water, and he recovered in three days or so." Addressing the reader, he adjusted the recipe for less urgent situations, "you compound the same with barley meal or fennel water."

The urgency of trauma might justify the physician's entry into the surgeon's normal domain. Abnormal growths, on the other hand, were relatively elective and therefore more readily relegated to surgery. In the compendia, however, they represent an uncertain intersection between medicine and surgery, in which physicians seemed to contradict themselves by expressly deferring to the competence of surgeons while criticizing them and, evidently, even carrying out their operations. Manual intervention included cautery, not only actual with hot iron but also virtual or potential with caustic agents. Platearius noted that, for pannus, "some apply powerful solvents and corrosive to the eyes, such as burned copper [cupric oxide] or the gall of a bird of prey, but I do not approve of these because the substance of the eye is tender and delicate, and easily dissolved by applying such things." Savonarola prefaced his entire section on therapeutics with the warning, "we should beware of strong corrosive medicines." Bernard may have been unaware of such caveats when he prescribed a medicine for film on the cornea, which "is cured with difficulty or never after it hardens." Burned copper and vulture's gall were among the ingredients in his eyewash, "and we should not look for a better one." He qualified his endorsement only slightly by adding, "it should be tempered if you wish to use it on delicate" patients.

In general, and in contrast with Gilbert, who mentioned "manual treatment with surgery" as part of apparently routine therapeutics, Bernard maintained a markedly conservative position on the treatment of the cornea. He did not recommend surgery for any of the eight distinct afflictions that he addressed, from ulcers to corrugation. With regard to the eighth, namely, scars, he cautioned, "as they are white, people struggle to cure them as if they were a spot, and the operation is worthless." A white spot, on the contrary, was curable, particularly in the beginning or in childhood. He found special merits in a remedy

> For small children, the juice of sparrow tongue, which Dioscorides calls 'poligonia', and which is remarkably similar to knotgrass. This is the herb that swallows bring to their chicks when their eye is pierced with a needle, and these recover their sight. And I have had it brought from the pleasure garden of the Most Serene King of Majorca.

This literally exotic remedy was one of a wide spectrum of topical applications, which constituted most of Bernard's ocular treatments. A considerable part, however, consisted of dietary adjustments and potions aimed at correcting any underlying humoral imbalance. These methods were consistent with the conventional doctrine that, in his words, some excess "melancholy is purged through the eyes, phlegm through the nose and palate, and choler through the ears." Sometimes the discharge collected on the surface of the cornea, causing white spots and the like;

sometimes it would "penetrate between two tunics, with cataracts as a result."

Cataracts

The compendia suggest that there was widespread confusion about the location of cataracts. Many practitioners, at least outside learned medicine, may not even have differentiated an external growth from a cataract behind the cornea. Gaddesden scoffed,

> This is a common affliction, and some wrongly believe that it is a spot (*macula*). If a man should be able to treat it, he will have almost countless money. I have seen many operators with the needle, who seemed to perform miracles, and who made more profit in one treatment than others in ten treatments of other diseases.

He further insinuated that they raked in money while operating on the wrong condition. First, he observed that an external growth could easily be identified because "the cornea is distinctly rough when it is touched with a round-headed instrument or with the short little brush that painters of books use." Next, he pointed out a cause of confusion: "when the eyelid is lifted and the eye is rubbed, some unevenness appears, and many surgeons are deceived by this, as I have seen frequently."

The compilers themselves were at odds or unclear about the exact position of cataracts behind the cornea. Some simply duplicated the traditional description, by Galen and others, of a watery opacity developing between the cornea and the crystalline humor. Others presented variations that suggested both a concern with anatomical precision and the limits of direct observation. The term *cataracta,* although introduced into Latin by Constantine in the *Pantegni,* did not gain currency in Salerno; it continued to compete with the original notion of water; and the condition itself remained unclear until the late 13th century. Johannes Platearius mentioned cataracts almost in passing, and he stated that they "develop between the conjunctiva and the cornea." Gilbert placed them "between the uvea and the crystalline humor" in one chapter, but simply "in the uvea" in another chapter. Even in the mid-15th century, Savonarola still noted the diverging allocations in Arabic sources; he wondered, "it is strange that the authors wrote confusingly and imprecisely about this location"; and in conclusion, he attempted "to settle the apparent disagreements" by allowing for two interpretations of water or cataract.

It is ironic that Gilbert, who surpassed other compilers in his treatment of optics, covered the subject of cataracts quite inconsistently in several places of the *Compendium*. After listing the condition as one of the kinds of film on the *exterior* of the eye, he ascribed the opacity to "moisture collected *between the tunics*." Then, most problematically, he added that, "in another way of speaking," cataracts referred to "blood filling the veins of the eyes and particularly of the *conjunctiva*, hence the name is derived from 'characters.'" Gilbert leaves us to wonder whether, with his penchant for physiognomy, he inferred this odd etymology from the treatise *On Moral Characters* by Theophrastus. Furthermore, he depicted cataracts as "standing water" (*aqua stans*), borrowing Avicenna's phrase, but he ventured beyond authoritative teaching and observation when he defined them as "wateriness and thick fumes that are mixed together." When Gilbert declared that the mixture prevented "the visual spirit from exiting" the eye (an echo of the extramission theory), he contradicted, at least implicitly, Avicenna's presentation of an obstruction that "prevents the images of visible things to penetrate to the lens."

Bernard combined both theories of vision when he depicted cataracts as preventing "the image of the visible object" from being cast onto the lens and the "visual spirit" from reaching the cornea. He also combined Galenic and Avicennan teaching and elaborated it into one of the first comprehensive and consistent discussions in Latin. He not only explicitly equated cataract with the more traditional term "water," but also extended the descriptive nomenclature to fumes and clouds. He also differentiated, perhaps more speculatively, between watery vapors that ascended from the stomach and more dangerous ones that descended from the brain. The appearance of such images as hairs, bugs, and flies signified that these vapors were beginning to accumulate in the opening of the pupil. Contesting this allocation, Valesco argued, "it seems to me, with all respect, that it is not a disease of the opening in the uvea," and he proposed that, rather, it was "classified with the diseases of the uvea on account of proximity." He also returned to a narrower circumscription of conventional teaching: "I declare, following Avicenna, that cataract is an extraneous moisture."

Authors formed a general notion of the moisture, and of the correlation between *aqua* and its descent or falling in *cataracta*, by the early 15th century. Yet when Valesco wrote the *Philonium*, he still managed to expand the understanding. First, he adopted three interpretations posited by the lexicographer John of Genoa, namely, as an underground waterway, a cloud, and rainfall. Then he developed the analogy in a remarkable exegesis that wove the first two meanings into the third as applied to the eye disease and that perceptively drew on meteorology and geology as well as on physiology.

> Just as a cloud or water is produced from vapors by thickening in the middle region of the air, on account of its coldness, so is a cataract in the eye from the coldness of the brain; and just as water flows through the veins of the earth from its original source to the eye of a spring, so sometimes this water descends between the layers to the eye. This is why the ancients named it in analogy with falling water, for just as a cloud or water in the air takes away the ray of the sun, so a cataract takes away the rays and images of the visible object, and these then do not reach the site of vision.

One reader of this passage, in a 1490 incunabulum copy of the *Philonium,* found it memorable enough to underline it and to write in the margin, "note how a cataract develops."

The manner and stages of the development were crucial for determining whether and how cataracts could be treated. They were "sometimes incurable, sometimes curable," in the sober summation by Johannes Platearius. If curable, "they are treated with a surgical instrument, that is, with a needle; the disease usually recurs, however, because the site hurts, pain triggers a flow (*rheuma*), and moistures run into the site." This assessment, in addition to skipping the presurgical option, was more rudimentary than the division into stages by subsequent compilers. Gilbert identified two stages of cataract. At first, when the patient saw bugs or small bodies, it was possible to cure the cataract by the application of pills and purgatives. But, "after confirmation, when the patient sees little or nothing, it can be treated by inserting a certain iron needle." Bernard proposed an almost threefold division of curability: "in the beginning, it can be cured by a good physician; after confirmation, however, only by the hand of the surgeon (*restauratoris*); and even by him not always but only when it is in an intermediate condition."

Gilbert proposed a test for determining whether the cataracts are curable, in one of many versions of instructions that may have originated with Galen.

> Order the patient to close the eyes, rub the eyelids with your thumbs and then, when the eyes are opened suddenly and the water becomes separated from the pupil unto the eyelid, it is not yet treatable by surgery; but if it remains congealed as before, it is treatable by surgery. However, if it resembles chalk, it is too coagulated and therefore untreatable, and it should

be left alone altogether. Also, if with one eye closed the pupil of the other dilates, it may be judged treatable.

A close comparison shows how Bernard was more methodical and precise.

> When the eye is inspected in a bright place, if the color of the water resembles that of a mushroom or of hail, or is black, it signifies that it is too hardened and unable to be pushed down, and there should be no operation. A second way to differentiate: let both eyes be closed and rub the diseased eye gently with the thumb, while the other eye remains closed; then let the diseased eye be opened fast, and if the pupil does not dilate, [the cataract] is no longer capable of being pushed down because it is too confirmed.

Bernard briefly cited the third, and possibly least reliable, dichotomy between a resilient cataract that was capable of being pushed down and a yielding one that was not ready.

The dietary and pharmaceutical prescriptions for the medical treatment of cataract were similar to those for vision, which we will consider shortly. Gilbert limited himself to purges with *hiera picra,* a ubiquitous compound, and *chochiarum* pills, a less drastic cathartic that included scammony and bitter apple (colocynth). Bernard provided more detailed guidance, beginning with "a very light diet." He advised not to eat any fish, "unless one wishes to thicken the cataract", and to "avoid all things that make vapors rise to the head." He reiterated elsewhere that eating fish accelerated the formation of cataracts, an idea Savonarola adopted. For medication, Bernard prescribed theriac in addition to *yera pigra,* for which he specified that it should be taken "many times but in small quantities." For the event that the patient should be rich, Gaddesden added such more expensive components as balm and gold pills. Bernard further wrote a formula for eyedrops, and he ordered that the patient should not only apply marjoram to the eyes but also smell it frequently.

"If the cataract is not cured by these means," Bernard concluded, "we should have recourse to the surgical hand," and choose "a diligent *restaurator,*" that is, surgeon. Other compilers were less definite in identifying the operator. Gilbert and Gaddesden (both perhaps reflecting an English context) cast a *medicus* in their respective (and clearly independent) scripts for the procedure, so that they must have at least assumed that either a physician or a surgeon might perform the operation. Savonarola maintained the ambiguity by referring to "treatment by instrument" rather than to surgery, and to the practitioner as *operator* rather than *chirurgicus.* In any event, since the compilers wrote chiefly for the young *medicus,* they laid down rules (*canones*) by which he would either proceed or, if not, guide the surgeon.

The first instruction was that the patient, prepared by inner and outer cleansing of the body, should be seated in a bright spot, facing but a little below the practitioner. With anesthesia out of the question, his or her head was to be held from behind by an assistant, and the knees to be "bent to the chest and tied," according to Gaddesden or, more gently, squeezed between the operator's legs according to Savonarola. With the patient's healthy eye closed and covered, and the affected eye held wide open and firmly turned toward the nose, the delicate procedure could begin. The tool varied, from a thin iron or bronze instrument in Gilbert to a gold needle, which was favored by some Arabic authors but rejected by Latin surgeons who preferred iron as less fragile. Bernard instructed to "make a hole in the cornea, pierce the conjunctiva until above the uvea, and to press the water down gently with the needle," which he described as "round-pointed." Valesco ordered, more circumspectly, "after making the Sign of the Cross in the Name of the Lord, insert the needle into the white of the eye with caution that it does not touch the red veins of the conjunctiva." The needle should be twirled while it was advanced gently until it reached the pupil and then, with firm pressure, pushed down the cataract. The operator might have to push repeatedly if the water resisted. In any event, he should maintain the pressure at least long enough for "one Have Mercy [Psalm 50] or three Our Fathers," by Savonarola's measure of time, or "five Hail Marys" for Gaddesden (both would range from two to four minutes in the more precise modern reckoning). The needle was to be twirled while being pulled out, with great care neither to damage the lens nor to draw out the aqueous humor.

This procedure, which has become known as couching, was the only one for which the compilers offered instructions. Other methods were used or tried in cataract surgery, especially by wandering practitioners. One alternative technique, which was mentioned in Arabic sources as possibly new and may have been practiced in medieval Europe, but which has drawn little comment from historians, was extraction. Gilbert reported that, "according to some, a sharp needle is entered through the pupil so that the water flows out." Avicenna had observed, "some men have different ways of treating water with an instrument: some make an opening in the bottom part of the cornea, through which they extract the water. However, there is reason for fear in this, because the aqueous humor leaks out when the water is thick." Avicenna's caveat may have contributed to the total eclipse of cataract extraction in the compendia. Bernard, for example, echoed the warning: "no opening should be made in the lower part of the cornea for extracting the water, because there would be a risk of draining the aqueous humor." Greater precision came, not surprisingly, from a surgeon. Guy de Chauliac mentioned—and disapproved of—extraction "by suction through a hollow needle." Savonarola, familiar with Guy as well as with Avicenna, was less decisive when he mused, "but what shall we say when the cataract is incipient and thin? There is room for speculation here; think about it."

Whatever the procedure and whoever performed it, knowledge and skill were both indispensable. Citing the surgeon-physician Guglielmo da Saliceto, Valesco warned, "in view of the danger to an organ as noble and delicate as the eye, no one should dare to try this operation unless he has been an apprentice (*discipulus*) first and has frequently seen the master operate." Gaddesden was equally stern in his remark that "neither the surgeon nor the physician knows this operation unless he has seen it performed." Moreover, if he has never tried it, "his hand will shake and he will botch the whole job. It is good to try first piercing the eye of a dog, cat, rooster, or calf, so that a man becomes used to doing this, that is, so that he knows how to enter the needle directly between the tunics without harm to the [aqueous] fluid of the eye." It is easy to imagine that the patient continued to need reassurance after the operation. Gaddesden advised, "the patient should be comforted with a good word, and his or her fear be allayed; and you should ask whether he or she sees with the cataract depressed." Even a positive answer was followed by a lengthy recovery, to be managed with great care. The patient, lying in a dark room for at least seven to nine days, needed to be "guarded from coughing and sneezing," according to Gilbert. Only a few authors deemed pain of sufficient concern to prescribe medication, but most insisted, by the authority of Mesue and Avicenna, on changing the dressings every third day and freshening the site with rose water, willow leaves, and the like. Savonarola commented, "the modern operators whom I have seen do not observe this, yet they succeed; but I believe that it would be fine if one does as these men say." This remark, with a note of some mild skepticism, implies that Savonarola was an onlooker to couching surgeries, notwithstanding his demonstrated interest in cataract as a serious threat to sight.

Vision Disorders

Cataracts, as the organization of most compendia illustrates, lay on the border between diseases of the eye and impairments of vision. These two areas were compartmentalized to a large extent, as we have seen, and the dichotomy becomes more apparent in a comparison between early Salernitan masters who concentrated on anatomical aspects and Gilbert, who devoted considerably more space to functional problems. Most compilers, however, agreed in dividing these problems broadly into loss, weakness, and corruption, a Galenic taxonomy that they also applied to the other senses. Beyond these three classes, they identified a host of extraneous factors that threatened every aspect of vision and, in response, a wide spectrum of measures for preserving, improving, and restoring sight in general. They all agreed that nothing was more harmful to sight than, in the ascending order of severity (and, possibly, moral implication) sleeping on a full stomach, overeating, frequent intoxication, and too much sex—or any sex according to a few. The prescriptions in the compendia also shared several ingredients, with fennel a favorite among the vegetable simples, and tutty among the minerals. Ever since antiquity, the most recommended panacea for the eyes was gall (*fel*), particularly of birds of prey but occasionally also of partridges, hares, and other animals. Biblical tradition supported the medicinal value of gall, with which Tobias cured his father's blindness at the command of an angel (Tob. 6:5-19 and 11:4-13). Galen remarked that "the gall of some animals is singularly praised by the physicians for the acuity of the eyes" on account of its beneficial property. The bitterness of gall was usually tempered by honey in external applications and in potions. Human milk was the only substance that surpassed honey for tempering strong simples, and it was only slightly less ubiquitous. Common, too, were specific instructions for preparing compounds; a recurrent one, to dry ingredients in the sun, no doubt aimed at imbuing them with luminous power.

The full catalog of threats to the faculty of sight was more extensive than the register of corresponding general remedies. Treatment was less effective than prevention, which included commonsense caveats about being exposed to smoke or dust, looking into the sun or fire, staying long in the dark like those in jail, and so on. There were also less physical threats, ranging from anger and sadness to intense study. Bernard worried about too much reading of small letters. More strangely, he also saw danger in sleeping with shoes on—Valesco's reiteration of the warning struck a reader of the *Philonium,* who underlined it and marked it with the word "nota" in the margin of the 1490 incunabulum. While such notions as this were probably rooted in popular lore, nutritional apprehensions about "thick" or "smoky" food and drink were based on physiological concepts. Some details about the connection between vision and diet afford a glimpse into daily life. Gaddesden, for example, mentioned the harmfulness of all things "vaporous, such as leeks and garlic; inflammatory, such as must and newly brewed beer; constipatory, such as pears before a meal, pastries, and old cheese; [and] viscous, such as eels and buttered fish." He abridged some "common verses" from the *Regimen of Health,* a guide to hygiene that has traditionally been characterized as Salernitan, for the conclusion of his dietary list.

> Leeks, wines, venery, wind, beans, smoke and fire,
> But staying awake most of all: these harm the eye.

Even if we are convinced that hygiene is essential to eye health, we may be surprised by Gaddesden's warning, "do not neglect washing the feet, and combing one's hair in the morning."

Compilers generally recognized the difference between the failing and the weakening of vision, although they did not always draw a clear line between *defectus visus* and *debilitatio visus.* They also seemed ambivalent about admitting helplessness while promising a cure. Nevertheless, they evinced sensitivity to the patients' ordeal of progressive loss (*minoratio* to *ablatio*) of vision, the corresponding descent into darkness (*obscuratio*), and the frightening prospect of eventual blindness. One way of allaying fears was to suggest that the condition might be limited. Thus, night blindness or nyctalopia ("noctilopia" in the medieval spelling) was set aside as a separate category. It was also brought closer to a natural phenomenon, by correlating it to the difference between nocturnal and diurnal animals. Gilbert differentiated among animals: "some see only at night and little or nothing in the day, such as jellyfish (*nocticula*) and toads; some, in twilight and little in the day or night, such as bats; and some in the day, night and twilight, such as cats." Some compilers, including Bernard and Gaddesden, simplified this passage, and they omitted not only jellyfish and bats, but also the finer points of Gilbert's rationalization. They also seem to have ignored an analogous question by Gilbert, "about the confusion of sight, as when someone is blinded when brought to a room with white walls after a long stay in the *ergastulum*" (Galen may have been the source of this reference to the *ergastulum,* the pit in which slaves were kept chained in Rome until Hadrian abolished the practice).

Notwithstanding such perceptive observations as this one, Gilbert and his peers were at a loss about many causes of the loss of vision and, hence, about appropriate treatments. The Salernitan masters, with their focus on practice, were keenly aware of this problem. Johannes Platearius noted, "a failure of vision happens in many ways, generally from the failing of the visible spirit." Bartholomeus admitted that, "sometimes, sight is darkened without any manifest cause." All authors recognized cataract as one of the most manifest causes, but many mentioned a counterpart with starkly contrasting latency. Savonarola juxtaposed cataract with *gutta serena,* a quiet drop or clear drop that could not be observed except by the result. He defined it as "a blockage which falls in the concave optic nerve," and which inevitably caused blindness. Platearius simply stated, "if sight fails from a blockage of the optical nerve, it is incurable," and compilers reiterated this verdict. "Gutta serena," which has become the label for the destruction of vision by an unidentified cause, makes us aware that glaucoma may have been one of the insidious banes that the compilers and other physicians might guess but could never understand, let alone treat.

Allusions, scattered in the compendia, might tempt some historians to believe in an early recognition of glaucoma. This belief would negate the dual fact that, in premodern nosology, diseases were not pathological entities but qualitative conditions, and in learned discourse, most definitions hinged on semantics rather than on empirical induction. This caveat does not mean that the allusions should be ignored: to the contrary, they contribute to a more nuanced understanding of medieval medicine, and of eye care in particular. Constantine, as we have seen earlier, in the third quotation from the *Pantegni,* applied the Greek root *glaucon,* meaning "bluish," literally in teaching that the color of the eyes changed to "a bluish grayness" (*glaucitatem*) when the lens moved forward from a natural position. A century later, Archimattheus of Salerno adopted a similar literal interpretation for an eye condition that he called "glaucosis" (the term, rarely used now, is still a synonym for glaucoma), but his explanation was humoral and qualitative rather than anatomical. The Salernitan master defined *glaucosis* as "having bluish eyes, either from abundance of glassy phlegm or from cold: this kind of color comes about when the fiery parts are condensed into airy parts and the airy into watery." The early allusions were quite vague and generic, in contrast with one precise 15th-century reference that is admittedly more tempting. Savonarola, in his—still qualitative—comments on "the loss of the function of sight" from a cause in the humors, explained that the tunics or nerves "are sometimes dried and wrinkled by intense heat, so that sight is destroyed completely, and this disease is called *glauconica,* and there is no remedy for it."

Compilers presented remedies for stopping or even reversing the advance of blindness, in spite of the acknowledged prospect of incurability. Some even seemed confident that one or other formula could be effective. For instance, Gaddesden claimed success with the combined application of a particular treatment, one of several in his chapter on blindness. The intricate preparation began with collecting the water flowing from "bundles of green branches of an apple tree" when they are burned, and then compounding it with fennel seed and parsley roots cooked in white wine. A very clean hemp stupe, soaked in this concoction, was to be applied, gently squeezed, to the eyes at night. The eyes were to be washed "with the same wine, two or three times a day; and this was "to be done until [the patient] sees." Gaddesden asserted, "someone was cured who had been unable to see for twenty-five years." His other prescriptions, however, as most of those by other authors, projected the same combination of resignation and determination that we have encountered in earlier chapters.

Bartholomeus recorded a gamut of recipes, from purges to eyewashes, for slowing down the advancing darkness. Johannes Platearius, endorsing and elaborating a recommendation in Constantine's edition of the *Viaticum,* advised that leeches should be placed on the temples. "If the failing of vision results from moisture which surrounds the brain itself, this excess humor should be purged by the appropriate medication. I have learned by experience that leeches applied to the temples are greatly helpful for this cause." Gilbert provided amazing details on this particular application and on the leeches to be used. First, he alerted the reader to the different appearances of poisonous and safe leeches. Then, he instructed,

> before they are applied, they should be rolled in ash so that they vomit if there is anything in their belly. Next, put ointment on the place where you want to suck blood; when the leech clings, cut its tail with a razor so that what it draws will go out through the tail, and so it will never be sated.

His instructions for removing the leech were equally precise: "drip tepid vinegar or something warm onto its head. Do not pull it off forcefully, or a broken tooth may be stuck and cause harm."

In his prescriptions as well as in his observations, Gilbert offered abundant proof that his excursions in the theory of vision were not mere academic exercises but complementary to his lively interest in sight as a health issue. Although both sides were not integrated, the numerous *dubia* that he raised were matched by the concrete details in his prescriptions.

For example, he added minute details to an exotic remedy, which, some 50 years later, Bernard mentioned casually in connection with *poligonia* and indirectly attributed to Dioscorides. Gilbert prescribed,

> Item, proven for failing vision, for defects and pains, and for the blind who do not see: take the chick of a swallow, blind it by pricking its eye with a thin needle, and place it back in the nest; when you return after three days and you see that it has recovered sight, take off its head, which you reduce to powder by burning it in a rough pot.

Such treatments inevitably remind us of the distance between modern and medieval sensibilities, but this should not make us overlook the amount of realism that was interwoven with their mysticism. This mixture is evident in the instruction with which Gilbert completed his swallow recipe: "take human gall or, if you do not have this, take the gall of a cat that has been nursing for thirty days, add two parts of opobalsamum [balm of Gilead] and castoreum [beaver gland], mix together, and put in the eyes." By now, we are aware that this and many similar recipes sprang not only from cumulative tradition and a different outlook on nature but also from the refusal to accept incurability.

The threat of blindness universally inspires much greater dread than the weakening of vision. The latter was, in comparative terms, even less frightening because the range of acceptable average sight was much wider than today. Gilbert and other authors actually showed greater interest in farsighted and nearsighted animals than in human analogies except for a few phenomena. One of these was the manner of people looking upward and, "when they wish to see better, placing their hand on one eye" in order to concentrate the power of vision. In any event, myopia was problematic for relatively few people, such as scouts and guards. Presbyopia, a problem for a steadily growing majority in the modern world, concerned a select minority that, of course, included the physicians. The compilers obviously shared this professional concern. They further echoed the conventional view that a decline in acuity was a natural accompaniment of aging, "on account of the incapacitation of the organ, the thickening and diminishing of the [visual] spirits, and the increase in undigested phlegm," as Valesco phrased it. He also adopted the idea that "combing the hair frequently is helpful, especially for the elderly, because it draws the vapors away from the eyes" to the top of the head.

A preoccupation with sharp vision was evident in the number and variety of Valesco's prescriptions and also in interjected references to his practice. He repeated, "and I add," to several of the recipes which he quoted from Avicenna, Arnau de Vilanova, Bernard, and others. While reporting that he had "tried, and used several times," such panaceas as theriac and mithridate, he assured for the entire register of remedies that "anyone of these, if used continuously when the body is cleansed and together with a good diet, noticeably preserves and restores vision." Gaddesden included himself among the beneficiaries of "a special water that I use for myself and my colleagues, and that I call 'aqua socialis.'" He claimed further,

> it is good for the elderly, the middle-aged, scribes, physicians, and those with night blindness and cataract; it is good for all weakness of vision, and it preserves the use of sight until the end of life. I have not found anything better for the eyes, for the patient feels improvement the second day that it is used. Therefore, this water should be given due honor.

He also offered a recipe "against diminishing vision from toil, old age, or coitus," which was to be applied in an eyewash or added to food as a powder. He promised, in a model of target advertising, that the medicament "makes one read small letters until the end of life, and see the contents in the urine, and the veins in the arms; therefore, it is good for barbers."

It is somewhat surprising that neither Gaddesden nor Valesco showed awareness of an aid to vision that was historic as well as mentioned in one of their favorite sources. The *Lilium medicine* was the first *practica* to name a magnifying tool that was the precursor of spectacles and eyeglasses. The tool appeared here on the cusp of a transition in reading aids, as may be seen from a closer look at the text and context. At the end of his therapeutic section on weakening vision, Bernard offered an *experimentum* that he prefaced with the boast, "until now it has never pleased God to reveal a better one." The recipe called for the laborious compounding of some 19 ingredients, and for placing the mixture "in summer, in the warm sun for forty days, shaking it every day in the same way as roseate sugar is prepared; in winter, in ashes of which the warmth equals that of a brooding hen." This would produce an eye drop "of such power that it would make a decrepit man read small letters without a beryl eye." The *oculus berellinus* was both remarkable enough for serving in a punch line *and* familiar enough to be mentioned casually. Indeed, as the pioneering work of al Hazen (Ibn al-Haytham, ca. 965–1039) on reflection and refraction became known in Latin Christendom, it found practical application in the magnification of letters by means of a hemispherical crystal that served as a supplementary lens. This "reading stone" was, most commonly, a green beryl (of which emerald is a variety), and the word is the origin of the modern German and Dutch words, *Brillen* and *bril*.

While Bernard was completing the *Lilium,* in 1305, the famed Venetian glassmakers in Murano, Italy, capped their progress in making crystal by fitting two glass lenses in iron frames and joining these for binocular use. The new device took hold, but the diffusion was slow, as the further fate of Bernard's original statement shows. The term "bericles" was still employed in 1377 by the French translator of the *Lilium* (who guaranteed that Bernard's recipe would serve "a decrepit man of seventy"). The word "antojos," on the other hand, which the Castilian translator chose around the same time, alluded to dual lenses held in front of the eyes. By the mid-15th century, Savonarola replaced Bernard's *sine oculo berellino*

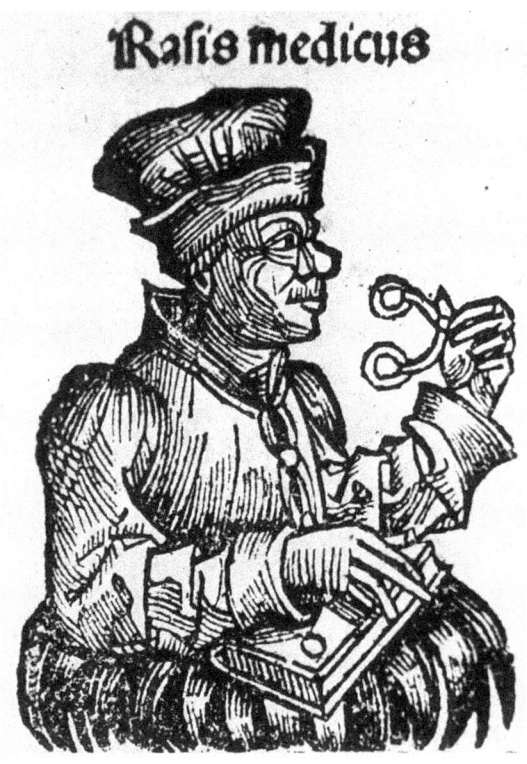

The physician Rhazes, in the gown and cap of a 15th-century physician, with a book and spectacles. Woodcut in the incunabulum of the *Nuremberg Chronicle*, published by Anton Koberger, Nuremberg, 1493, fol. CXCII. (National Library of Medicine, Images from the History of Medicine # B08255)

with *sine ocularibus*. Moreover, he unequivocally extolled the benefits of using eyeglasses or, more precisely, "glass eyepieces" (*ocularibus vitreis*). He explained,

> they preserve the essence of what is seen and they do not allow the eye to become tired in seeing minute things, and so the spirits are not dissolved. This is well known to goldsmiths from experience when they plan to make something fine and clever, and particularly by those who craft stones for rings, because they use them all the time and this is why the eye does not tire, for when a thing crosses from a clearer to a denser medium, it appears bolder.

It may be noted that Savonarola discussed eyeglasses before proceeding to medicinal remedies for weakened vision.

The third class of vision disorders, namely, the corruption or malfunction of perception, occupied relatively little space in the compendia. The major reason was that several aberrations were either discussed as symptoms of cataracts or classified with headaches, drunkenness, and impairments of faculties of the brain. We have come across the "seeing of flies" of *scotomia,* for example, as an error of the faculty of imagination. Some compilers expressed wonder about extraordinary aberrations of vision that they probably inherited from Pliny's *Natural History* and more mythical sources, and which they correlated with the thesis of extramission. Gilbert entertained a *dubium* about the impact of the seeing subject on the seen object. He posited that, in the process of vision,

> change takes place within the eye, but change occasionally arises *from* the eye. This is evident in a menstruating woman who, when she is uncovered and viewed by an entire army, infects a mirror and whatever she looks at, by the infecting spirits of the eyes and through the infection of the air.

Gilbert then moved on to another hoary myth, which is worth quoting because it dovetails with the werewolf mythology that we encountered in the preceding chapter. The impact of the glance is also evident in a man who is "infected when he is seen by a wolf before he sees the wolf"; on the contrary, if he sees the wolf first, "he is not infected because the air and spirits going out from him destroy the approaching infection." Gilbert, Bernard, and others introduced a third logically related myth, about the basilisk that "kills by its mere glance," in their chapter on venoms. In sum, notwithstanding the broad and deep implications that they share with evil eye lore, these myths bear less on the physiology of vision than on notions of infection and poisoning. Nevertheless, they illustrate the crucial role of air, as a medium, in an understanding of vision that did not rely on humors.

Ears and Hearing

The separation between vision physiology and the humoral framework, and the distance between eye anatomy and nosology, was paralleled in the compilers' chapters on hearing and the ear. The Salernitans generally discussed neither the process of hearing nor the instrument as such. When descriptions began to appear, they were strikingly simple, and they lacked many of the details that were available in the translations of Greek and Arabic authoritative sources. The following sketch may illustrate the imprecision.

> The instrument of hearing is composed of rocky bone, extended nerve, a concave optic nerve, and quiet air. In addition, there are pockets and sinuous coils in the opening, and cartilage that appears on the outside in the shape of oyster shells. It should be understood that hearing occurs when the exterior air moves the quiet air that is naturally present in the concave nerve.

This synopsis, in Bernard's *Lilium,* represents the average depiction of ear anatomy.

Even when authors gave more thoughtful accounts, they hardly correlated these with nosology. Gilbert, for one, left anatomy in the background and kept diseases separate, notwithstanding his intelligent parallels with the physiology of vision and his perceptive illustrations. He drew no practical inferences, for example, from a comparison between the blinding effect of bright light and the deafening impact of such sudden loud noise as thunder. Another concrete observation was occasioned by an anatomical feature that was known but of no medical consequence, when he explained that the temporal bone was extraordinarily dense in order to let sounds "strike more forcefully, for vielles and zithers resonate better when the strings are hard and dry." The idea of percussion as the essence of hearing held the potential for fruitful further exploration. At the same time, it is clear that anatomical and physiological specifics, already inherently fewer than for vision, became simplified even further because they seemed of limited relevance to the treatment of ear problems and hearing disorders.

Physicians realized that the inner ear, even more than the eye, lay beyond their diagnostic and therapeutic reach, and they evinced growing apprehension about venturing too deep into the ear canal. By virtually limiting their attention to the outer ear, they assumed, paradoxically, the surgeon's prerogative. Furthermore, they participated in manual interventions, as the compendia suggest. The dichotomy of competencies, however, is also documented in the physician's manual, particularly in the prevalence of humoral explanations and medicinal treatments, and in the trend to delegate actions that were deemed indecorous. Earache was one issue that, whether the cause was internal or external, lay unequivocally in the physician's sphere. Even when it resulted from trauma, it was treated with medication. The compilers presented pain, more saliently here than in other instances, variously as an ailment, a symptom, a criterion for treating certain complaints differently, and even as a cause of such a real disease as deafness. "Pain of the Ears" was the comprehensive heading for nine or more ailments and defects in the *Passionarius* and other compendia from Salerno. These ailments, which ranged from earache to deafness, received separate chapters in most of the later manuals.

Another difference between the Salernitan masters and their successors lay in the therapeutic response to earaches and more tangible problems, both by instilling medication and correcting the body's complexion. The Salernitan authors liberally recommended eardrops for every ailment. Their prescriptions teemed with such terms as "instillation," "infusion," and "injection"; ingredients ranged from vinegar and pepper to *nitrum* (niter, or natron, or hydrated sodium carbonate, or potassium nitrate) and hellebore in Gariopontus, or to "a little opium" in Bartholomeus. They showed no reservation, and they even seemed to ignore a basic caution about injecting medication, which was voiced in the *Pantegni* and emphasized in later manuals, perhaps under the influence of Avicenna. Gilbert cautioned, "nothing should stay long in the ear, and I say the same thing for injections into the womb or by rectum." Bernard maintained perhaps the most conservative attitude toward the procedure. He specified, "a medicine should not stay in the ear for more than three hours." As a general rule, he taught, "if it is possible to treat with compresses and plasters, this is what we should do, while putting off an injection as long as we can, because whatever enters will be harmful after it has performed its task, unless the ear is cleansed with extreme care." In another instance he declared, even more forcefully, "I do not approve that anything be instilled into the ears since many other methods may be found."

Grudgingly, Bernard accepted the conventional method of introducing wormwood and other bitter simples for killing worms in the ear, as taught by Constantine. He stopped short, however, of the aggressive advice of Gariopontus, "if these do not help, instill live sulfur and live calcium with honey." Bernard preferred to "extract the worms with care." Even for this more careful extraction, his enthusiasm seemed limited. His description of the procedure was banal in comparison with Gilbert's instructions to "take a fragrant apple that is fully ripe, to warm it near a fire so that it smells sweeter, and apply it to the opening of the ear at night; in the morning you will find the worm in the center of the apple because of the delight of the smell." The compendia convey the general impression that worms in the ear were a widespread problem, common enough for Gaddesden to mention an "auricular worm"—in the literal sense rather than the metaphorical musical earworm. In addition to entering from outside, worms were also engendered inside unclean canals. Some authors attributed the latter to spontaneous generation, but it was consistent not only with poverty and neglect of hygiene but also with rural life. This is indicated in a vignette that should neither be ignored nor overrated by the historian. "Note," Gilbert remarked, "that grains of barley grow in the ear of some people, and they produce worms." This remark, while repulsive and evocative of gothic depictions of dark Middle Ages, should not obscure the caring of such a physician as Gilbert, who continued, "as soon as the worms have been killed and extracted with pincers, we should proceed with cleansing medicines."

The effect of a rural setting on ear health is evident across the compendia. Gariopontus observed, "something might fall into the ear cavity by accident, such as a grain of wheat, a bean, a straw, or a bristle." He recommended making the patient sneeze, a conventional remedy that Johannes Platearius supplemented. Sneezing should be induced "with the mouth and nose pressed close," so that the force of the air expelled the object. If this was of little avail, other methods included the insertion of "a smooth thin twig tipped with turpentine or something sticky" or, as a last resort, suctioning by the "repeated application of a cupping vessel." Compilers displayed the greatest ingenuity in devising methods for extracting water from the ear. Constantine instructed to "insert a reed of which the head has been dipped in oil and heated in the outside in an oven." Platearius preferred to use absorbent *lana pinnula concarum*, meaning "sea wool" or the silky filament from "the sea shells in which pearls are found"; if the rare and precious substance was not available, a cotton wick might suffice.

Bernard suggested several additional attempts for drawing out the water "after the body has been cleansed," each of them with fascinating ramifications. In one attempt, the practitioner was to "apply a small reed to the ear and let some lowly (*vilis*) person strongly draw in the air by mouth through the head of the reed." In a somewhat puzzling excursus on the recourse to "suction by a lowly person," Gaddesden related, "I saw someone do this; he had a reputation as if he was a healer of all the deaf because by this method he extracted, as if it were in an instant, all the material collected in the ear." For a more impressively ingenious approach, Bernard ordered the practitioner to take

> the reed with which children draw water and shoot it a long distance—it is called "ladoira" [syringe] in our dialect—place the end in the ear, and then suddenly draw back the stick which is inside it: nature, which does not permit a vacuum, very strongly draws the water out.

Yet another attempt consisted in warming the reed at the outside end, in order to evaporate the water. Bernard warned, however, that the situation was very difficult if the water or, worse, anything else was deep inside.

The deep penetration of water, worms, or other extraneous matter into the ear was the potential cause of serious problems, among which acute pain, inflammation, and loss of hearing were the most critical. Dizzying and desperate pain in the ear, and the patient who suffered it, called for the practitioner's resolute response. Bernard admitted, "if the pain is fierce and intolerable, we are forced to apply cold drugs after the administration of phlebotomy" (about which more anon). For unbearable earache, he prescribed drops of the opiate, *philonium*. In keeping with his conservative outlook, however, he insisted that the drops were to be preceded by rose oil and other protective simples, tempered with woman's milk, and followed by cleansing castoreum, if harm should come from the sedative. He admonished sternly, and with some surprising finger-pointing, "we should be diligent and careful, because I have seen many die in the hands of the restorer." This reference to the restorer suggests that even the administration of eardrops may have been among the manual tasks that physicians delegated to surgeons. Be that as it may, Bernard added an anecdote in order to prove the possibility of a cure with strictly external medication.

> It happened to me once that an old restorer suffered an intolerable earache. General purges and particular procedures had been performed in

accordance with the teaching of Galen, Avicenna and all the other authors, and they did not help at all. Then I applied chamomile oil to the ears and made sachets of chamomile and, in truth, he was cured.

The anecdote further served to justify recourse to multiple administrations: "therefore, when medications do not help, it is good to apply many and diverse things as long as they are regulated by reason."

The widest therapeutic array was aimed at ulcers of the ear, abscesses, bleeding, and sanious discharge. It drew, consistently and predictably, less on anatomical specifics than on complexional principles. Topical applications were fewer than treatments that aimed for restoring the humoral balance in the body or in the head. Laxatives were prescribed for expelling harmful vapors that rose from the stomach and *caputpurgia* for draining congestive or putrid humors from the head through the nostrils. Various prescriptions for bloodletting were less precise in their purposes, for

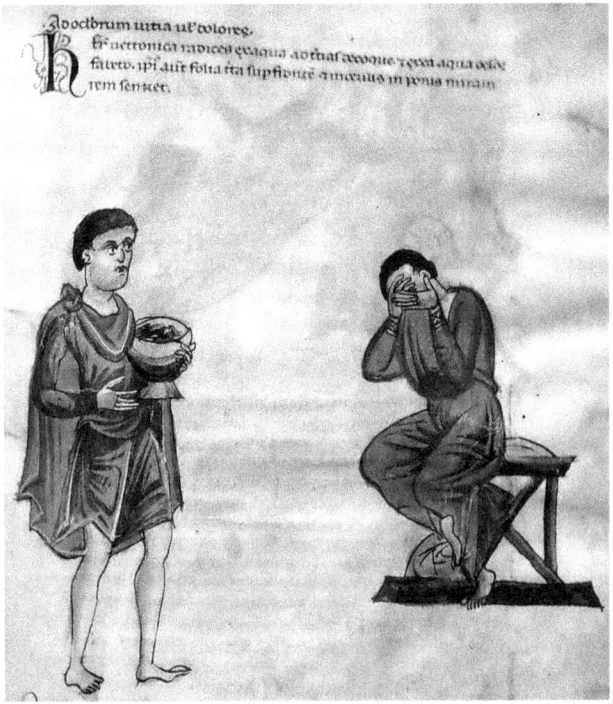

A healer brings herbal medicines for "ailments or pains of the eyes" and "ailments and pains of the ears" to a patient in agony. Drawing in a 13th-century manuscript (but obviously copied from a much earlier model) of *Apollodorus de Herbis*. (Wellcome Library, London. Wellcome Images M0007391)

instance, those by Gariopontus for "cupping on both shoulder blades, and incising both 'horns of the head' [? *cornua capitis*] with iron," for chronic bleeding from the ears. Some practitioners, who in Bernard's estimation too readily resorted to bloodletting, drew his characteristically conservative disapproval.

> I say, briefly and without discussion, that phlebotomy should not be done in the veins behind the ears, because it would cause sterility, as this is where the 'juvenile' [jugular] veins are. It is acceptable in the veins of the ear lobes, from the age of seven until the patient is of an age that phlebotomy can be done in the arm. People beyond the sea (*ultramarini*), however, are more accustomed to this bloodletting than we are.

It may be noted that, in one statement, Bernard managed to combine an application of Hippocratic anatomy, an allusion to geographic–cultural difference in medical practice, and a limited concession to acceptable remediation.

The borders of acceptable therapeutics were necessarily flexible when authors, their claims of success notwithstanding, were uncertain about deeper causes and effective responses. The limits of effectiveness were undeniable for earache, but they were conspicuous and readily acknowledged for hearing disorders. Most compilers adopted the Galenic scheme in ranking these disorders, in descending order of seriousness, as complete loss, in deafness; weakening, so that "one hears only shouting"; and corruption or malfunction, "when one hears sounds, noises, and tunes within the ear." A wide variety of external and internal factors could be responsible for any category, but the immediate cause lay in the instrument itself, when the auditory nerve was blocked, injured, affected by thick humors, or harmed by cold. This interfered with the dual task of this nerve, which was closely analogous to the task of the optic nerve. The two-way function of the auditory nerve was to convey the *spiritus* of hearing from the brain and to transmit to the brain the sound that was produced in the encounter between moved air from outside and the quiet air inside. Blockage of this channel resulted in deafness or utter silence, *surditas*. Deafness at birth was compounded by muteness, which gave the populace the impression of mental deficiency, and authors the occasion to ponder, "hearing is the gate of intelligence." Bernard underscored the auditory nature of his era, as well as the vigor of his humanities background, when he quoted verses from the 12th-century *Cosmographia* by Bernardus Silvestris, to the effect that all the knowledge of Athens, Rome, Chaldea, Liberal Arts, Law, and Medicine had "found refuge in hearing," so that all learned wisdom "would perish if man were deaf."

There was general agreement that deafness ranked with blindness as a bane to humanity and, even more, as a challenge to the physician. Bernard summed up the consensus:

> congenital deafness (*surditas nativa*) is not cured, and long-standing deafness, which means for longer than two years, is beyond hope. Deafness from severed nerves is incurable. Deafness from a hard aposteme is curable. Deafness that alternately increases and decreases is remediable.

This terse review is instructive on several levels. It echoed yet subtly modified traditional tenets, for example, by tightening up the teaching of Johannes Platearius that "deafness which has lasted for two or three years is rarely or never cured." The summation further narrowed the scope of reasonable attempts, by identifying conditions beyond hope. Inversely, it suggested that successful treatment might include the spontaneous healing of a hard aposteme. In addition, the limits of the practitioner's abilities and duties were sometimes blurred, at least for the modern reader, by the inherent ambiguity of *curare* as referring both to care and to cure. The most significant aspect of Bernard's overview is the use of the qualified predicate "remediable," which pointed to a fourth dimension of medical care. Remediation, strictly speaking, was less than outright cure but more than mere palliation, and it complemented prevention as the most fruitful part of the physician's task.

Prevention and remediation were less easy in practice than in theory, however, even for relatively minor hearing disorders. There were many external and internal factors that defied correction. Continued loud noise, which gradually destroyed hearing, surrounded such people as "residents of mill-houses, who speak loudly and hear only shouting." This observation by Gilbert may surprise us if we have never heard the grinding of millstones, and it illustrates historical change in general as well as the difference in prevalent noises. The difference is dramatically underscored by the medieval adage that pealing church bells, which were part of everyday life, caused not only momentary but sometimes long-lasting tinnitus, that is, ringing in the ears. Gaddesden differentiated other causes and forms of tinnitus, with a touch of poetry.

> If it results from wind, the sound resembles that of a trumpet; it also seems to rise and fall, as in the bubbling of must [in making wine]. If the wind

tends to be humid, it sounds like rain; if thick, it sounds like a mill; if dry, like the breaking of trees.

Gaddesden further cited the view that "tinnitus is the herald of deafness." The threat or the vexation of tinnitus made it tempting to prescribe opiates and other sedatives. Bernard argued, however, "it should be understood that, whatever the authors may say, it is better to put away the narcotics than to apply them in this case." This plea also overruled the underlying notion that cool narcotics counteracted overheating, to which the ears were prone because they were the natural drain for the waste of yellow bile, the hot humor.

The Nose and Smell

A conventional though rarely quoted doctrine assigned the draining of waste for each humor (except the blood, which might have excess volume but not waste) to a different facial organ: yellow bile to the ears, black bile through the eyes, and, most important, phlegm to the nose and palate. This construct, which has more ramifications than we can pursue here, framed many discussions of the nose, and particularly the ranking of its functions and malfunctions. The joint mention of the nose and palate is one of many instances in which, aside from their respective purposes, the nose and mouth constituted a unit. They also shared the distinction of being portals into the body below the head, unlike the eyes and ears. Some nasal and oral ailments, therefore, appeared in more than one section of the compendia—and will be distributed over this and the following chapter. Our concentration here is on the initial appearance, if not as much in the literal sense as Gilbert took it, with his penchant for physiognomy. While pondering the *dubium,* "why the nostrils are wide in someone who is angry," he speculated, "hence, when Moors see a captive with flaring nostrils, they argue that he is angry and they feel hatred for him."

The other compilers adhered more closely to the conventional introduction of an organ or body part. Bernard, for example, introduced the nostrils (usually plural in Latin) as

> composed of many things: first, the bone called 'sieve' [ethmoid], which is perforated, and the front of the cerebral membrane which is perforated toward the ethmoid bones so that nature may expel the superfluities through those sites and draw the breath or air to the head for tempering the arterial blood of the brain itself; second, two extensions going out from the

ethmoid bone in the form of the tip of a nipple, and this is where smell is judged when the fragrant vapor is carried to the site through the air; third, cartilage and flesh on the outside.

This sketch exemplifies, again, an anatomical description dominated by teleology and humoral physiology. It defines the threefold task of the nose, in descending order of importance, as the discharge of superfluous humors, respiration—which will be examined in our next chapter—and olfaction.

Draining the humors, and phlegm in particular, was the primary purpose of the nose although, perhaps surprisingly, blockage was not perceived as a major threat even in cases of nasal polyp. The principal affliction was *rheuma,* the excessive running of fluid from the head. Authoritative tradition divided *rheuma* into three forms, although Gerard of Cremona's translation of Avicenna's *Canon* suggested that the nomenclature was unstable, and not every author adopted the taxonomy. Gariopontus did not mention *rheuma* and, instead, recognized three divisions of catarrh. Such Salernitan masters as Petrocellus and Johannes Platearius simply ignored the triple taxonomy. Ironically, most compilers adopted it and, in support, quoted two lines from the *Salernitan Regimen of Health.* These "magisterial verses," as Savonarola called them, specified that flux to the chest should be called *catarrhus,* to the throat *branchus,* and to the nostrils *coryza*—which is still the term for a head cold. The generic *rheuma* was much more serious than the ordinary runny nose, and Bernard advised that it

> should not be neglected, because it is almost the mother of all illnesses: this is clear because it causes deafness or tinnitus in the ears, cloudiness in the eyes, foul odor or polyp in the nostrils, paralysis in the tongue, quinsy in the throat, consumption or pleurisy in the chest, nausea or vomiting in the stomach, loose bowels in the intestines, arthritis in the joints, and so on.

Savonarola gave the sweeping list focus by adding, "sometimes it runs to the legs and makes them swell, as in Duke Ludovico de Bertania." The many and diverse effects of the flux lent urgency to an understanding of the causes that determined the treatment but were very elusive.

External causes of *rheuma* ranged from northern winds to postprandial naps, presumably in a drafty spot. Due to seasonal influences, catarrh was more likely in autumn and coryza in spring. Another steadily noted cause lay in strong aromatics, such as musk, crocus, and onion mentioned by Avicenna; Latin compilers added lily and wild mint. These were harmful because they "dissolve the vapors in the head," according to Bernard. Gaddesden proposed, somewhat differently, that "all but a few aromatics" are so warm that they cause a headache, and "all pain attracts *rheuma*," Galen taught. As the few cold aromatics that might be responsible, Gaddesden itemized roses, camphor, water lilies, and violets. The association between aromatics and headache, and the mention of roses in particular, together with the constants and variants in correlations with nasal discharge, is intriguing because they might hint at allergic reaction, a possibility to which we will return when considering asthma in the next chapter. An essential internal source of *rheuma* was either the production of excess vapors by an overheated brain or the condensation of stomach vapors rising to a cold brain. Compilers borrowed an analogy from Avicenna for explaining the latter as similar to the rise and flux of distillate from an alembic. The usual dietary correctives and a host of medicinal treatments, from inhalants to steam baths, corresponded to the wide spectrum of suspected causes. Johannes Platearius taught that the correspondence should be observed with care and remedies applied repeatedly. Gariopontus, on the other hand, insisted that "all care should be applied to the head," but he also prescribed oral medications. Gaddesden, considering that *rheuma* resulted primarily from cold causes, cautioned, "poultices and rinses are not appropriate unless they are wiped and dried off immediately, before they cool off, and this is something that practitioners commonly do not know." He offered "pills which I make all the time for either case," that is, whether the cause was cold or warm. "Should the cause be cold, and the patient rich, one may add some musk, to a weight of three or four grains." Savonarola also prescribed musk, together with other aromatics "that are noble substances, for the noble"; maintaining equity, he recommended that "the poor should smell dried nigella [of the Ranunculaceae family] in a linen cloth, for this is a unique medicine." Other lozenges contained ingredients that were popular for centuries, such as licorice for cough, sugar candy for soothing the throat, and calamint for facilitating the ejection of phlegm or mucus.

Rheuma had a counterpart in the flow, usually more abrupt, of blood from the nose, which did not originate primarily in the brain but in the nasal veins or arteries themselves and therefore drew more directly on the blood supply of the entire body. Compilers normally devoted a separate chapter to nosebleed, to be treated by introducing a styptic tent into the nostrils, pouring cold water on the head, and other commonsense measures. They also reasoned, however, that bleeding from the nose could be a natural form of bloodletting and that it was good if it occurred on a critical day and brought visible alleviation to the patient. Savonarola even argued that in some cases it was appropriate to cause bleeding "by introducing leeches into the nostrils and stirring them somewhat." He appeared more sanguine (pun not intended) than other authors, with a minor editorial exception, in estimating the amount a person could lose safely. Bernard set the normal limit at four pounds, the boundary of danger at eight pounds, and the certain threat of death at the moment of fainting. Savonarola, on the other hand, claimed that "from a person of average health and age, up to twenty-four pounds could drain before he or she would die (Avicenna has a different figure, up to twenty-five)." He supported his claim with anecdotal evidence: "in my days I have seen a pregnant woman from the Zabarella family of Padua losing about twenty-two pounds of blood through the nose, and she gave birth and survived, as did the baby."

Sneezing paralleled nosebleed in double ambivalence, as it could be a natural or induced phenomenon, and it might trigger a healthful or unhealthy flow. Its taxonomy was more protean, however. While sneezing usually also received its own chapter, it might show up in a strange context as, for example, between the chapter on inebriation and the chapter on epilepsy in the practical part of the *Pantegni*, between lovesickness and epilepsy in the *Viaticum*, and between inebriation and incubus in Valesco's *Philonium*. It was either associated adversely with *rheuma* or classified alternately under transient movements of the brain or nerves, as akin to spasm; under respiratory events, as akin to coughing; with digestive expulsions, as akin to hiccups or vomiting; or even with reproductive matters, as aiding delivery or causing abortion. As a symptom, it indicated coryza when it was "frequent and accompanied by mucus," according to Valesco; it pointed to pneumonia or other problems of the chest when it was accompanied by fever. Sneezing could be stopped, if necessary, by holding the nose, vaporizing and inhaling such warm herbs as chamomile or anise, applying ointment to the nostrils, rubbing the face, or even provoking anger or any other strong emotion. When it was beneficial, as for migraines, Petrocellus instructed to take euphorbia and some other simples, "to reduce these to a powder, and to blow them into the nostrils" (euphorbium is still a homeopathic medicine for sinus relief). Compilers were aware but seemingly somewhat disdainful of such less complicated methods as sniffing pepper or smelling lilies.

When we keep in mind that the mechanism of olfaction remains incompletely understood to this day, we appreciate the repeated acknowledgements in the compendia that the elusive nature of the sense of smell matched the evanescence of odors. The *Pantegni,* by emphatically correcting the anatomical description, gave the impression that misunderstanding was widespread.

> Some have viewed the channels that appear in the nose as the instruments of smell, because no smell is perceived when the nostrils are obstructed and it will be perceived immediately if they are opened. But this opinion is false, for these [channels] only bring smell to the frontal brain. The instruments of smell are two little parts, resembling teats, which descend to the ethmoid bones where the dura mater is perforated.

The shift from the nostrils to the olfactory bulbs was a significant correction, but the olfactory process itself remained sketchy. In the *Pantegni*, smell was represented as "a fume resolved from odoriferous bodies and mixed with air, which is drawn through the nostrils by the olfactory bulbs and transmitted through their perforations to the brain."

Physicians could be satisfied with a rudimentary conception of the sense of smell, because it had little bearing on the role of odoriferous substances in the diagnosis, etiology, or care of disease. They showed little concern with the loss or weakening of the faculty, unlike for the other senses. They were preoccupied, instead, with the corruption of the sense, and less with the distortion of odors than with an internally generated problem that they termed "fetor of the nostrils." The compendia suggest an increase in this preoccupation. In Avicenna's *Canon*, the condition was discussed rather concisely, attributed to vapors from below or humors from the head, and committed to routine remedies. Constantine's *Viaticum* mentioned, more dramatically, that "people sometimes suffer horrible fetors in the nostrils" from a host of causes. The chapters grew more elaborate and intense in the 14th and 15th centuries, which may reflect a growing proximity among people, particularly the nobility and upper bourgeoisie. Bernard expressly limited himself to the corrupted sense "when the nostrils and breath smell offensively to the subject and others." He deemed it "a very bad and mortal sign" when, in the absence of anything fetid, the patient thought to smell "something like rotten fish." In less extreme and more quotidian situations, "if the stench could not be removed, it should at least be covered up, so that no one will notice it. For, if the physician suffered from this, it would be very disgraceful and especially when he is dealing with nobles."

Bernard and his peers drew most of their prescriptions for nasal stench from the deodorants that they inventoried in their section on cosmetics. Saliceto, however, treated the condition as a genuine disease, which called

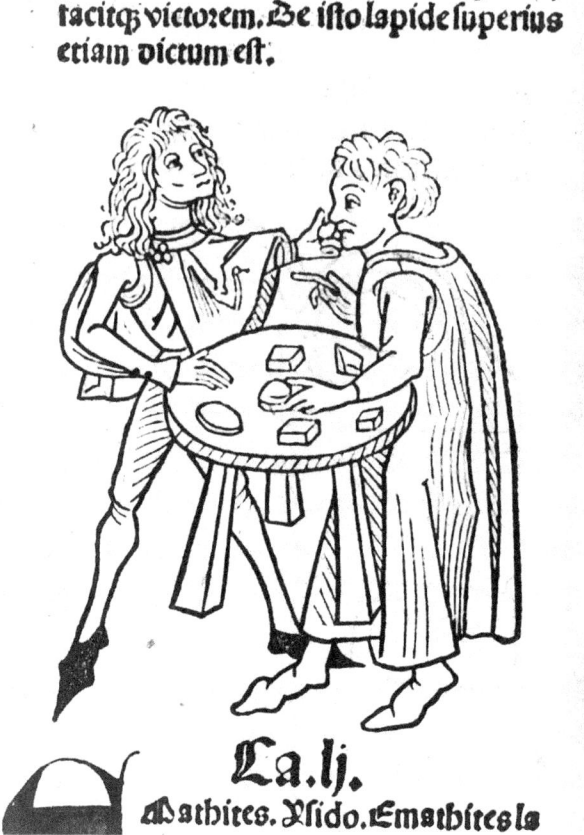

A lay healer treats a patient's nose, with hematite for bleeding. Woodcut in an incunabulum of Jacob Meydenbach, *Ortus sanitatis*, Mainz, 1491, fol.gg4v. (Wellcome Library, London. Wellcome Images L0013762)

for specific medication, even though he devoted several chapters to deodorants in the *liber de decoratione* of his *Summa*. He called on personal memory to highlight a special remedy.

> This is what we did in our day. We made a certain lady, who was well known to us, rinse the nostrils with the best wine which could be found, every morning, and it did her good. We did nothing else, and by this method her illness was blunted in time. But when she stopped the rinsing for some time, the illness immediately manifested itself.

For a further glimpse into the social scene, we may note that Savonarola cited Saliceto's reminiscence but changed, perhaps inadvertently, the patient into a nobleman.

The Mouth, Taste, and Touch

It may surprise the modern reader to find that offensive nasal odor figured more prominently in most compendia than the corresponding oral problem, which appeared as a mere extension of the former in several manuals, including Valesco's *Philonium*. One exception, worth noting because it may suggest an urban setting, was Savonarola's *Practica*. Savonarola asked the reader, "nobody should bite me if I happen to become long-winded on the treatment of this condition, because this affliction is too obnoxious and horrible and the patients are too solicitous in seeking a cure." Other compilers gave prominence to *fetor narium* and referred back to this subject in their discussion of *fetor oris*. Even when, from at least Constantine and Petrocellus on, they recommended rinsing the mouth after meals with odoriferous wine or pure wine, their expressed concern was with dental health rather than social decorum. The lack of personal anecdotes about halitosis may be another indication that the physicians' concern with public impact was less than for other odors. Gilbert alluded to a more private effect of bad breath when he remarked, from a typically male perspective, "women put great effort into covering up, and they should keep a bit of laurel leaf, or a little musk under the tongue so that they do not deprive men of the desire for intercourse." He also bore witness to a social context when he advised, "let a *pomum ambre* be made and be carried all the time in the hands or in the bosom." The pomander, a device that continues to fascinate historians, was used not only for concealing unpleasant odors but also for warding off pestilential miasmas. Gilbert's recipe called for 15 ingredients, but he still added, "if the patient is rich, gold and ground precious stones may be added."

Guglielmo da Varignana reported, "it is written that keeping gold in the mouth removes the odor," but then he moved from secondhand to personal testimony, "we have experienced that wine from a wormwood decoction, together with lemon rinds, removes a bad smell which comes from the presence of something putrid in the stomach." Valesco reminded the reader that remedies should include cold aromatics if bad breath was due to a warm cause and warm aromatics for a cold cause. "Some practitioners, however, are deceived because they order warm aromatic spices, such as cloves or galangal or ginger to be given to anyone who has bad breath, whereby they increase the warm humoral imbalance, and the patient gets worse." This warning portrayed, at least implicitly, the *practicantes* as lacking both the knowledge and the observance of complexional equilibrium, which were paramount for *physici* or *medici*. In the same vein, the compilers implied the superiority of learned medicine over case-by-case (*casualis*) empiricism when they tied such a relatively lesser subject as *fetor oris* into a wider nosological network. They associated bad breath not only with tooth and gum disease, but also with the brain, stomach, and lungs—so that halitosis will reappear in later chapters of this survey, in connection with the diagnosis and therapeutics of other ailments.

While references to oral odor pervaded nosology, the principal parts of the mouth were treated in relative isolation from the rest of the body. The lips, teeth, and tongue each constituted a virtually self-contained subject, even though neither the complexional origins nor the diagnostic significance of their ailments were ignored. The chapters on diseases of the mouth normally opened with "fissures of the lips." Cold north winds were cited among the principal causes and greasy salve among the common remedies of chapped lips. Gaddesden prized sweet almonds, either ground and pressed into oil or "chewed and sucked, as I have experienced often enough for myself when riding horse against the wind or in the hot sun." Fevers were, predictably, prominent among the internal causes. However, if cracking of the lips followed a tertian fever, it was "the sign of a good turning point" (*crisis*) according to a long-standing tradition. Bernard noted that "the common people" (*vulgares*) also held this view, albeit on less than scientific grounds, "because a patient has recovered after they see sores on the lips, and this is how they get some notion."

The compendia leave the impression that dental problems were among the most irksome afflictions of the mouth, and perhaps of the entire body. Neglect of oral hygiene was a universal cause, regardless of the extensive coverage in regimens of health and in spite of the emphatic pleas by nearly every author of a *practica*. Constantine urged, for example, "take care to wash the teeth" and "cleanse the gums and mouth with a rough cloth." Petrocellus commanded, "care should be taken of the teeth and gums, with exceptional discipline." Bernard taught that the teeth "should be cleaned with sage wine, and then be brushed [*fricari*, the origin of "dentifrice"] with a mild wine and lemon rinds." He further warned, "if one is negligent in this, slime and residues collect in the teeth, and these become the cause of harm." The harm took many forms, from tooth decay to rotting gums. The medical responses were, here again, based on humoral physiology, while anatomical specifics seemed almost incidental. The casual regard for these specifics and for exploring them is conspicuous in Bernard's summation, "it should be understood that there are thirty-two teeth in a complete set; those in front are called incisors, then come the canines, and then the molars; and they are divided into heads and roots, *as is evident in anatomy*." Even in more detailed descriptions of the teeth, the anatomy was based almost exclusively on Avicenna, for instance in Valesco's *Philonium*. It should be noted, however, that while admittedly compiling information from as many authors as possible, Valesco also injected notes of originality. First, in a direct address to the reader, "I tell you, I have seen people who have only thirty teeth, including myself with sixteen in the upper mandible and fourteen below." He continued, curtly dismissing an urban myth, "what is being said about those born after the Great Mortality [the Black Death], that they have only twenty-eight teeth, is false and makes no sense."

Valesco declared that dental ailments "are twelve or thirteen in number, in so far as I have been able to collect from the sayings of the authors." He followed the conventional order by beginning with toothache, which must have been so commonplace that it was a part of domestic care and a fertile field for roving quacks. Savonarola observed, "I have seen that patients suffering from this ache commonly do not approach physicians except in great need, that is for the most intense pain, and after first trying many things." In addition, he was troubled by the relationship between dentistry and medicine. Prefacing his chapters on the teeth, he admitted, "I have been agonizing whether I should pour a considerable amount of time or take an easy and passing look into something that is considered to have become a barber's affair and is treated mostly by vulgar entrepreneurs on street corners." When turning to remedies for toothache, he called the subject "a mess among people because anyone, man or woman, publicly proclaims to be a master, and to be armed with many or almost infinite and, as they say, the most efficacious remedies."

Rather than abandoning sufferers to empirics, Savonarola and other compilers treated toothache as a full-fledged subject of learned etiology and therapeutics. They reported that it was caused by humors from the brain or vapors from the stomach that, in the words of Johannes Platearius, "cause pain when they flow into the nerves of the teeth." Remedies included bloodletting from the cephalic vein and opiate mouthwashes, to which Platearius added, "I believe that it is very beneficial to apply an external poultice with hellebore." If this still did not help, "the ultimate remedy is skillful extraction with forceps." He revealed that he had tried his own hand at the operation. "Some say that the tooth can be extracted easily and painlessly with lees of olive oil and wolf's milk [a kind of euphorbia] compounded with flour paste, but I have learned by experience that this is false." About three centuries later, Valesco reinforced the sense of skepticism with a practical call for humility, when he advised, "in cases of dental ailments, you should not claim to know fully which medicine will stop the pain immediately; if you do this, it will be embarrassing to have been deceived so frequently."

It is ironic that helplessness did not prevent physicians from claiming to know medicines where they were arguably most helpless, that is, for most afflictions of the tongue. Treatments covered the entire gamut, from topical applications for sores to purges for head discharges and stomach vapors. On the other hand, anatomy and general nosology merely adopted or even simplified Galen's teaching. Savonarola gave an inkling of an outlook that made most compilers gloss over anatomical details. He argued that anyone who wished to scrutinize the complexion of the tongue, a compound organ, needed to know thoroughly how each of the components was constituted and interacted with the others, "something that, I think, should be left to the speculator rather than to the practitioner, at least in this case." Hence, descriptions tended to be general, derivative, and framed by teleology. The tongue was described as having a spongy texture, ample blood supply, and "sevenfold nerves" for serving the sense of taste and the more noble faculty of speech. The superiority of speech over taste, not only in general but as a particular medical issue, was due to a vast range of reasons, which ranged from practical importance to underlying valuations. It is worth keeping in mind that, among the five senses, taste ranked close to touch in moral ambivalence. Both were viewed as useful and dangerous at the same time, deemed most susceptible to pleasure and pain, and associated with the hard-to-control impulses of *appetitus*. Constantine juxtaposed taste and touch, as well as pleasure and pain, in close connection with sex. The sense of touch was ascribed to the entire body but, to the surprise of the modern reader, it was not discussed in relation to the tongue or of the lips.

The compilers focused on speech, as the principal function of the tongue, even though medicine was of little avail for the loss or corruption of this faculty. They all agreed that muteness was incurable if existing at birth and difficult to remedy if supervening later, but they still listed several remedies. Their most remarkable consensus, however, was in attributing speech defects less to cerebral or neural malfunction than to "some damage to the instruments of locution," as Galen taught. Tightness of the frenulum or ligament underneath made the tongue tied and, in the most literal sense, "express a concept with difficulty," as Bernard phrased it. Constantine and others called for an incision "to restore the movement around the mouth"—something surgeons still do in lingual frenectomy or frenuloplasty. Softening or heaviness of the tongue made patients stutter or mispronounce words: the standard example for the former was "saying 'do-dominus' for 'dominus' [lord]"; for the former, "saying 'Aristoles' for 'Aristoteles.'" Both problems were aggravated by excess salivation. This must have made one patient particularly grateful to Gaddesden, who boasted, "this is the cure which I applied to a nobleman, bachelor in civil law, who was hampered by much moisture: I made him a lot of very dry gargles and did rubs of the extremities, and every night I gave him frankincense."

Next to the primary functions of taste and speech, the auxiliary role of the tongue in digestion received little more than an afterthought. The digestive function surfaced, almost casually, in a simile when Bernard mused, in the style of Galen, "the tongue is like a hand for speaking and chewing and swallowing, which reaches out to the esophagus and the trachea." In fact, swelling of the tongue and other abnormal conditions were likely to appear, not only as symptom but even as problem, in different sections, for example on poisons. Along parallel lines, the tongue was mentioned in connection with snoring and apnea in chapters on excessive sleep (*subeth*) rather than on the mouth. This is at least partially due to the fact that the role of the tongue in breathing was barely recognized—and is still incompletely understood—and that the compilers almost overlooked the mechanism of respiration in their preoccupation with respiratory diseases, as we will see in the following chapter.

Uvula to Diaphragm and *Passiones Spirituales*

The uvula is shaped like a teat, wide above and narrowing to a point. It is located between two openings. It purges the head of phlegmatic moisture. Sometimes it loosens, droops, or swells, which causes cough and difficulty in swallowing or breathing. It swells on account of blood and other humors, or of a fume rising from the stomach. Patients suffer considerable pain when swallowing food, or even when swallowing saliva. Sometimes an aposteme develops on the uvula, which can be seen when the tongue is pressed down with a finger.

If the uvula is swollen below and white or livid, it may be cut, but not when it is red because, as Hippocrates says [*Pronostics* 3.23], inflammation and hemorrhage would follow. One should wait until the upper part becomes thinner and the lower enlarged, and then incise after administering a purge, opiates, and strong drying gargles. The incision should be done, with forceps made for this purpose, in the thinner part with care not to touch the root. Cauterization is better, with the end of a cane or reed, or with the glowing tip of a gold or iron rod. Some churchmen, however, cut a healthy uvula for the purpose of improving the voice, and the patient incurs permanent hoarseness.

We understand that the uvula prepares the air for the heart, cleansing it, bringing it into balance, and moistening it; that it purges the brain and drains the discharged phlegm; and that, therefore, an incision is made at the risk of all these functions and to the detriment of the mouth and chest. The uvula should not be neglected or overlooked.

An excerpt from one of the Salernitan Masters at the head of this chapter would have maintained the chronological sequence of our introductory quotations, but Salernitan manuals were so focused on therapeutics that they contain very few quotable and meaty observations. However, the *Compendium* of Gilbert the Englishman, from which these lines are excerpted, bridges the gap. While incorporating the legacy of the Salernitan schools, Gilbert personified the coming of age of the medical university, at Montpellier in particular. He benefited from a second wave of translations from Greek and Arabic sources, and he probed the theoretical and therapeutic dimensions of medicine. Moreover, in some ways—and with the exception of organization—he represents the ideal compiler by his articulateness, interest in the broadest spectrum of medical learning, and personal comments. The quoted lines open the chapter "On the Uvula," which is the first of "Book Four, On the Diseases of the Respiratory Parts" in his *Compendium*. They can only sample the richness of the chapter, let alone of the entire manual. A collation with other writings suggests an equally rich background, and it points to a paradox. First, it reveals the profound influence of Albucasis, Haly, Mesue, and other Arabic authors, a crucial element that is latent in the chapter itself but abundantly evident in the surgical manuals of the time. On the other hand, a comparison with the authoritative texts also indicates the degree of Gilbert's independence, which we have already seen manifested in the preceding pages.

The Gullet, Throat, and Neck

The excerpt from Gilbert largely reproduces the core of traditional teaching, but it also includes some noteworthy variations, as we will see. For centuries, authors gave the uvula a prominence that may seem disproportionate to the modern reader. They viewed it as a sentry between the mouth and the rest of the body. Their seriousness in determining the uvula's functions stands in striking contrast with their sketchy anatomical descriptions. The part was named *uva*, "grape," or *uvula*, "little grape" for its pendulous appearance or, as Johannes Platearius speculated, "because it contains much moisture, like a grape"; Savonarola believed that "it is called *uva* for the similarity with a seed of a grape." The common comparison with a teat (*mamilla*) made sense if one thought of such mammals as a goat or a cow. Petrocellus strangely misinterpreted the stated resemblance—or, quite possibly, a scribe took some liberty—when he claimed, "as the ancient physicians wrote, the uvula has many openings like women's nipples." Many associated the uvula with bilateral glands that were prone to inflammation. These glands, which they located at the base of the tongue, in the gullet, or at the entrance to the throat, corresponded to the tonsils as well as the adenoids of later nomenclature. Called "the almonds" (*amigdale*), they were thought to supplement the sublingual glands as sources of salivation.

An overview of compendia from the 11th to the 15th century leaves the impression that the itemized functions of the uvula increased, though not uniformly, in number and precision. They were not systematically spelled out in the *Canon,* while the *Pantegni* taught that the uvula "was necessary for a threefold reason," that is, to "make the voice beautiful and strong, lighten the entering air and temper its coldness, and intercept dust so that it does not enter the throat or lung." According to the *Practica brevis* of Platearius, "the task (*officium*) of the uvula is to purge the head of excess moisture." Gilbert, in his *Practica,* spelled out the task as "preparing the air for the heart, cleansing it, bringing it into balance, moistening it, and conducting it, as well as purging the brain and channeling away the discharged phlegm." In the *Lilium,* Bernard specified, "the uvula has five uses (*iuvamenta*), first because it protects from smoke and dust"; second, it tempers the air going to the lung and heart; third, it assists in forming the voice, "like the finger of a flute player on the flute hole"; fourth, it prevents air from entering the stomach when one speaks and food or drink from entering the lung, "and this is why it is not good to eat and talk at the same time"; fifth, "it prevents rheumatic matter from descending abruptly into the chest and stomach." By the time of Valesco's *Philonium,* the number of tasks grew to six, most of which he attributed to Galen, although he elaborated the task of protecting the *meri* or esophagus—one of the subjects of our next chapter.

Elaborate attention for the care of the uvula paralleled the detailed speculations on its role. Apostemes and relaxation or swollen drooping were perceived as threats to breathing, speech, and digestion. Chapters on quinsy and other diseases of the throat addressed the therapeutic challenges, which included infections of the tonsils. For the uvula itself, regular medication with lozenges, rinses, and the like was quite sufficient according to Bernard. Surgery, however, was an option, with serious implications. Resection of the uvula was already practiced in the time of Hippocrates, as we know from *Pronostics* 3.23, which was cited by Gilbert (see the introductory quotation) and by almost every compiler. In fact, therapeutic and even preventive uvulotomy was common in European medicine until the 17th century; it survives in African cultures; and, as a medical fashion, it may be compared with the more recent propensity for tonsillectomies.

Complete removal of the uvula (now called uvulectomy) was a special object of apprehension. The *Pantegni* warned, "some die from a radical excision because they take in too much air, which cools the chest and lung." In his *Practica,* Petrocellus predicted more ominously that the incision would "bring a person to ruin, and make patients become consumptive or die rabid." Platearius urged to perform the operation "with the greatest caution, after administering purges, phlebotomy, opiates and, as I have read in the *Pronostics,* when fear of suffocation is not at all an obstacle." Gilbert, as we have seen, denounced some churchmen for removing a healthy uvula and thereby ruining a voice that they had expected to improve. The victims themselves may even have sought the operation. Bernard warned, "let them beware, who have their uvula incised in order to sing better, for without a doubt they will never afterward give a beautiful performance with their vocal instruments."

The warnings in the compendia give the impression that uneducated operators performed most of the unnecessary incisions. In general, the admonitions have an undertone or an accent of skepticism toward lay practitioners. Thus, Valesco presented precise guidelines for incision, "on the premise that neither the aforesaid remedies nor any other reasonable measures help," but he concluded, "this is where those illiterates (*ydeote*) fail who excise radically." In addition, he reported a precautionary example of malpractice.

> I was called to a church official (*presbyter*) who had an aposteme on the uvula. After seeing him, I intended to proceed as I have described in this chapter, to seek a barber and to make all the necessary preparations. Meanwhile, in my absence, another presbyter came, and he resected the entire uvula with forceps.

As might be expected, the result was disastrous.

> The patient lost so much blood and so many fluids ran to his chest that, with the great tightening of his chest and lung, he was barely able to breathe. In the end, he could not expectorate and purge his chest, and the third day he choked to death. Therefore, be forewarned about the error of illiterates.

Valesco sighed, "may God spare us from evil."

Quinsy was viewed as the most serious affliction of the throat. The term now specifically designates an acute inflammation that causes a purulent abscess around the tonsils (peritonsillar abscess), but the Latin predecessor, *Squinantia,* had a far broader meaning. The category extended from a sore throat to acute infections of the pharynx, with numerous variations among authors. Platearius and others identified three kinds, all of which were caused chiefly by an imbalance in the blood. The first was accompanied by little external swelling but intense pain, very high fever, and diminished voice; it was deemed incurable and deadly, on the authority of Hippocrates, and it suffocated the patient in a few days. The second kind, manifested by some external swelling and less pain or fever, was barely curable. The third, *squinantia* proper, was recognized by heavy external swelling, low or no fever, and moderate pain; it did not become deadly unless the swelling turned inward. Nevertheless, the word remained identified with choking and similar fatal conditions, and even Platearius documented the lethal potential in a family anecdote.

> If suffocation is already imminent, a piece of wood or instrument should be placed properly inside the mouth and fixed to break the membrane of the aposteme, but this must be done with the greatest care. I have never done this, but my father of blessed memory [Johannes Platearius Sr.] did it when he was playing dice with a certain Salernitan. This Salernitan was suddenly attacked by quinsy, and when he began to choke he was unable to speak and showed the painful site with his finger. My father, knowing the treatment, placed a wedge between the patient's teeth and pushed a key inside. The membrane of the aposteme was broken so that a great quantity of blood flowed and the man was liberated.

This episode is testimony to the bravery and determination of a practitioner, the cool head and resiliency of a patient, and the importance of luck in medicine—for both the practitioner and the patient.

It is ironic that *squinantia* provided Gilbert with an occasion to distance himself from his teachers and to pronounce his own preference. When the treatment included phlebotomy from the saphenous vein, "the Salernitans cut laterally, but it is safer to cut lengthwise so that the tongue does not become disabled for forming speech." While the quality of speech was important, the sonority of the voice was valued even more highly. This esteem was underscored by frequent references to Galen's idealization, "the voice is the noblest voluntary action, proceeding from the noblest action of the soul, that is, from the movement of thought and deliberation." Valesco was more methodical than other compilers in drawing the difference between speech and voice and in describing physical details that "anyone who wishes *to look into anatomy* will be able to know in advance." Before we infer that he was alluding to dissection, however, we should realize that he derived all his descriptions explicitly from Galen and Avicenna and that these led him to conclude, "from this it is manifest that the uvula and the epiglottis are not the same thing." Nevertheless, the mechanics of voice gave Valesco an opportunity to demonstrate his perceptiveness. Observing that "art imitates nature in the formation of voices," he drew a detailed comparison between the production of music by the parts of the musette (*museta*, a small bagpipe) and the production of voice by the thorax and lung, trachea, epiglottis, tongue, and palate. Valesco also proved perceptive about acoustics by noting, "trumpets and other wind instruments sound better near the surface of water because of reverberation: the sound, unable to penetrate the water, bounces off the surface."

Compilers generally devoted a separate chapter to various impairments of the voice, which they assembled under the title "On Hoarseness" (*De raucedine*). Immediate causes of hoarseness were external or internal. External causes were either dietary or environmental, and they ranged from salty foods to smoke and cold winds. Valesco cited the example of "wine merchants who stay in very humid cellars and caves." He further discussed a rumored direct cause, when he addressed the staple academic question or *dubium* about man becoming hoarse when seen by a nearby wolf. A first answer, congruous with notions of infection that we saw in the preceding chapter, proposed that the voracity of the wolf contaminated the air. Dismissing this explanation "proposed by philosophers," Valesco combined an external and an internal cause. He argued, "there is another and better answer, for someone who sees a wolf in close proximity tries with great effort to shout, and the sudden crying affects the vocal instruments, so that humidities are abruptly drawn to these organs, soaking them and quickly causing hoarseness." Internal causes of hoarseness could be reduced to a temporary, chronic, or constitutional deficiency of the patient's vigor. This was the case for "children, the weak and convalescent, the incarcerated, the religious, and the like," in Bernard's telling juxtaposition. In the old, moreover, hoarseness was incurable because their constitution was humid by nature.

The fundamental cause of an impaired voice was a complexion that was too dry or, more critically, too humid. Savonarola observed, "excessive dryness is harmful, and this is why trumpeters pour water into their trumpets; excessive humidity is harmful, and this is why a violin for which the wood was cut during a full moon will never sound well"—the strongly humid influence of the moon was most evident in the tides. Furthermore, "teachers (*doctores*) who lecture with a loud voice, and people who tire themselves in speaking and shouting often incur hoarseness because the exertion makes them sore and warm, so that moist matter is drawn to the epiglottis and windpipe." Savonarola was more precise than others in identifying different abnormal qualities of the voice, from tremulous to thick. Thus, he described a raspy (*aspera*) voice as caused by dilation and drying out of the windpipe surface, "as in forceful shouting and blowing, especially after eating, and this occurs mostly in hunters who are shouting after the dogs and wild animals." He also raised two *dubia* about a thin voice, whether it could result from sleepiness or from sexual intercourse. The medical advice to avoid the likely causes was easier given than followed, and compilers filled a considerable number of folios with remedies that ranged from lozenges and inhalants to bloodletting. Bernard urged to "administer tailed pepper (*cubeba*) night and day, morning and evening, without mercy, as if it were child's play." He seems to have been an authority on the treatment of hoarseness. Valesco cited "the pills that Bernard de Gordon presents," and he turned a "medicament of Gordon" into his own by specifying a dosage: "to this medicine I add four drams of tailed pepper."

Valesco was the compiler who, among physicians, provided the greatest amount of information on the swelling in the neck that was called *bocium gule*. This affliction was classified among the apostemes due to phlegm, in juxtaposition with scrofula. It also tended to be left to the attention and care of surgeons, which was the case for scrofula as we have seen in chapter 3. In any event, and with due caution about a retrospective diagnosis, the medical manuals leave little doubt that the condition came close to the swelling of the thyroid gland, now known as goiter, which is due to iodine deficiency and which is often associated with regions distant from a seacoast. Bernard, for one, linked the condition to geography.

> Some diseases are regional, such as consumption in mountains and diarrhea in valleys; in some regions there are trees with fruits which, when eaten, produce *bocium gule* by their inherent nature, and in others the water by its nature produces obstruction of the liver and a foul [skin] color.

Earlier, without reference to diet but with sharper geographical focus, Gilbert noted, "*bocium* most frequently affects the gullet of inhabitants of mountains." Valesco combined the regional, dietary, and genetic aspects when he presented the condition as prevalent in an area of the Pyrenees with which he was intimately familiar. He reported that *bocium* was "a disease proper to certain regions such as Saurat in the County of Foix, and this is on account of the diet or of the cold water which they drink. In addition, sometimes it is a hereditary disease and it is passed on."

The actual presence of the affliction is reflected in Gilbert's remark, "certain old wives know how to remove [the swelling] with the appropriate herbs. We, however, should seek to remove them this way," that is, with an *experimentum*, a treatment with empirical concoctions. He admitted, "if these do not help, we must have recourse to surgery." He seemed to consider radical resection possible albeit very difficult, and to accept cautery as a feasible alternative. Another author, totally averse to any surgery, warned in his *Summa medicine* (attributed to Arnau de Vilanova), "you should fear to incise or to cauterize a *bocium colli;* external and internal *bocia* may be attenuated with the use of mineral waters, especially those that have a tartaric (*tartarei*) or sharp taste." Valesco took an intermediate position. While he deferred to surgeons as most qualified to treat *bocia,* he prescribed several ointments and plasters, and he referred to his chapter on scrofula for more remedies. He vouched for their effectiveness by calling on his experience, "we have cured *bocia* by resolving them this way, and we have received honor and gained profit from it. However, praise be to God. Amen."

The Chest

Many compendia contained a section that, even if it was titled "On Respiration," covered the entire chest and ranged from asthma to *zona* (shingles). The section focused, nevertheless, on the *spiritus* and the spiritual instruments as shielded by the thorax—from the Greek word for the hoplite's breast and back armor. Notions of the fortified chest paralleled the metaphors of the cranium shell protecting the instruments of animation and of the pelvis basin holding the instruments of nutrition and procreation. The ribs and muscles that encased the strongbox received relatively little attention, in contrast with the breasts, which decorated the exterior and which, in the framework of Aristotelian and Galenic teleology, were a hallmark of humanity. The concentration on the lungs and respiration, on the other hand, was disproportionate if viewed (anachronistically) from a vantage point after William Harvey. The heart, though ranked as the most or second most noble organ, had a considerably lower profile than the lungs or even the breasts. This disparity reflected the faulty understanding of the function of the heart but, even more, perceptions and actual health conditions. Even if cardiac disease was more widespread than diagnoses could have determined, it was less omnipresent than pneumonia, tuberculosis, and other respiratory ailments. Fatal heart attacks, while recognized and feared, were eclipsed by the everyday threats of throat infections, prolonged coughing, and all sorts of breathing difficulties—not to mention intestinal illnesses, pestilential fevers, and multiform trauma.

The Lung(s) and Respiration

Compilers discussed lung diseases and respiratory disorders at length. Yet on the whole, they covered these issues less thoroughly than other ailments of the body and with a marked tendency to gloss over anatomy and physiology. They were largely silent on the detailed descriptions by Aristotle, Galen, and Avicenna, with which they were no doubt familiar, at least in the convenient summary by Constantine. It is particularly remarkable that Gilbert, who normally introduced each body part by explaining its structure and function, skipped the explanation of respiration. Valesco similarly abandoned his habit of heading each discussion with a clearly marked section on the anatomy of the eye, throat, stomach, and other organs. The scant coverage in the manuals may be explained by the dominance of humoral and teleological constructs and, in this instance, by the concern with internal diseases for which anatomical knowledge seemed of little therapeutic interest. Even when Savonarola represented one of the few exceptions to the pattern by covering pulmonary anatomy, he pointed out that the composition of the lung was "simple with regard to the understanding of the physicians." He further gave the impression that the information had limited practical relevance, by concluding, "from this, you know in practice where sanies or blood of the chest is brought to the outside, for any kind of material collected in the chest is forced to the lung by the strength of the expulsive faculty and then expelled by coughing."

The basics of lung anatomy and physiology remained consistently simple from Constantine to Savonarola. A salient point is that, even after dissection became part of the medical curriculum from the 14th century on, the lung (*pulmo*) was envisioned as a single organ. Antonio Guaineri even stated that the mediastinum "divides *the lung.*" The compilers' rudimentary sense of anatomy may be gauged from their conception of three pulmonary membranes, namely, the mediastinum, the diaphragm, and the pleura. The pleura (from Greek for "side") "covers the ribs, according to Mundinus." While Savonarola cited the pioneering anatomist Mondino de' Luzzi (Bologna, ca. 1270–1326), neither he nor any other compiler mentioned the actual lung cover, that is, the inner layer of the pleura. The lung itself, lobed as it were into two or more panels, "enfolds the heart"

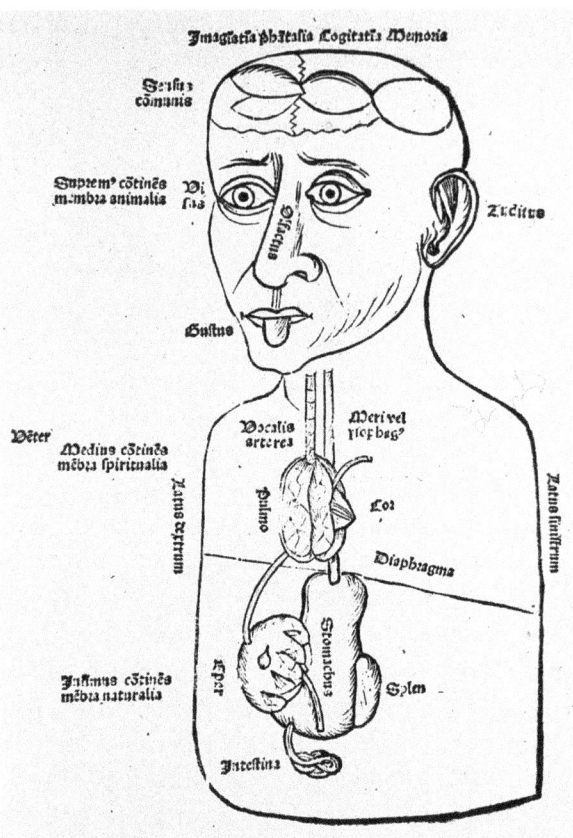

Anatomy of the head, thorax, and torso, including the *membra spiritualia* (left margin), and showing one lung (*pulmo*) wrapped around the heart (*cor*). Woodcut diagram in Johannes Peyligk, *Compendium philosophiae naturalis* (*Compendium of Natural Philosophy*), Leipzig, 1499, sig Q1v. (National Library of Medicine, Images from the History of Medicine # A013188)

in order to keep the source of natural warmth both from overheating and from choking on fumes, the by-product of generating warmth.

The vital task of the lung, in conjunction with the chest muscles and with the attractive and expulsive faculties, was to dilate for drawing in cool air and to contract for drawing off the heated air and the noxious fumes. The trachea, a two-way conduit, was known to bifurcate and then to ramify until, in Savonarola's description, "the branches are small, called 'hairlike' (*capillares*); these are interwoven as in a net, and so they constitute the substance of the lung." The exchange of air is made possible by the soft and airy tissue that resembles a sponge or, for Constantine, "coagulated foam." From the capillaries, air enters into porosities or interstices where it is tempered so that it will not be too cold for the heart. This cool air enters the left heart ventricle through the venal artery (the pulmonary vein), which also brings the warmed air and waste fumes to the lung. From the right ventricle of the heart arises the arterial vein (the pulmonary artery) through which blood nourishes the lung.

Pneumonia and Pleurisy

The two labels that head this section for the sake of simplicity are not synonymous with the parallel terms in the compendia, for the distance between modern and medieval terminologies was greater in this area than in many others. *Peripneumonia* or *peripleumonia* was a rather open term for an infection of the lung, a category that occasionally overlapped with *pleuresis* in spite of formal distinctions. Overlaps and confusion were due to imperfect anatomical understanding, to interactions and apparent similarities between infections, and even to continued difficulties in forging a Latin medical vocabulary. In *peripneumonia,* for example, the prefix *peri* meant "around," as Johannes Platearius pointed out, so that the category could include *pleuresis,* as an infection surrounding the lung. Gilbert actually argued, "both apostemes differ little in causes, signs, and treatment," yet he also described differential diagnoses of an "ulcer *in* the lung." Bernard evinced a similar ambiguity between equating and differentiating both diseases: "the treatment of *peripleumonia* is almost the same as that for *pleuresis,* except that in *peripleumonia* we need to administer stronger medicines."

Bernard subscribed to the traditional view that *pleuresis* could evolve into *peripleumonia,* which then took one of two courses, "either killing within seven days or changing into consumption." Gariopontus taught that *peripneumonia* was the more acute and dangerous of both diseases and that it "kills swiftly because, once the lung is compromised, it is unable to be healed with the incessant motion of the air inside." Notwithstanding this alarming assessment, compilers devoted less space to *peripleumonia* than to *pleuresis*—which, paradoxically, may come closer to the pneumonia of modern nosology. *Pleuresis* generated the most intense debate on definitions, diagnosis, causes, and cures. The category was divided into a true kind, which affected the pleura, and a not true kind that affected the two other membranes. There was much discussion about adding more divisions, which made Savonarola scoff, "some take pleasure in the multiplication of names, which should embarrass the physician."

A sense of urgency may have contributed to Savonarola's impatience. He wanted his reader to

> know that in our city of Padua, and in Treviso and Venice, sometime around March in the year 1440, there appeared a bad *pleuresis* which was contagious and which killed very many; yet, I have not found it written by our authors that it is contagious, and several people believed that this one had been poisonous.

While giving no clues that would allow speculation about the nature of this respiratory epidemic (pneumonic plague?), he explained that it was due to a "virulent" (*furiosa*) cause and it occurred "in the beginning of a spring that had been preceded by a very cold winter." The mysterious disease may have struck the region earlier. Guaineri of Pavia, who died in 1440, defined *pleuresis* as "a disease that attacked us in conjunction with evil dispositions of the times." In fact, contemporary circumstances may have induced him to address *pleuresis* at length in a 21-chapter *tractatulus* that may have existed by itself before becoming incorporated into his *Practica*.

Medical authors were aware that it was easy to misinterpret symptoms and signs and that it was often necessary to rely on guessing. For assessing a particular case of *pleuresis,* Bernard realized, "the physician needs to know, at least by some conjecture close to the truth, how much distance there is between the onset and *status*." He found it necessary to add "a sawlike" (*serrinus*) pulse (that is, with beats alternating between strong and weak) as a fifth differential symptom to the four that Galen identified. The four distinctive symptoms of *pleuresis* were a constant fever, breathing difficulty, cough, and sharp pain in the side. These signs, Guaineri emphasized, "are inseparable, as all the ancients confirm." An accurate diagnosis was crucial not only for immediate treatment, but also for foreseeing whether the disease would change into a more lethal one. Diagnosis closely dovetailed with prognostication because, as Guaineri proposed, "this disease most commonly runs by critical days. The moribund patient often dies on those days, so that you will compute them carefully if you wish to gain honor."

The recognition of prognostic signs was more complex than the evaluation of symptoms, and it had greater consequences for the attending physician. Guaineri blamed fellow practitioners for basing their prognostication on one single method, as I saw in the case of a squire of the duke of Savoy who was suffering from *pleuresis*. When I was called to him on the seventh day, his urine looked normal. This led some Jews in charge of his care to assure that he would recover. When I returned to the patient I found him having great difficulty breathing, high fever, and little expectoration, with the sputum somewhat livid.

Presenting himself as an example of correct protocol, with a touch of condescension that reminds us of Galen, Guaineri showed his presumably inexperienced reader how to prognosticate properly.

Relying on all these signs rather than on the good quality of the urine, I judged that he would die. On the eleventh day, when the Jews had visited him they said that he was resting and sleeping. I found him departed to another world, however, while they were still standing there with his "good" urine.

The ability to foresee a fatal outcome had an immediate practical benefit, according to Bernard. If aggravation instead of relief followed the physician's faultless care and the patient's medication, "it is a very bad and mortal sign, and in such cases we should not persist."

The advice to cease treatment was ambiguous. It left the practitioner between the classical admonition, to flee when death was at the door, and the ethical command, to continue palliative care. Furthermore, Bernard's sober resignation toward the terminal stage of *pleuresis* stands in contrast with his intense interest in correctly medicating the initial phase. On the whole, "drugs should be used sparingly, in order not to diminish the [patient's] strength (*virtus*), because this is what cures diseases." Therefore, "no strong medicine should be given in *pleuresis,* whatever the ancients say, and some moderns boast of holding this doctrine. Without need for discussion, it does not seem reasonable." On the other hand, Bernard rejected two moderate and inferentially contemporary practices. Against some who "try to cure *pleuresis* with 'attracting' medicines, by cupping and mustard plasters," he argued, "I disagree, both because the [offending] matter is not easily drawn from that location, and because there is fear that the forceful drawing may make the aposteme increase." He expressed reservation toward others who "spend much effort on mitigating symptoms such as derangement, insomnia, thirst, constipation, diarrhea, and the like: I would agree with them, were it not that such bad symptoms do not occur if the disease is curable and the patient is well managed from the start."

Bernard's most insistent and rationalized position regarded the administration of *repercussiva,* substances that beat back the offending matter. He rejected the use of these medicines in principle, "because they are administered either internally, in which case they cause thickening and more putrefaction, or externally, in which case *repercussio* is prevented by the slanting of the veins and the density of the ribs." He seemed prepared for a partial concession that, "if they were to be of some value, as Heben Mesue held, this would be at the very beginning." This might be possible "if one were right there and received from God the great favor of knowing the onset and of carrying repercussive medicines in his bag." However, "it is not clear how such things could coincide, so that I greatly wonder why good Heben Mesue was dozing." Savonarola chided Bernard for "ridiculing Mesue," but he accepted the premise, because "patients do not seek the physicians' counsel or help at the very beginning" of their illness. Guaineri defended "our very holy Johannes Mesue," as referring to the first phase of *pleuresis,* which could last four days, rather than to the very first moment, which is "a fleeting thing, far removed from the physicians' ken." Therefore, in addition to misinterpreting the words of Mesue, "good father Bernard de Gordon bites him too sharply."

Guaineri's interest in such debates was limited, however. He concluded his defense of Mesue against Bernard by remarking, "let us move to the common act of practice, and leave these good men and most outstanding practitioners in paradise, where all their quarrels have come to rest." His preoccupation with practice extended into surprisingly mundane details of patient care. To a delicate damsel who was unable to take any of the normal medicines, he offered a special potion, "which she took with pleasure and which worked wonderfully." He frequently and proudly replaced recorded prescriptions with some "confection, which I usually make, and which is very pleasing to the taste." One of his dietary recipes for *pleuresis* was more reminiscent of cuisine than of the clinic.

> I have a properly cooked chicken deboned and then wrapped in a white cloth, placed between two trenchers, and pressed: from this flows a juice that is clear as water, easily digestible, greatly nutritious, with few superfluities, and delicious to the taste.

Casual remarks also illustrated Guaineri's appreciation of comfort. He reported that "the ancients order to roll patients from side to side" for dislodging pleuritic matter, but that it is better to rock them in hanging beds, which "we Italians call hammocks."

Asthma

Unlike *pleuresis,* which was consistently assigned to a specific place and agent, asthma was, and largely remained, an open-ended concept. The original term was vaguely suggestive of wheezing but generally synonymous with shortness of breath and, we should note at the outset, often paired with cough. The compendia are ideal signposts for following the early vagaries of asthma as a disease category, with chapters that attest to successive—though not linear—attempts to move toward a more definite meaning. One of the early Latin manuals, the *Passionarius,* adumbrated the attempts by shifting from synonymy to juxtaposition. Gariopontus stated, "a most burdensome problem of the lungs afflicts asthmatics *and* those who have a hard time breathing (*asmaticis et suspiriosis*)." He followed Galenic physiology in attributing the problem to "thick and cold phlegm stuck in the cavity or opening of the lung"; he applied basic Hippocratic holism to the inference that, therefore, asthma occurred mainly in winter and in old age. He observed that it affected "those who work with metals," or resulted from "dust, a bad odor, plaster, and the like." This intriguing allusion, which recurred in many texts, draws our attention to the fact that compilers did not perceive what modern medicine has come to recognize as allergy. Occasionally, when mentioning adverse reactions to aromatic substances, they hinted at rose fever—a forerunner of hay fever—and other forms of hypersensitivity disorder. Bernard, for example, prescribed a syrup for the constriction that might be caused by the roses in rose sugar, a favorite remedy for consumption. For Gaddesden, roses were among the aromatics that caused headaches and rheum. Valesco made equally intriguing references to various triggers. He mentioned "the air of pits in which crops are kept" as a cause of asthma; further, foods could harm the respiratory organs, "as is evident in people who frequently eat chestnuts." These and other observations, however, were scattered like straws in the wind, and they did not lead compilers beyond general associations between breathing difficulty and various factors in the air.

Copho presented asthma as a generic equivalent of breathing difficulty. He tried to provide clarity by presenting four distinct kinds, "namely panting, dyspnea, bloodsucker, and orthopnea." Johannes Platearius, on the other hand, simply stated, "asthma is the same thing as dyspnea" (which is now the term for shortness of breath). He then specified three kinds of asthma, "according to the different location of the excess moisture." If the lung was pressed from outside and thus unable to expand for inhalation, the condition was "called 'bloodsucking', in analogy with the action of a leech, because the patient labors in drawing air just as the leech does in drawing blood." If moisture filled the pulmonary tubes and did not allow the lung to contract, the patient labored in exhaling and suffered from heavy breathing or panting. The third form, Platearius proposed, was "called 'orthopnea', that is, 'straight' dyspnea because the patient suffers equally in inhaling and exhaling." The threefold classification proved so fluid that it was possible for the author of the *Salernitan Regimen of Health* to invert the definitions and to identify panting as labored inhalation and, more strangely, bloodsucking as difficult exhalation.

In the course of the 13th century, the need to integrate Avicenna's definitions compounded the confusion in the taxonomy of breathing problems. Gilbert stated broadly that these problems resulted "from every defect that can afflict the chest." He noted that some author switched the terms and that "other kinds of breathing difficulty are better known for the dangers that they entail, so that they are included in other diseases." In the end, definitions and distinctions mattered little for Gilbert because, "the treatment of asthma does not differ from the treatment of cough." Bernard, however, aimed for greater precision in defining, differentiating, and explaining various forms. While accepting a substantial overlap between asthma and dyspnea, he distinguished them, respectively, as noisy and noiseless. Valesco expanded on Bernard, as he did so often. He described the breathing of asthmatic patients "as if they had puppies or little birds in their throats." The sound, he explained, was due to a constricted trachea near the lung, "for it becomes sharper when the opening of the organ is narrower, as is evident in effeminate men and children, and in artificial song instruments."

The awareness of instrumentality in considering asthma held greater potential for anatomical inquiry than many other diseases. This awareness was eclipsed, however, by a preoccupation with definitions, categories, and analogies. Bertruccio demonstrated this preoccupation, as well as the ambivalence of terminological precision, when he proposed that breathing difficulty

> is called "asthma" when it affects inhalation, soundlessly and with little coughing; 'oregmon' when there is much sound at inhalation; "orthopnea" when it affects both inhalation and exhalation and is accompanied by sound. You should know, though, that the physician does not care about this difference in names when there is little difference in reality.

Bernard, who was fond of repeating the Galenic dictum, "there is no need to argue about names," nevertheless preferred to pursue nominal distinctions rather than functional differences. Not settling for the standard forms, he expanded the taxonomy by specifying that asthma and dyspnea shared *five* kinds between them. To the three categories of *sansugium, hanelitus,* and *orthopnea,* he added a fourth, "doubled panting, as by someone smitten by love, or by crying children who, while continuing to pant, also draw draft after draft." A fifth kind was "like the panting of someone being strangled." In all five kinds, cold and humidity constituted the root cause, and the airways were directly involved. External factors now included "the air of caves and mines and metal smelters, the ingestion of poison, and working with quicksilver"; internal causes ranged from rheum to "anything that can exert pressure on the diaphragm," but there was no correlation with such mechanics as constriction.

Bernard tried to provide physiological perspective, by contrasting involuntary and voluntary interruptions of respiration, in his *clarificatio.*

> It should be understood that breath is retained at will or by coercion. If by coercion, the immediate result is death, on account of the lack [for the heart] both of refrigeration and of ventilation expelling excess fumes, so that a human dies quickly like those who are strangled.

Holding one's breath at will, on the contrary, was possible for quite a while, "because natural evaporation continues even though it is not perceptible." Expanding this idea, Valesco contrasted the continued evaporation in voluntary retention of breath with strangulation, in which fatal fumes accumulated on account of the victim's "distress, effort, and struggling." It is worth noting that both Bernard's and Valesco's explanations diverged from Constantine's teaching, which they were elaborating, about the ability of "any animal to hold its breath in a hot spot, deep under water, or in a smelly place." Observation brought Constantine to a different conclusion about an autonomous halt in breathing: instead of positing that evaporation continued, he believed that "the heart flees toward the lung in order to cool itself a little, and thus an animal is able to survive in such places as long as there is air in the cell of the lung."

Long-term survival was considered unlikely for asthma, with the exception that children sometimes outgrew it, "cured by the change of age," as Guglielmo da Brescia (Brixiensis, Corvi, or Aggregator, 1250–1326) reported in his *Manual of Practice for Every Disease from Head to Foot.*

Brescia condensed Avicenna's teaching—that asthma combined a prolonged course with sharp paroxysms—into the axiom, "this disease may be called both chronic and acute." In view of the mortal danger, the dire prognosis, and apparent incurability, Bernard admonished, "the physician should beware of vain promises." At least, "we should proceed very diligently" with treatment that, in any event, was mostly palliative. Valesco suggested that palliation could be mundanely simple when he advised, "it would not be without benefit for asthmatic patients if they are able to sing or raise their voice from low to loud, whether in church chant or in cantilenas: their chest and lung would be stimulated and it would promote the expulsion of their superfluities." At the same time, Valesco like most compilers recorded dozens of prescriptions, with a preference for domestic remedies. In order to promote the patient's expulsive power, for instance, "I strengthen nature by giving some chicken broth with three egg yolks and a little ginger." He even overruled the sovereign authority of Avicenna, who "orders to administer narcotics, whereas I prefer to apply a relaxing compound of chamomile and sweet clover." The diversity and the number of these remedies may give the impression that they were specifically for asthma, while most of them actually duplicated those prescribed for cough. Valesco confirmed this reality, as Gilbert had earlier, by declaring, "I say briefly that, when it comes to treatment, asthma and cough are very similar." Bernard was perhaps the most explicit in teaching, "hoarseness, cough, and asthma are three diseases that are treated with almost identical medications; hence, the discerning physician will check in the chapters on hoarseness, then on asthma, and then on cough."

Cough

Johannes Platearius, who placed cough together with asthma in the same chapter, defined *tussis* as "an obstruction of the air in the trachea, which occurs sometimes from a disease and sometimes in conjunction with a disease (*per compassionem*)." In the latter case, it was a *sinthoma* that accompanied another disease, including "a stomach problem or a liver tumor, as in patients with dropsy." Definitions of cough identified a dual essence. It was, most simply, a movement of the respiratory organs for the purpose of expelling harmful superfluities. On a deeper level, cough was a joint action of the psychic (animal) faculties of sensory reception and motor command with the vegetative (natural) faculty of expulsion (the latter is broadly analogous to the autonomic nervous system of modern science). The authors faced various difficulties, however, in trying to understand the mechanism, capture the significance, and cover the range of the phenomenon. The combined action of the faculties provided a rudimentary rationalization of the involuntary movement, analogous to sneezing, but it did not explain the intricacies of a reflex. More important, while noting that expulsion consisted of alternating bronchial dilation and constriction, and that the chest and lung moved together, compilers said little or nothing about the role of the intercostal muscles and the diaphragm. In an indirect mention, suggestive more of clinical experience than of anatomical precision, Bernard remarked, "cough can follow a disease of the liver, by pressure on the diaphragm and consequently on the lung."

The most basic difficulty was to determine what coughing meant for medical theory and practice. The formal question, whether the act is within or against nature, generated exhaustive debate. Most versions of this *dubium* may seem utterly speculative and exemplifying scholastic dialectic, but they sprang not only from intellectual curiosity but also from concerns with etiology, diagnosis, and treatment. Conventional doctrine, buttressed by Galen's teleology, defined coughing as "a movement in accordance with nature." In the first place, this movement was not only purposeful, for the protection of respiration, but also a manifestation of natural vigor, in expelling harmful matter. Furthermore, it was orderly because it was governed by three faculties, in contrast with a spasm or other random movements. An additional definition differentiated between a natural and contra-natural cough. The movement was natural when it expelled only noxious elements and brought relief. It fell outside nature—and in the realm of disease—to the extent that it interfered with normal or natural functions, was triggered by unnatural causes, indicated a lesion or aposteme, or caused another illness. Valesco chose this differentiation for concluding the question, "whether involuntary cough is always a movement outside nature." He discussed the *questio* in detail and in typically academic fashion, proposing no fewer than five positive and five negative answers (*sic et non*). In one of his arguments, he recalled that "my master John de Tournemire" of Montpellier taught that one kind of cough results in "manifest relief" while another brings the patient nothing but "vexation and trouble."

The types, causes, and effects of coughing were bewildering in their variety, which corresponded to enormously diverse and often inconsistent therapeutics. Temporary episodes usually resulted from external factors, which ranged from dust and smoke to corrupt and pestilential air. These factors were relatively open to recognition and correction. They might even be identified "from the report of the patient and his companions," for example, "if he caught a cold" while fishing or while bathing in the stews, as Valesco pointed out. Chronic coughs, on the other hand, resulted from such internal causes as an unbalanced complexion or a localized infection, and they required complex treatment. The elaborate first stage consisted in the management of the seven nonnaturals, which began with providing clean air and an easy diet. Constitutional factors, including age and habit, called for a compatible regimen. Humoral imbalances required correction by contraries, so that "anger suits those who are cold, and fear those who are warm, while joy is commonly beneficial," according to Bernard.

The contrast between a warm and cold complexion had a counterpart in the distinction between a wet and a dry cough. The obvious criterion here was the production or absence of sputum, although both types left room for ambiguity in occasional allusions to a qualitative condition aside from the material factor. Be that as it may, Valesco warned that a nonproductive cough often belied the presence of offending matter in the lung, so that "young physicians mistakenly think that it comes from dryness, whereas Bernard de Gordon declares that dry cough has six causes." These causes were as varied as ulceration in the lung, a dry complexional imbalance, and fumes from an infected stomach or liver. A chronic dry cough, Bernard noted, was particularly exhausting for the elderly and for patients with dropsy, and worrisome in general "because it leads to consumption"—about which more later.

A wet cough could be due to the moist or phlegmatic complexion of an individual, location, or moment. A slightly more specific etiology added a material cause, namely, *rheuma*, which Bernard called "the mother of nearly all diseases." In this case, the flow, also called *catarrhus*, consisted primarily of phlegm that ran from the brain or throat into the pulmonary airways. The mucus could be too thick and viscous to exit or, on the contrary, so thin and watery "that nature is unable to catch it." While it might evaporate during the day, mucus accumulated in nocturnal cold and inactivity, so that "coughing is more persistent during the night" and likely to "deprive the patient and his / her neighbors of sleep." Reaching into cosmic etiology, Valesco asserted, "patients who cough from an abundance of phlegm are troubled more when the moon is in the sign of Cancer, especially at full moon, because this sign dominates the chest; sometimes those who are thus afflicted die at that time, as if they were suffocated." Abundant rheum might cause "a moist cough that is almost desperate and incurable," for which Bernard prescribed progressively aggressive purgatives, from a plaster on a shaved head to cautery on the forehead; "if it is not cured by these, let it be cured by all-knowing God."

For most running of phlegm from the head, compilers listed milder cures that fell within the range of age-old and universal remedies. Patients inhaled steam from boiling water in which licorice, chamomile, and similar soothing simples were steeped. They held in the mouth, as long as possible, all kinds of lozenges. Some of these were sweet, compounded from rose syrup; others, however, were tartly expectorant, with such ingredients as tragacanth, cubeb, and myrrh. "If the patient is too delicate," Bernard allowed, "myrrh may be replaced with figs and cleaned raisins." Savonarola elaborated, "we can leave out the myrrh, because people are too self-indulgent and delicate, and abhor bitter things." If these medicines proved insufficient, resistant phlegm was dissolved with the help of a digestive syrup and then drawn out by means of a purgative concoction of damascene prunes, tamarinds, and the like.

The proportion of exotic substances in the recipes, together with the attention for delicate patients, reflected the social level on which learned physicians spent most of their efforts. Nevertheless, the compilers did not ignore the larger part of society, in which coughing was no doubt pervasive. Their chapters on cough included, more frequently than most other chapters, special treatments for the poor. Bernard devoted two full paragraphs to "the cough of the poor." After offering a dozen prescriptions for cases in which "the coughing person (*tussiculosus*) is a pauper" from a cold cause, he still apologized, "if I have overlooked any, let the diligent and friendly reader add them." He began with "the first proven method (*experimentum*), which is to hold one's breath strongly and frequently, and [the patient] will be cured immediately." This remedy may make Bernard seem callous, until we find it mentioned by Savonarola with the addition, "this is from Avicenna." All three authors, in fact, were merely following Galen, as we learn in the *Philonium*. Valesco quoted, verbatim and at length, Galen's teaching that retained breath "not only prevents coughs from a bad cold complexion, but it is even medicinal because it increases and fortifies the warmth that is kept within the instruments of respiration." The initial impression of callousness on the part of Bernard and Savonarola might be reinforced by their recommendation that poor people suffering from cough take powdered sulfur in a soft-boiled egg. They offered this as an ultimate cure however, and Bernard admonished elsewhere that a recipe that contained sulfur "should not be administered to an emaciated or weakened patient except in great urgency and in near-despair." Moreover, sulfur was an ingredient in numerous recipes since antiquity; one of its particular properties was to counteract a cold and humid imbalance, which was a cause "from which, very frequently, the poor incur" a cough.

While showing a special affinity for poverty, cough was "a common and often lengthy illness." It became an urgent concern, for rich and poor, when it was accompanied by the expectoration of pus or blood. *Empima* and *hemoptysis* received separate chapters in many compendia. Coughing up pus signified infections in the chest or lung, of *pleuresis* and *peripneumonia* in particular, but it was also seen as a *cause* of consumption. Savonarola cautioned,

> it is common for patients to come after suffering, for forty days and more, from a cough with sanious discharge which they ascribe to the cold air, not knowing that they have empyema; they say that they wish to be cured of this cough. They have become consumptive, however, by a negligence and ignorance into which also some physicians tend to fall—I have seen several.

Therefore, he urged the young practitioner: "[A]pply yourself to finding the source, by asking when the patient first felt pain, and by considering whether at that time he / she felt stiffness, pricking, or warmth." In other words, careful attention to the patient's history might be crucial to avoid the slide from episodic discharges of pus to the merciless advance of consumption.

The differential diagnosis of empyema presented several challenges. Superficial similarities led to confusion with *ptisis,* with various consequences. Savonarola expressed alarm at finding that

> sometimes, physicians are deceived into thinking that a patient with empyema is consumptive, so that they consider his illness incurable. And then, when recovery follows the purging of purulent matter, they suffer embarrassment. Therefore, they should carefully consider the signs of consumption and empyema.

It was almost equally difficult to differentiate between the expectoration of pus and the less worrisome spitting of phlegm. A method, which was recommended for centuries, echoed diagnostic techniques beyond the spectrum of medicine. "You will find out," according to the *Pantegni,* "by dropping the sputum into a vessel filled with water and waiting for an hour: it is purulent matter if it sinks to the bottom, but phlegm if it floats." For a supplementary test, the *Philonium* added, "purulent matter reeks when thrown onto burning coals, whereas phlegm does not." Valesco underscored the importance of differentiating when he directly correlated diagnosis and treatment, in a personal reminiscence.

> A burgher in Montpellier, about sixty years old and of lean built, had much phlegmatic material flow to his chest cavity. Since it was white, as if it had been purulent, a judgment was made and some said that he was becoming consumptive. Masters Bernard Foresterii and Francis Connilli, both of happy memory, and with whom I was present, were called to his side. They said that he was not consumptive since he showed no sign of consumption.

Consequently, the masters simply prescribed distilled water with such herbs as fennel and parsley, "which he used, and he was completely healed." The treatment and outcome would have been far different if the patient had been consumptive.

Coughing up blood was the most consistently mentioned symptom of consumption, but it could result from an enormous variety of other causes. In identifying these causes, the compilers illuminated some noteworthy beliefs and practices. Expectorated blood could originate in almost any part of the head, chest, or abdomen; it might even result from the retention of menstrual and hemorrhoidal bleeding. External factors ranged from dietary excesses to screaming and to all kinds of trauma. Some suggested causes were more mysterious or even shocking. Bernard claimed that someone might spit blood after "sleeping on the ground in the moonlight, and especially when the rays enter through a narrow window and strike the head." Many authors, including Galen and Avicenna, mentioned a more nightmarish cause, namely, the swallowing of a leech. It is difficult to determine to what extent they were reporting a common occurrence or repeating a cliché. Compilers showed a degree of independence, however, for their citations of this report noticeably abridged and expanded the classic sources.

Most surprising, perhaps, is the apparent indifference of the compilers to the graphic—if seemingly incredible—precision of Galen's advice to the diagnosing practitioner (*De interioribus*, IV.8). Galen noted that, in cases of spitting blood without obvious cause, "it is necessary to make an extremely thorough examination (*superscrutari diligenter*)" of the nasopharynx. "A leech," he observed, might be stuck there and "grow day by day so that, if it was small and hidden at first, it becomes clearly visible after three or four days." Platearius explained that the victim might know this from "an itch in the uvula and palate," and the practitioner "from communication with the patient who admits to having drunk murky water from a pool or swamp." Bernard elaborated that the physician needed

> to be diligent in his inquiry. For example, you can ask the patient whether he has been used to drinking nothing but water, is a thirsty person, has been traveling overnight, and has been drinking from wells or river edges: if this is the case, it is safe enough to conjecture that he has ingested a leech; then you should examine his mouth in the sunlight and carefully check whether anything is stuck to his palate or throat.

The matter-of-fact responses, which may give the impression that the occurrence was not uncommon, extended to the casual details in remedies. Platearius, for instance, recommended that "the patient should repeatedly inhale the smoke of live sulfur and afterward drink vinegar with salt, and so the leech will be ejected upward or downward; note that it cannot live in the stomach or intestines because of too much boiling."

Prescribed treatments for hemoptysis from other causes, while greatly diverse, were often simple and optimistic. Platearius recommended that the patient be given, "with the food, a powder made of two parts hematite stone, a third of roses, and a fourth of cinnamon." The mineral form of iron oxide and often red, hematite, from the Greek word *haima* for "blood," was credited with the special power of restraining hemorrhage. An even more obvious remedy for hemoptysis, mentioned by Platearius and most other authors, was phlebotomy or *minutio,* that is, diminution of the presumably superfluous blood. One general hemostatic agent, however, was not to be used against the spitting of blood. Valesco admitted, "we do not include arsenic here, because we fear condemnation when we wish to administer it internally by mouth; we can apply it externally, though, because it dries and scarifies effectively." Encouraged by Galen's expressions of self-confidence, Valesco told his fellow practitioners not to despair about patients who coughed up blood from a lung infection, as long as it was recent, because "several have been cured completely." Even if the infection was chronic and incurable, patients "do not necessarily die, but they can live for a long time, especially when they have no fever. In my time, I have seen many like this, men as well as women." A direr prognosis loomed, as Bernard stated, "if fever accompanies the vomiting of blood, which is fatal: I have not seen anyone escape if the amount was considerable."

Consumption

Ever since the time of Hippocrates, authors viewed the triple combination of fever, cough, and hemoptysis as a hallmark of consumption. A notable exception would have been Gariopontus, if he actually stated, "consumption is a dangerous and very malignant disease of the lung, *without* any spitting of blood." This statement, however, seems to be an interpolation, and it was far more categorical than the declaration in a preceding chapter of the *Passionarius,* "we know consumption from fever with cough and with expectorations that are bloody, bluish, or purulent." Beyond the three standard characteristics, the *defining* criterion of consumption was, of course, the progressive wasting of the body. As a disease category, consumption may be considered the forerunner of tuberculosis, with due recognition of the significant differences in understanding and treatment and, in particular, of the paradigm shift with the introduction of bacteriology. In Latin medicine, *consumptio* remained a generic physiological term, while *phthisis,* the Greek word for decay, yielded *ptisis* as the label for the disease and *ptisicus* for the patient.

Ptisis was commonly defined, on the authority of Galen, as "an ulceration of the lung and a consumption of the entire body." Outside this core statement, and sometimes even within it, formulations and explanations varied from compendium to compendium. Johannes Platearius, for example, presented a slightly variant version, "*ptisis* is the consumption of the substantial moisture of the body, which results from an ulcer of the lung." The divergence, while almost imperceptible, was twofold, for it replaced the juxtaposition with an effect-and-cause link between consumption and ulcer and, more significant, it inserted the Galenic concept of the *humidum radicale*. Furthermore, this version led straight from the definition into an explanation.

> [*Ptisis*] sometimes comes from a catarrh from the head that strikes the lung and ulcerates it by hollowing it out, as the saying goes, "a drop hollows out the stone etc. [by falling not twice but many times]." Or it comes from dryness when the substance of the lung becomes arid and thus fragile, as may be seen in the vine tendril that, by the end of autumn, becomes so dry that it is easily broken by a light wind.

In this interpretation, which was both more concise and more lucid than most, Platearius drew on traditional wisdom, daily observation, and analogy as aids for explaining elusive phenomena. At the same time, he opened a window onto a panorama of uncertainty about the nature and causes of *ptisis*.

On the most elementary level, in a science constructed on definitions and semantics, the characterization of *ptisis* as an ulcer of the lung allowed for nosological confusion and, consequently, for misdirected treatment. It blurred the difference between *ptisis* and *peripneumonia,* which was virtually synonymous with *ulcer pulmonis.* Several authors avoided the ambiguity simply by applying the phrase, "an *ulceration* of the lung," thus identifying *ptisis* as a more extensive condition. Nevertheless, a clear distinction between the two diseases called for additional criteria—in a continued process that demonstrated the possibly fruitful role of confusion as a stimulus for inquiry. In their concern with placing the standard definition in a precise framework, the compilers kept adding explanations and differentiations by which, ironically, they often compounded the confusion. This risk was foreshadowed in the need to account for pulmonary ulceration in the first place, beyond analogies with a gouged stone and a dried tendril. Gariopontus and others proposed that the ulceration resulted "from dripping rheum, persistent drainage from the uvula, or catarrh that went bad and flowed into the lung." Even trauma joined the growing spectrum of causes of *ptisis,* for example, when Platearius claimed that "by jumping or shouting or the like, a vein in the lung bursts, blood rushes forth, and turns into pus."

A complementary challenge was to explain, in turn, how an ulcer of the lung could cause the breakdown and consumption of the entire body. Platearius argued, in a tightly constructed syllogism,

> the purpose of the lung is to draw in air from the outside by dilatation and to deliver it to the heart for the mitigation of the innate warmth; when the lung is ulcerated, it feels the lesion and refrains from moving, so that it does not dilate properly; hence, it does not provide sufficient air to the heart, which gradually overheats; hence, fever arises—specifically, that hectic fever which accompanies *ptisis* and which consumes the body's substantial moisture.

Gilbert greatly expanded the physiological account. First, he posited a double failure of the ulcerated lung, which "neither sufficiently draws the air for mitigating the innate warmth in the heart nor cleanses the heart of smoke or fumes generated in it." Then he specified that "overheating of the spirit" in the heart led to "a consumptive heat in the whole body, while it is possible that, at the same time, the strength of the heart is diminished.

The liver, too, fails in strength and neither digests the [radical] moisture nor delivers it to the body in due measure."

The *Lilium medicine* shows how the catalog of possible causes had grown by the early 14th century. First, to the possibility that *ptisis* resulted from "rheumatic matter running from the head," Bernard added the qualification that this flux might be "bloody or choleric, sharp and corrosive, or salty phlegm." Then he speculated that a second cause might be a bursting oral abscess; a third "the retention of menstrual and hemorrhoidal blood, with the corrupt vapor rising to the lung"; a fourth, a festering disease of the chest, "as in the case of *pleuresis, peripleumonia,* the spitting of blood, the accumulation of purulent matter, and the like." He ended with a sweeping fifth category that included

> excessive exterior warmth, cold that ruptures the veins, a fall or a strike, windy air, staying long in mine caves and next to furnaces in which metals are melted, working with quicksilver, and all such things that tighten and injure the chest and lung, as is also the case with autumnal air.

Gaddesden interwove two-sided etiology (in an odd echo of the chicken-and-egg conundrum) with imaginative etymology, for adding a sixth kind of cause: "*ptisis* takes its name from *tussis* [cough] because it is caused by cough, and also the other way around."

Causation was a criterion for some conceptual differentiations between *ptisis* and such more comprehensive categories as hemoptysis and, most notably, hectic fever. Gaddesden summed up conventional doctrine in the firm declaration, "every *ptisicus* is *ethicus* but not the other way around." The chronic overheating of the body in hectic fever could be due to other factors, aside from pulmonary ulceration and failure. The logic of this taxonomy was endorsed by Bernard, who argued, "the proper subject of [*ptisis*] is the lung, not the heart or the liver, for the purulent ulcer is the entire primary cause, and the body is consumed primarily by the hectic fever that follows the ulcer." There were, nevertheless, large grey areas between *ptisis* from pulmonary infection and consumption from other causes. Thus, nutritional deficiency or malfunction rather than respiratory disease seems to have been responsible for Valesco's observation that, "often, *ptisic* patients have swollen feet and extremities, and this is due to weakness of the digestive faculty, extinction of the natural warmth, and bad complexion in the liver."

The authors combined physiology, anatomy, logic, and semantics in forging more complex taxonomies. They even divided the meaning of *ptisis* itself into two interpretations. "In the strict sense," Bartholomeus taught, "it is an affliction of the lung; in the broad sense, it occurs in the elderly who are consumed by age." With greater precision and consideration of anatomy, Bernard proposed that *ptisis,* "in the proper sense, is due to an ulcer of the lung; in the broad sense, it may come from an ulcer in the trachea or the pulmonary canals or, even, in the linings of the chest." A more consequential distinction was between the ulceration of *ptisis,* as consuming "the substance of the lung," and *peripleumonia* as affecting the pulmonary membrane or, by extension, the chest. This differentiation had direct implications for practice because, as Valesco pointed out, "ulcers of the chest heal faster than ulcers of the lung."

The most urgent need to discriminate came at the bedside, in making the diagnosis and prognosis that determined treatment. The practitioner needed to interpret the signs that indicated the patient's predisposition, actual condition, and prospects. In true Hippocratic fashion, the compilers associated predisposition particularly with age, constitution, and season. They varied, however, in some interesting details. The most vulnerable age was in the years that were dominated by warmth and that ran from 18 to 25, according to the *Pantegni,* but from 18 to 35 according to compendia from the *Passionarius* to Savonarola's *Practica.* The *Pantegni* described the constitutionally predisposed as "thin, narrow of chest, having raised shoulder blades, and frequently affected by a warm catarrh." The *Lilium* included "a long neck and twisted legs" in the profile, with a bad diet and autumnal air as compounding factors. In the *Philonium,* Valesco with his characteristic touch depicted the predisposed "with raised shoulder blades, as if they had the wooden wings of a Saint Michael." As compilers continued to adopt and adapt signs of predisposition to *ptisis,* it is surprising that they largely ignored a trait that was mentioned in the *Pantegni* and which a modern reader may find most interesting, namely, that "this disease comes to patients from people around them, and from fathers and grandfathers."

A considerable number of signs were seen as indicating the actual presence of *ptisis.* The most decisive ones, as listed and explained in the *Pantegni,* were "continuous low fever, rising during the night and after meals, because this disease resembles lime, which becomes warmer when water is poured on it; sometimes there is excessive perspiration, lack of appetite, redness of the cheeks, and hollowness of the eyes." The latter was due "to the consumption of moisture," while a more puzzling symptom, "soft blisters on the heels," was attributed to "the removal of the natural warmth and 'spiritual' power from the foundations." Bernard, among others, added such notable diagnostic details as persistent cough and "pain in the left shoulder blade and the left breast." He even claimed that it was possible to differentiate *ptisis* from *peripleumonia* and to trace the source of hectic fever to a pulmonary ulcer by means of a strange *experimentum*, of which I have not been able to identify the origin: "if a thread is dipped in the water of dragon's blood [a bright red resin] and strapped around the chest, where it dries fastest, there is the focus (*minera*)." Earlier, Platearius also added several signs for making the diagnosis as precise as possible. He believed that "many err in their diagnosis by judging empyema patients as *ptisici* when they do not have *ptisis*," and he highlighted this allegedly common error with an anecdote.

> For verifying this matter, my father made this experiment: he made the patient breathe with open mouth. If he perceived that his/her breath smelled very bad whereas it did not before, as would be the case in some people, he judged the *ptisic* patient to be incurable. From the fetid breath he conjectured that the substance of the lung was corrupted. On the other hand, if the breath was not fetid, he did not despair about [the patient's] wellbeing.

The Platearius family demonstrated—admittedly to an exceptional degree—that, whatever the speculations and techniques, differential diagnosis was a thoroughly practical matter.

Prognostication was an equally pragmatic and often even more urgent concern. Not only the treatment of the patient but also the fate of practitioner depended on knowing where this chronic disease was headed. A prediction depended on the interpretation of signs that not only overlapped with the symptoms but also ranged more widely, from clinical manifestations to codified omens and cosmic factors. These signs indicated the further course, likely complications, and, most important, the outcome of the disease. The first year after the onset was decisive, although Platearius made an interesting distinction in age. Patients under 40, the disease either leaves or kills within a year; "the elderly, over forty, it does not kill as fast so that, with the benefit of medicine, they are able to live until the end destined for them by God." It was not always easy to recognize the moment at which the disease became confirmed, after about a year in most cases. Bernard claimed that, in judging the transition, countless practitioners were deceived when they examined the patient's sputum, for example, by not knowing whether a bad smell was due to *ptisis* or empyema. In the water test, moreover, when the sputum did not reveal telltale purulent matter by sinking to the bottom, it might be kept afloat by "viscous phlegm, and then the physician would be deceived unless he separated it with a stick."

Bernard urged, "we should be very careful in the prognostication of *ptisic* patients," and he added an avowedly folksy expression, "because they die talking." When a patient's color turned from abnormal redness to pallor, and his sputum became noticeably salty and smelly, "avoid him, because he is about to die," Gilbert warned. On the other hand, he assured that, "as long as none of these signs appear, there will be room for hope." Valesco proved more sanguine when he explained his remark that fetid sputum was "most often a fatal omen." He elaborated,

> I expressly say "most often," because I had a fifty-five-year old monk in my care who was completely *ptisic*. He had such bad breath that no one could stay at the table with him. And yet, by the grace of God, he was fully healed with the treatment described in the chapter on *ptisis,* to my greatest amazement. Praise God who heals those whom He wishes.

He recalled this personal experience, which obviously left a deep impression, not only in his chapter on bad breath but again, more vividly as we will see, in his section on the treatment of *ptisis.*

One of the most distressing symptoms was that, while living with the illness for a year, the monk coughed so violently that he seemed to eject part of his lung with the sputum—a sign that both the ulcer and the lung had hardened, according to authoritative tradition. Cough was an essential reason why a purulent ulcer of the lung was impervious to cure. Bernard placed it at the top of his list of no fewer than seven reasons. With most authors, he emphasized the baffling dilemma about forceful coughing as the only means for cleansing the ulcer: "if suppressed, it will lead to death by suffocation but, if not suppressed, it will enlarge the wound and burst a vein." *Ptisis* also defied cure because few medications addressed the humoral imbalance of this composite disease, and among these even fewer were able to reach the deep site. In his most perceptive explanation, Bernard speculated that the incurability of *ptisis* "could be due to physicians, among whom few know sufficiently how to differentiate; in addition, out of disgust for sputum, they do not want to apply their eye." Making matters worse, "patients do not wish to show themselves to the physician until the disease is confirmed, as long as it does not bother them too much."

Here again, as for other diseases in the compendia, avowals of incurability coexisted with a sense of continued obligation. Valesco memorably demonstrated this sense. Right after affirming that the pulmonary ulcer "is mostly incurable," he admonished, "nevertheless, since some are apparently cured, it does not seem right to abandon patients altogether as hopeless, for sometimes man begins a work and God continues and completes it." He gave the most poignant testimony of the coexistence of despair and determination when he recounted the case of the monk in his care, "who completely presented all the signs of *ptisis*, and whom I and many others judged close to dying. Because he was my friend, however, I placed him under treatment with diet and medicines, and by God's command he was cured." Even if authors credited complete recovery to divine intervention, they implied that there were various forms and degrees of successful treatment. Bernard pointed out that "it is possible to palliate *ptisis* for a long time in children, the elderly, and those who are stout." Compilers left little doubt that palliation was not limited to these groups and that it did not preclude the hope of curing. They expressed a sense of confidence when assuring that, at least "in the beginning, if the blood dominates or the body is plethoric, the *ptisic* patient should not be afraid to have phlebotomy." An equally aggressive method seems to have originated in Salerno. Gariopontus reported that, "in the newest treatment, patients are to be cauterized on the chest." Gilbert specified, "the newest advice is to apply cautery to the clavicles."

In general, therapies for *ptisis* were more conservative than for the diseases that we have encountered previously, and few resorted to heroic medicine by manual intervention or magical remedies. Basic and constant care consisted in the adjustment of the nonnaturals for reversing, slowing down, or minimizing the effects of pulmonary ulceration and bodily wasting. The regimen (which was tailored, by default, to the male patient) banned bathing and anything that would similarly drain his strength; depression and all emotions that disturbed his composure; and, above all, sex which depleted his entire substance. Valesco insisted on total abstention, "nay, if he has a wife or a female companion, he should be completely separated from her, for this act takes away the nourishment of the organs." In the realm of emotions, "let him avoid anger and sadness, and play some game in which he can neither incur a loss nor win a profit." For distraction, and for restoration of mind and body, Gariopontus recommended massages, especially of the neck and chest, in addition to gentle walks, pleasant scents, and good air.

In covering the six nonnaturals, compilers allotted considerable space to the patient's diet, as usual, but they gave uncommon prominence to good air and milk, two factors that have been central in the treatment of consumption from antiquity to the 20th century. They singled out certain foods as being both nutritious and medicinal: honey was the vehicle of all medicines for the respiratory organs; more surprising, crayfish were called blessed medicine, to be consumed in chowder or gargled in a broth. Dietary details, however, paled in comparison with the emphasis on the environment, in an exemplary combination of Hippocratic inspiration and common sense. Season, clime, and air were paramount concerns in the effort to manage chronic lung disease. Clean and dry air was not the normal environment of towns or most plains, so that "it should be sought by artifice," Bernard stated. He supported this statement with a citation and expanded it with an interesting thought. He referred to Galen, who "led his *ptisic* patients to a certain mountain near [*sic*] Sicily that has a continuous fire at the top," with an eye on "the dry air which goes out toward the middle of the mountain, both for the patient's sake and on account of the milk from those pastures." Bernard returned to reality by adding, "since we do not have such a mountain available, let us at least obtain anywhere what we can: we should choose the highest mountain and let them live there, and provide pastures and animals according to the particular possibilities."

Age-old mystique surrounded milk. Galen glorified milk as designed by Nature and given by God as the ideal food, drink, and medicine, all in one. It perfectly matched the particular ills of *ptisis:* its essence of cheese repaired the ulcer, its essence of serum purged the purulent matter, and its essence of butter restored what was lost to consumption. Summing up the continuity of tradition, Valesco prefaced his section on the treatment of *ptisis,* "let us begin with milk, as the Arabs did, Rases, Haly, and many others." It is important to note that milk was equally prominent in the treatment of hectic fever and that authors from Galen to Bernard underscored the logical connection by their cross-references. Whatever the treatment, a universal directive was that the milk should be drunk before it cooled off or spoiled, or should be boiled instantly. Platearius and others recommended placing "heated river pebbles or iron into it." Bernard refined the recommendation by suggesting, "we should boil it on a fire and add a little salt and honey"; he even added instructions for a bain-marie or double boiler: "it should be poured into a bowl that has been washed out with hot water and stands above another bowl which is filled with hot water."

In the conventional ranking since at least Galen, the milk of asses was considered better than that of goats, and the latter better than that of sheep or cows. The compilers showed no interest in Galen's claim that, to enforce his preference, he "brought a she-ass into the house in which the patient lay." For the rest, they adopted his general rating, which was based chiefly on the degree of thinness and digestibility. They suggested adapting the choice to the patient's taste or distaste, and they explained the ranking by the inherent properties of each kind. For nutritional value, Savonarola reasoned, one might choose cow milk; for purgative power, he preferred horse milk—apparently the only author to do so. For natural perfection and appropriateness, however, he echoed the consensus that nothing was better than human milk, which "should be taken from the breast, if possible." This recommendation was already of long standing by the time of Galen, who reported that "the ancients prescribe that *ptisics* suck a woman's breast, and I agree because they chose it as closest to human nature and they wanted it to be taken before it would be corrupted by the air." In another chapter, he specified that the ancients "enjoined patients to apply their lips to the woman's nipple and to suck or, if unable to bear this, to transfer the milk from the nipples to the stomach as fast as possible, while warm."

Galen's descriptiveness led more than one compiler to embroider in ways that are somewhat intriguing. One example will suffice. Valesco suggested, "in case that the patient is not squeamish and wishes to take the milk from the breast of a young and beautiful woman who produces good, thick, and white milk, this would no doubt be the most beneficial because it is natural to a human." The requirement, that the donor be young *and* beautiful, raises a host of questions, not only about esthetics but also about physiology. These questions gain poignancy in a collation with a vignette that Valesco inserted elsewhere. He recalled,

> it happened, in Paris, that the *ptisic* son of a certain burgher was healed by taking milk from the breast of a young girl; after taking the milk, he made her pregnant with a male fetus, and thereupon she took him as husband: praise God, the Most High!

Two medical caveats usually accompanied the recommendation of any kind of milk. One, which was also part of hoary lore, warned that milk and wine should never be taken together. The other, which drew on *Aphorism* 7.66, banned the giving of milk to patients with high fever, which it would inflame further as if it were poison, according to Johannes Platearius.

Against consumptive overheating and loss of moisture, Platearius offered "an electuary of my father," with licorice and sugar as the main ingredients. Most of the medicinal simples were parts or extracts of plants, from an extended spectrum that ran from the domestic birthwort and maidenhair to the more exotic cottonseed and hyssop. Knowledge of their properties was critical for medicinal treatment. The properties had to match the quality and extent of the ulceration, suit the particular patient and circumstance, and complement each other. Further knowledge was required, in addition to art and experience, for mixing the simples into syrups, potions, powders, pills, and lozenges. Mindful of this challenge, Bernard ended several lengthy paragraphs on compound medicines with the thought, "even though these would be sufficient for the experienced, let us continue in greater detail for the sake of the young." In a general conclusion to his chapter on *ptisis,* he mused,

> this is not a simple but a complex disease, so that we should not continue with one method of medicating but work alternately with cleansing, drying, softening, and nourishing agents, partly with this and then with that, sometimes more and sometimes less, and I leave this to your diligence.

The complicated accounts and treatments of *ptisis* typified not only the complexity but also the comprehensiveness of respiration as a subject in the compendia and in medieval medicine in general. In fact, the instruments and workings of the *spiritus* subsumed much of the vital role of the heart.

The Heart

The heart occupied a relatively limited portion of the Latin compendia. A systematic comparison with the coverage of other organs or functions would be worth pursuing beyond the confines of this survey, but a tentative tally reveals a significant disproportion. On average, the heart occupied less than one-fourth of the pages that were assigned to the chest. In the general subject matter, it received almost 10 times less space than the brain, 8 times less than the sensory organs, 10 times less than the stomach and abdomen, and about 5 times less than the reproductive organs. The limited visibility of the heart in the manuals—even if these represent only part of the spectrum of medieval medicine—points to one of the most striking contrasts between premodern and modern priorities. Moreover, a comparative glance at postmedieval manuals leaves the impression that, notwithstanding the fundamental impact of Harvey, changes in the valuation and care of heart health were limited until the rise of cardiology and the surgical breakthroughs of the past two centuries.

While designated chapters on the heart were markedly few in the average *practica*, they were either oddly placed or entirely omitted by several Salernitan compilers. Bartholomeus, for example, incorporated heart problems entirely into his chapters on fevers. Petrocellus inserted four brief chapters on pulse, cardiac illness, and heartache between a chapter on hoarseness and three on cough. Other Salernitan masters simply skipped the heart as a separate subject. Copho proceeded directly from asthma to hiccups and intestinal worms; Gariopontus switched from respiratory to digestive problems; and Johannes Platearius ended the section "on spiritual diseases" with hemoptysis and then immediately moved on to Book Four, "on the diseases of the stomach." The odd arrangements and the hiatus in Salernitan manuals resulted primarily from a preoccupation with therapeutics. The low profile of the heart in later compendia was due more to the structure of their content and the underlying conceptual framework, as various components of heart health were dispersed across the subject matter rather than assembled systematically into one dedicated section.

Compilers commonly summarized the essence of cardiac function in their chapters on fevers. "Properly speaking," Bernard taught, "fever is a disease of the heart that has become overheated and inflamed" and sends warm spirits through the blood to the entire body. Important aspects of the heart were also scattered across separate discussions, of the pulse, bloodletting, and so on. A recurring theme was the anatomical and etiological relationship between the heart and the stomach, which occasionally gave rise to confusion. Constantine collected a number of "accidents of the heart" that originated in the mouth of the stomach. When Bartholomeus reviewed *causon,* the burning fever raging especially in the chest, he devoted several paragraphs to "cardiac or diaphoretic disease," in which he appeared to equate excessive sweating and heart disease. Petrocellus attributed the equation to the Greeks, in contradiction to Galen's actual definition of *kardialgia* as "a biting pain in the orifice of the stomach"; later authors classified *cardiaca diaphoretica* as a stomach issue or, at least, as an extraneous variety of heart disease. Bernard described a particularly intense stomachache as "a difficult affliction, *as if it were* cardiac." Tradition bequeathes a more literal interpretation in the popular term, "heartburn." Petrocellus emphasized the distinction by drawing a clear anatomical picture. In a didactic tone that was appropriate for novice readers, he proposed, "you should understand cardiac patients (*cardiacos*) this way: their heart is ill, not their stomach, for the heart is one thing and the stomach another. The stomach is the mouth of the belly, but the heart is the origin of the veins, arteries, and pulse."

The rudimentary character of this clarification may suggest that Petrocellus was addressing a reader on the most elementary level, below that envisioned in the average manual. Nevertheless, it paralleled the limited extent of the compilers' investment in cardiac anatomy and physiology. Gilbert, Bernard, Gaddesden, and others omitted descriptions altogether. The few who provided some information treated it as secondary if not tangential to their concentration. Moreover, long after human autopsy became practiced more widely and dissection entered the medical curriculum, some continued to depend explicitly on written sources, comparative anatomy, and hearsay rather than on direct observation. The paradox was evident in Valesco's paragraph on the aposteme that the heart could suffer in a membrane, "as Galen says in the fifth book of his [work *On the Affected Places,* then known as] *De interioribus,* chapter one and two, in the column where he says, 'I had a certain monkey.'" After noting that Galen discovered tumors in the capsule of the heart, first in his monkey and then in a rooster, Valesco correlated Galen's findings with a recent human autopsy by adding, "Master Jean de Tournemire, my teacher, also reports the case of a certain count."

Even for the most obvious and commonplace descriptions, compilers—arguably in keeping with their role—tended to cite authoritative teaching by book and chapter or column. We have seen this tendency illustrated by Valesco, whose citations were the most frequent and precise. For example, "the heart has the shape of a pyramid," he declared, "as Galen says in the fifth book of *The Usefulness of the Parts of the Body,* in about the fourth column"; further, "the lung is nourished by the thin vaporous blood that comes from the right ventricle through the arterial vein, as Galen says in the sixth book of *The Usefulness,* at the end of the fifth column"; and so on. Savonarola cited his sources with similar precision, but he introduced more details about the shape, ventricles, texture, location, and other aspects of the heart as secondhand information. Demonstrating the prevalence of book learning over insights gained from dead bodies, he noted that the heart had a retentive capacity, "and therefore retained blood is found in it after death, as is stated in [Galen's] book *On Wasting* [*De tabe* or *De marasmo*]."

Savonarola attested to the second sense in which the knowledge of human anatomy was derivative, namely, by depending on animal dissection. He asserted that the three leaflets of the tricuspid valve "are difficult to see in dissection because once *the animal* is dead, the heart becomes so small that they are not easy to see." He further devalued the role of direct observation by reporting from hearsay, "it is said," that there are 11 *hostiola* in the heart—with the number of little orifices actually referring to the valvular leaflets. "These," he stated, "are barely apparent in humans, and I have added them for the sake of persons who struggle in vain in anatomies." His apparent disinterest in dissection was balanced by his dismissal of speculation. Thus, when positing that the heart is "of a fiery complexion," he added, "I do not believe Averroes who pronounced it warm and moist in complexion, but I leave this to the theoreticians." On balance, however, between hands-on experience and speculative dialectic, Savonarola offered a remarkably comprehensive and uncommonly methodical summation of teaching on the heart as it was available by the mid-15th century and "of interest to the physician."

While Savonarola and other compilers found the anatomical descriptions and complexional theories only tangentially applicable by the physician, they adopted traditional cardiac physiology as the foundation of all practice. The defining purpose of the cardiovascular system (to use an anachronism) was to generate, maintain, and temper the natural warmth that, in combination with the radical moisture, was the essence of life itself. The heart was commonly seen as "the source of warmth" and called "the principle of life." Savonarola compared it with "a king in the center of his realm." Inspired by Aristotle, Valesco likened the heart "to the sun which, standing in the middle of the planets, gives brightness to the fixed and wandering stars while, by means of light, beam, and influence, it instills (*influit*) in lower things the power to blossom, bear fruit, and reproduce." The heart similarly, "gives life to each member and to the entire body by influencing the arterial blood and the spirit." Valesco added perspective to the idea by inserting Ptolemy (as transmitted through an Arabic adaptation) into a citation of Galen.

> As it goes for the influence of the planets and of the movements of celestial bodies on the terrestrial, so it goes for the influence and movement of the heart on the other organs: according to Ptolemy, if the movement of heaven and the influence of the celestial bodies ceased, the terrestrial world would swiftly fail; in the same way, when the movement and influence of the heart cease, the other organs fail and die with it: this is what Galen says in *On Disease* [*De morbo et accidenti*], Book Five, Chapter One.

This comparison merits special attention because it exemplifies the traditional view of cardiac function as influencing rather than imparting motion or, more precisely, causing circulation.

The heart radiated warmth and instilled *spiritus* throughout the blood. Pulsation facilitated this task, but it had a more vital dual role. In unison with pulmonary movement—for it was, as it were, wrapped in the lung—pulsation drew in fresh air to prevent the overheating of the heart, and it vented the fumes produced by the three digestions (which were introduced in our first chapter). On the whole, this physiological construct was more qualitative than mechanical, although a quantitative or even an anatomical factor might emerge incidentally. In one of the more curious instances, based on an observation by Avicenna, Bernard mused,

> it is a wonder where dogs get their boldness and speed, for they are cold and dry animals, whereas boldness comes from heat, and heat is highly mobile. I say that they are bold because the ventricles of their heart are narrow and tight, which warms the blood and makes it boil, so that they become angry. Hares, on the contrary, have wide ventricles from which already limited warmth escapes easily and, with their cold complexion, they are very fearful.

For humans as well as for animals, cardiac physiology bore implications that extended from the surface of anatomy to the edge of emotions. It hinged on the construct of complexion, however, for health as well as for disease.

According to Savonarola, "as far as the physician is concerned, there are four complexional conditions that commonly affect the heart." He distinguished these conditions from trauma and aposteme, which he gave short shrift in the last lines of the chapter because they were beyond hope and ended almost always in death. The treatable affections were weakness of the heart, rapid pulse, tremor, and syncope. They were to be treated with largely identical medicines, because they were similarly rooted in humoral excess or complexional imbalance. Among the humors, blood and yellow bile were deemed the most likely agents. Yellow bile was linked to rapid pulse and, particularly, to syncope, because of its fiery nature but, almost as much, because of alleged experiential proof. Gilbert and others were convinced of the dangerous potential because "Galen *proved it* when his monkey suffered a fatal syncope: after she was cut open, yellow bile was found in the mouth of her stomach." Among complexions, an excessively cold or dry one was most directly opposed to life. Savonarola left it to "the theoreticians," however, to determine at what point the primary qualities lapsed from a normal, healthy condition.

The most decisive difference among the four affections lay in the extent of the imbalance: when it was moderate, it resulted in a weakening of the heart; when more extreme, it caused one of the three more critical problems. Two of these were mere variations of the same effect, namely, an increase in the speed and frequency of heart movement, which was constant in tremor and intermittent in rapid pulse. The fourth and worst problem was syncope, which occurred when the bad complexion

> has a stronger and more intense effect, so that it hinders and chokes the movement, burying the spirits inside or driving them together toward their origin. If it wins a final victory, extinguishing the spirits and the warmth of life, then comes death.

Applying the reduced taxonomy to a simplified discussion, Savonarola concluded, "once you have the treatment of tremor and syncope, you will have the whole treatment of heart weakness and rapid pulse. Hence, following the leader, I will forego dealing with the latter two."

Most compilers followed the leader (*ducem*), Avicenna, in their coverage of *egritudo cordis* or *cardiaca passio*. Literal translations of these section titles are misleading, because the phrases "heart disease" and "cardiac disease" suggest chronic conditions. The modern connotation was largely absent from the compendia, except for the consensus that "if [heart disease] lasts long, it means death." Varignana proposed that "the heart does not suffer lengthy diseases," although he implicitly allowed for a prolonged affliction by including sadness among the heart diseases. In any event, the two principal ones, tremor and syncope, were seen primarily as acute, even if the former was recurrent or relatively persistent and the latter more sudden and brief. Both were frequently lumped together, as differing only by the strength of the cause and by the intensity of the treatment. They also lay in a continuum of causation, as summed up by Bernard, "every bad complexion exceeds and weakens the virtue, a weak virtue leads to tremor, tremor to syncope, and syncope to death." Inversely, as Valesco declared, "death, unless caused by violence, does not occur without a preceding syncope"; Gilbert insisted that syncope "cannot occur without disease of the heart." Here and elsewhere, the phrase *passio cordis* referred to tremor while, in turn, *tremor cordis* often served as a comprehensive label for virtually all heart disease, and it was routinely juxtaposed with *cardiaca passio* as synonymous, notwithstanding the pervasive confusion with diaphoretic disease.

Aside from placing the root cause in a complexional imbalance, some compilers offered more complete explanations by attributing tremor and syncope to a drastic rise or drop in the innate warmth, a loss of vital spirits,

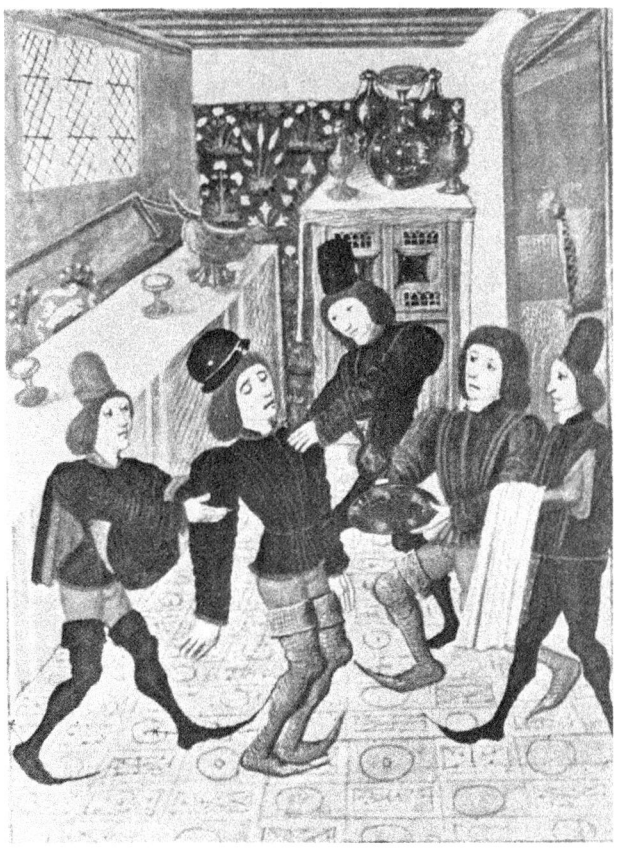

Syncope. Valesco's patient and patron, Gaston de Foix, dying of a heart attack. Miniature in a 15th-century manuscript of Froissart's *Chroniques*. (Wellcome Library, London. Wellcome Images L0009917)

or a suffocating condensation of fumes. These changes, in turn, could result from one or several more tangible or incidental factors inside or outside the body. Serious threats to the heart arose from disorders in other nearby organs, such as the stomach; connected, particularly the brain; or both, nearby and connected, as the lung. Even intestinal worms and, often related, utter malnutrition were held responsible. The most dreaded internal factors were extreme pain and sudden swings in the affections. Excited joy was the most dangerous, affecting the heart more immediately than sadness and more destructively than anger. Compilers highlighted the deadly potential of rejoicing but not, as might be expected, the stereotypical association between rage and cardiac arrest. Their emphasis was apparently due to authoritative tradition, for most of them quoted Galen's teaching that, in exultation, all the warmth escaped abruptly and the heart collapsed. Anger, on the contrary, as Bernard elaborated, did not force the heart to contract at once, even when it brought the blood to a boil.

The recognized external triggers of cardiac crisis were numerous and diverse, ranging from heat to cold, from exhaustion to overindulgence, and from poison to pestilence. In one of the most detailed inventories, Valesco brought together the causes that drew special attention from several compilers. He noted that, in the administration of bloodletting,

> syncope can occur in two ways: in one, the dissolution of the natural warmth follows the draining of too much blood; in another, fear forces the natural warmth and the spirit inward, so that the phlebotomized patient faints before two ounces of blood have come out.

Colic, wounds or ulcers, and torture were sources of pain that could trigger a heart attack. In "epidemics of anthrax and buboes," it often happened that "the painful site sends corrupt vapors to the heart." Illustrating his extensive etiology with personal memories, Valesco recalled a snowbound journey on which he saw people near death from the cold, and a visit to a grain cellar in which someone had "suffered a syncope and died suddenly."

The sudden and often deadly incidence of syncope diminished the relevance of prescriptions. In Bernard's prognostic litany,

> if someone has suffered heart tremor for a long time and a syncope occurs suddenly, business is finished. If someone suffers a prolonged syncope and the face becomes livid or dark, he will never walk on earth again. If syncope comes suddenly, has no evident cause, and lasts, it is over (*consummatum est* [words of the dying Christ]). If a sternutatory is administered to someone in syncope, as by injecting powder of white hellebore into the nose, and the patient does not sneeze, there is nothing further to advise but that the crucifix and thurible be brought in [for a funeral].

Bernard later clarified that, if a sternutatory had no effect in the seventh and final attempt to treat an ongoing syncope, "the physician should flee without taking leave of the host" an admonition with a classical pedigree.

Here again, Bernard and most compilers demonstrated a paradoxical combination of predicted abandonment and persistent care even though, on the whole, their prescriptions carried an undertone of helplessness. For tremor, for instance, they hesitantly admitted that cupping and bloodletting might be beneficial for relieving humoral pressure, but they also recognized the debilitating effect. Syncope was decisively distinguished from apoplexy, yet it received such similar treatments as forcefully rubbing the extremities and shouting the patient's name, which were no doubt contraindicated. Perhaps the most startling carryover from apoplexy was Bernard's prescription, copied by Valesco, to force open the mouth of the unconscious patient and to "rub the tongue and gums with theriac and musk potion (*potione muscata*)." Virtually every treatment of tremor and syncope included the use of aromatics. The smelling of "cold" camphor or "warm" cinnamon would promptly correct the critical excess in, respectively, complexional heat or cold. "For either imbalance," Bernard assured, "the following are valuable: pure gold leaf, pure silver leaf, pearls, corals, ivory shavings, bone of stag's heart, hyacinth, emerald," and a handful of other simples.

"For gold in phisik is a cordial, / Therefore he lovede gold in special," was the final stroke of the physician's portrait in the *Canterbury Tales*. Chaucer's gibe was far more informed than we might infer from the vague exegesis by some historians. Rather than merely echoing a widespread notion about a tonic that quickened the pulse, the verses alluded to a medical doctrine that was both specific and universal. A century earlier, Varignana declared, "all the authors assure that gold is beneficial in every heart condition." Since at least Avicenna, gold headed the list of "heart medicines (*medicamina cordialia*)," followed by silver, pearls, other precious substances, and more ordinary ingredients that included hyacinth and bugloss. These simples were closest to a perfect balance and therefore possessed special properties for cardiac conditions. It should be emphasized that, at least in this context, precious substances were not prescribed as a measure of the patient's status but, rather, in consideration of the vital urgency. The prescriptions lacked the alternative for a medicine "if the patient be poor," which other therapeutic sections offered. In reverse, Gilbert prescribed some syrups as an alternative remedy for tremor, "if the patient is of the nobility." Recourse to cordials was a measure both of the insufficiency of ordinary simples and of the nobility of the treated organ. These criteria make it unlikely that we will encounter gold in the *materia medica* for treatments below the belt, in the next chapter.

From Gullet to Gut:
Passiones Nutritivorum

> As disease of the stomach is my subject for this book, and as the stomach is cured of many afflictions by the induction of vomiting, it seems right that I begin by writing first about vomitives. I have seen many who fell ill immediately after taking great amounts of food and drink. If I had not promptly made them vomit, they would have fallen into a dangerous illness or fever, and they might have died; they were liberated instantly, however, by the induced vomiting. It is good for those with a stomach full of phlegmatic and viscous humors; for those with a fever from excessive fullness; and for those who suffer from heaviness of the body.

This is how one compendium moved directly from chapters "on afflictions of the lung" to a section or a "book on thirst, vomiting, and all the diseases of the stomach." The *Breviarium practice,* compiled around 1300, was spuriously attributed to Arnau de Vilanova, perhaps due to confusion with the name Reinaldus by which the author identified himself. After being drawn to the text by the attribution to the stellar Catalan master, one discovers that the *Breviarium* lacks both the sophistication of Arnau and the substance of such compilations as Bernard's *Lilium* or Valesco's *Philonium*. As a straightforward guide to *practica*, however, it enriches our survey and this chapter with a valuable glimpse into compendia that were less polished than the academic treatises but also more reasoned than mere lists of remedies. While it is idiosyncratic in organization and thrust, the *Breviarium* eminently demonstrates the challenge of maintaining a head-to-foot arrangement for the body in general, and of following any order below the diaphragm in particular. The compiler of this manual was less preoccupied with the formal organization of the subject matter than most of his contemporaries, so that he will let us see more plainly how difficult it was to deal with abdominal diseases in an orderly and comprehensive fashion. The contents of the abdomen, in contrast with the head and chest, were too chaotic and multifunctional to allow for a single target, a logical sequence, or even a simple descending order. Moreover, the subjective and (literally) lowly experience of abdominal functions eluded rationalization more persistently than it did for other regions of the body. Digestive problems, on the whole, were more ubiquitous, constant, *and* varied than breathing difficulties; stomachaches were more bothersome than headaches, and—to return to the introductory excerpt—vomiting was more disagreeable than coughing.

Vomiting may seem a strange topic for opening this chapter. However, it occupied a central place in the section on the "organs of nutrition." This prominence is a distinctive feature of many compendia. In general, it confirms a preoccupation with processes that eventually became viewed as symptomatic, dismissed as subjective, or ignored as marginal. Compilers devoted separate chapters to commonplace concerns that ranged from such mundanely casual issues as hiccups and flatulence, to such potentially serious conditions as thirst and loss of appetite. They presented several of these phenomena, moreover, at the same time as symptomatic, problematic, *and* therapeutic (as they presented coughing and sneezing in their section on the "Passiones Spirituales," surveyed in the preceding chapter). *Vomitus* played these multiple roles more constantly than any other phenomenon. It appeared in the diagnosis, prognostication, and treatment of nearly every digestive problem—and, beyond, of diseases from ephemeral fever to kidney stone. In addition, it received an impressive number of pages as a subject in its own right. Widely varying considerations of vomiting will document the compilers' treatment of the upper tract, and it will add perspective to their chapters on the lower tract. As a tangential benefit, some of the observations on *vomitus* or *emesis* will illuminate medieval attitudes, while others will suggest sensibilities that are not commonly associated with the Middle Ages.

From the Throat to the Stomach Entrance

Discussions of vomiting incorporated the fundamental notions of digestive anatomy and physiology. They spanned the digestive tract from the esophagus to the entrance of the stomach and into the base of the stomach. Furthermore, they covered processes from ingestion to retention and regurgitation, and they hinged on the basic impulses of appetite and rejection. Compilers largely ignored the pharyngeal phase of the digestive process, between the mouth and the esophagus. Some were even silent on the esophagus, including Gariopontus, Petrocellus, Gilbert, and Reinaldus or Reinald as may be seen in the excerpt that opens this chapter. Many lumped the esophagus together with the stomach entrance or introduced it almost in passing before hastening on to the problems of ingestion. The medical nomenclature itself may still have been in flux by the early 15th century, when Valesco found it necessary to spell out the terminological congruence. He declared, "the path from the gullet to the stomach was called esophagus (*oisophagos*) in Antiquity, stomach orifice (*os stomachi*) by those who came after Aristotle, and *meri* in Arabic." In an amusing instance of anachronism, most likely drawn from an encyclopedic source (as might result today from recourse to Wikipedia), he credited Galen with the information that *meri* is the Arabic term. His summary description, too, was drawn from an encyclopedia, in this case the 13th-century *Catholicon* of John of Genoa.

For more information about the anatomy and function of the esophagus, Valesco and the other compilers were satisfied with rudimentary descriptions and with references to Galen and Avicenna. Direct observation was a very distant source in their description of the esophagus as consisting of "tissue and two parts which are called 'tunics' by the anatomists"— these were authors *on* anatomy, rather than performers of dissection as one might infer. The inner tunic or layer contained longitudinal villi or muscle fibers, and the outer layer had latitudinal villi, which Gilbert called "transversory," Savonarola "transversal," and later anatomists "circular." In a rather simple scheme of esophageal peristalsis (as the mechanism became known *after* the Middle Ages), propelling swallowed matter downward was the task of the longitudinal muscles, expelling harmful substances the task of the latitudinal muscles. The role of faculties (*virtutes*) in these actions eclipsed the contribution of stimuli and reflexes. The vegetative or "natural" (*naturalis*) faculty of motion controlled deglutition or swallowing, in conjunction with the psychic or "souled" (*animalis*) faculty of sense that made the action at least partially voluntary. Emesis, on the contrary, was mostly an involuntary process, controlled by the autonomic natural or vegetative faculty. It was further defined not only as automatic but also, paradoxically, as unnatural. Valesco, for example, in a combination of everyday experience and learned rationalization, proposed, "swallowing is an easier movement because it is in accordance with nature, while expulsion is a more difficult movement because it is against nature." The dichotomy of his formulation epitomized a conundrum that placed vomiting at the center of the discourse on ingestion and to which we will return shortly.

When he concluded his summation of authoritative doctrine on the *meri,* Valesco admitted that much of it was "for teaching the young." Compilers focused more on the function and malfunction of swallowing than on the underlying ills of the instrument, for which they offered little more than generic treatment. The esophagus was vulnerable to internal obstruction, by a tumor or ulcer; to such nearby ailments or trauma as quinsy or rib fracture; and to a general bad complexion as in fever or old age. Even a potentially lethal injury might be of less interest than the symptom and the symptomatic cure, as would appear from Savonarola's recounting of a high-profile case.

> In my days, the lady Marchioness of Mantua suffered an excoriation of the esophagus and she was in so much pain that she was unable to swallow anything. As a result, she neither ate nor drank anything for six days or so. Her own and famous physicians applied many medications, but to no avail. Our Cermisone was called in, and he gave her tepid egg white to swallow, which she did without trouble. He continued this for six days, giving twenty egg whites and more a day. In the end she became able to swallow the yolks as well, and so she made progress and was liberated.

The mention of Antonio Cermisone (d.1441, Padua) was one of the rare instances in which Savonarola praised a contemporary. The anecdote itself was unusual by its insertion in the midst of constant references to Avicenna, and in a context where he claimed, "I am trying to be as brief as possible," and admitted, "I have gone over this material lightly" because most of it would be covered more fully in subsequent chapters.

No two compilers treated the subject matter in the same order, and these pages will follow an amalgamated sequence that aims for clarity and consistency. While the esophagus received uneven attention, a wide range of concerns with the digestive tract and processes converged on the entrance to the stomach. Authors conventionally identified the orifice or "mouth of the stomach" (*os stomachi*) as the seat of the appetitive faculty, and as highly innervated and sensitive. Nevertheless, they placed the source of appetite itself in the stomach, as responding to a feeling of emptiness. The response in hunger was an "appetite for the warm and dry"; in thirst, an "appetite for the cold and moist." Beyond these elementary notions, the topic of *appetitus* elicited elaborate contemplation, led into many directions, and overlapped with other aspects of health. The psychic as well as the vegetative faculty governed appetite, which therefore depended at least in part on free will. The voluntary aspect, by which appetite overlapped with desire, deepened moral implications that were already present in swallowing. The term for gullet, *gula,* also meant gluttony, craving, even greed. Gilbert, with his penchant for physiognomy, believed that "in a glutton (*guloso*) you see a big mouth." In their comments on the healthy management of hunger and thirst, physicians tended to moralize, to quote such familiar adages as "we eat to live and do not live to eat," and to invoke the authority of the philosophers Plato and Porphyry as well as of Galen.

According to the template that was applied to every human faculty, the appetite could be weakened, corrupted, or destroyed. Valesco, who proved particularly fascinated by questions about the concept of *appetitus,* listed no fewer than 15 causes for a weak appetite, from a bad complexion to a weakened sensitivity. Under the 12th one, he grouped the *accidencia anime* or emotions "and the sexual urge when it cannot be fulfilled, for once it is fulfilled it causes appetite, according to Galen." Medication could restore a failing appetite, if no fever was involved, as Valesco demonstrated with a dramatic episode from his own practice.

> I had in my care a knight who was wounded in the scrotum, and the sword had penetrated through the rear at the end of the thigh around the pudenda, with an incredible flow of blood and loss of appetite. For almost two days he remained without food and drink, and when he forcibly took some chicken broth at some point, he felt pain and sourness in his stomach. At last I arranged for him to take claret made with sugar and aromatic spices; he began to take some food and drink right away, and by the grace of God he was restored to his earlier health. This is because he had no fever.

Here, once again, a vignette with kaleidoscopic reflections enriched the *Philonium.*

Valesco's recall of this case with a happy outcome appeared in the midst of his references to Hippocratic and Galenic teaching, and thus it epitomizes the interweaving of personal thoughts with authoritative tradition that enlivened so many compendia. The event itself illustrates not only the horror of sword injuries, but also the possibility of escaping fatal infection, fever, and hemorrhage after suffering a massive wound. It also shows a physician continuing his care in a seemingly desperate case—without making a fuss about his perseverance. The story further proves that recovery was possible, even though the treatment may have had little to do with it. Perhaps most important, the account proves that Valesco did not merely repeat what he read in the sources but, rather, adjusted his treatment. Earlier, for failing appetite in general, he had cited Bernard's prescription of "a hen roasted in lard with cloves and sprinkled with rose water and muscat wine"; but in the anecdote he adapted the recipe, first to chicken broth and then, when his knightly patient could not even tolerate this, to a pleasing aperitif.

The appetite could fail perilously, but it might also be restored fortuitously. The outlook was least favorable when the faculty, corrupted in itself, deviated from the paths of nature and reason. Canine or voracious appetite was one form of such corruption, due to a spoiled humor, most often phlegm or black bile, which had become absorbed by the stomach orifice. Another possible cause was a bad cold complexion. The association between cold and hunger, an everyday experience, was reinforced by ethnic stereotypes. Savonarola and others observed, "inhabitants of colder regions have a more intense appetite, so that Germans, English, and others, eat more than Lombards." Cold might affect the orifice or the stomach directly, as in a case reported by Reinald. His master "treated a certain Genoese who suffered a canine appetite, due to a bad cold complexion of his stomach, and who had been in the care of many physicians." After these failed to cure him, the master

> made him dip bread in the lees of oil and, after he had eaten this bread, gave him thick sweet wine to drink. This way he had his taste brought under control, and he was cured of this illness in short time. I once saw someone who made a pound of cow fat to be melted together with a pound of oil, in the manner of an ointment; he ate all of it and became so disgusted that he went five days without eating, and thus he was cured.

The latter remedy, if allegedly effective, was unappetizing enough to suggest that there was no easy cure for canine appetite. The impression is reinforced by Savonarola's comment that "some, following Rhazes, apply cautery to the side opposite the stomach orifice; in my time a certain physician wanted to do this to a noble man, but all the experienced physicians disagreed with him, among them our Marsiglio of Padua" (Marsiglio de Santa Sophia, d. ca. 1405, not to be confused with the philosopher Marsilio de Padua, d. ca. 1342).

Platearius and several others equated canine appetite with the more worrisome affliction of *bolismus* (analogous to bulimia nervosa). Gilbert asserted, "canine appetite or *bolismus* is an ugly stomach ailment, in which one vomits in order to eat, and we read that Nero perished of this disease by the wrath of God." Most compilers, unlike Gilbert, treated *bolismus* as different from canine appetite. Savonarola offered a pointed definition of *bolismus*, as "a hunger in all the parts of the body while the appetite in the stomach is totally or almost totally removed." Petrocellus defined the condition as a failure of mind and body, in which even a large amount of food caused neither satisfaction nor weight gain, and which "occurs especially to travelers." Bernard singled out "those who travel across snowy places," and he added,

> this is why common folk say that the person has stepped on a certain herb that has the property of increasing the appetite. The truth, however, is that such people are exhausted in body, filled with nausea, and weak in stomach, so that the stomach begins to have appetite (*appetere*) when it becomes cold but, because of the general exhaustion, the appetite falls as soon as it arises.

The failing faculty "should be aroused by pricking the extremities, gentle whipping with small twigs, and aromatic scents," after which warm syrups and plasters should counteract the cold.

Savonarola urged the use of stronger methods because he was convinced that "canine appetite, if it lasts, leads to *bolismus, bolismus* to fainting hunger, and fainting hunger to death. Hence, be vigilant." Some authors blamed fainting hunger, *fames syncopalis,* on weakness of the stomach orifice, others on weakness of the stomach. The patient was "unable to tolerate fasting" without suffering "inanition," that is, utter depletion of vitality. After the syncope itself was overcome by forceful stimulation, the weakness was addressed simply with the use of meat broth and bread dipped in wine. When extreme hunger resulted in vertigo, short of syncope, Bernard prescribed a similarly mild remedy, "to take a mouthful of bread dipped in the juice of quince or astringent fruits." This prescription seems at odds with Gilbert's warning that "in no way, something acidic or astringent" should be given to patients with debilitating hunger; he considered it helpful, on the contrary, to give "greasy things if their will desires (*si voluntas appetit*) to eat these."

In a retrospective diagnosis of Nero's *bolismus,* Gilbert explained that the response to an excessive appetite combined voluntary and involuntary elements, psychic and vegetative faculties, and moral and natural implications. The role of volition vanished, however, when the appetite was perverted or destroyed. The perversion caused a craving for "coals, chalk, stones, soap, and the like," in the words of Platearius. The craving, which corresponds to what is now known as pica, was associated primarily with pregnancy. Reinald claimed, "I have seen numerous pregnant women who used to suffer from this disorder, in the first, second, and third month, on account of the menstrual blood that is not completely turned into nourishment." Savonarola added the conventional explanation that the excess menstrual blood "becomes spoiled and, coming to the stomach, corrupts it, causing this appetite." This *bolismus* was not limited to pregnant women, however. It also occurred in mental illness, specifically in mania and melancholy, and even in men who might seem healthy. "If it occurs in men," Valesco observed, "we obtain the signs from them if they are willing to say the truth, which is quite rare; nevertheless, they display signs because they all have a bad color." Summoning his own experience, he elaborated,

> in my day I have seen many men and women eating earth and ashes, and many of either gender eating sour things such as green figs and bitter things such as unripe apples and prunes. I saw one noble woman who kept eating millet secretly for fifteen years, and she became dark blue, that is, blue-green like someone with stomach and liver disease; until the end of her life, she was unwilling to reveal her illness.

The treatment of perverted appetite, especially in pregnant patients, included "light vomiting" according to Savonarola, with the caveat, "you should be careful not to incur blame, and it is safer to treat them with medicines that strengthen the stomach and dissolve the material, such as *diaconiton* [an electuary made with quinces] with spices, and the like."

The weakening and the perversion of appetite, while discussed in detail, were far less serious concerns than its loss and inversion in *fastidium*. Authors associated this strongly averse reaction to food and drink both with the nerve-rich stomach orifice and with the stomach. *Fastidium*, "which the Greeks call 'anorexia,'" according to Petrocellus, could accompany any disease. Authors showed an inkling of the psychological implications, even if their understanding of the disorder fell far short of modern insights into anorexia nervosa. Platearius advised,

> patients with *fastidium* should be surrounded by people who are eating with the greatest delight, to whet their appetite. Also, diverse dishes should be placed before them so that variation whets their appetite, for sameness is the mother of satiety.

The assertion that "a variety of foods stimulates the appetite," contradicted a more widespread adage, "a wide choice of foods is unhealthy for a person, and that of spices is worse." Savonarola gave the adage a faint moralizing undertone when he stated, "in those who lead a delectable life, the use of diverse and delicate meats causes vomiting." The recommendation by Platearius of a varied menu also ran counter to more specific warnings that it would cause head lice, intestinal worms, and even leprosy.

It is understandable that practitioners would contradict prevailing doctrine when treating patients who suffered a total loss of appetite that might become chronic and ultimately fatal. Some compilers found the prevention of this danger, by means of good eating and drinking habits, important enough to insert a set of general dietary rules into their discussion of disgust or related subjects. In his chapter on a hypersensitive stomach, Savonarola formulated such broad canons as "the patient's dishes should be small in quantity, rich in nutrition, and good for the stomach." In his chapter on *fastidium*, Bernard spelled out basic guidelines and a daily diet, although he promised, "by the grace of God, we intend to publish a longer treatise on *The Regimen of Health*"—a promise that he fulfilled three years later. A good diet began with wine that was "well aged and odoriferous"; the water, from "a gushing well, which runs eastward," should be taken "far from the spring so that it has been purified by ventilation and the powers of the stars"; the meats should be from birds or quadrupeds, domestic or wild, ranging from poultry to pheasants and from pigs' feet to young deer; fish should be scaly and "from clean waters that run far from cities"; fennel, parsley, and several other herbs were recommended while one "should avoid all legumes except pea soup"; most surprisingly, all fruits were also to be avoided, "with the occasional exception of roasted almonds, two nuts after fish, or half of a cooked pear or quince."

Bernard repeated the guidelines in his treatment of "a cold and moist stomach," before proceeding to particulars for one whole week. The day-by-day menu, with a touch of gastronomy, affords a colorful glimpse into the daily lives of patients who could afford the care of a learned physician.

> On Sunday, use hens in a broth of ginger and saffron, and roasted pork, from the side of the pig, with green sauce without vinegar but with cinnamon; for supper, have one little bird, roasted with a marinade of wine and salt. Monday, leaf vegetables, that is, borage, spinach, and parsley, should be mashed together and eaten with salted meats and fresh ribs from young sheep; and take a roasted partridge with cinnamon sauce; for supper, pork that has been roasted with onions placed on top. Tuesday, slightly salted pork backs with leeks and mustard; for supper, young rabbit roasted with pepper sauce. Wednesday, young rabbit with seasoned broth, and roasted

partridge. Thursday, mutton in a marinade and chicken in bread. Friday, peas with parsley and sage, and roasted fish, which should always be from the sea and cooked in pure wine. Saturday, if he or she eats meat, use veal from very young and tender suckling calves, with good pepper sauce, and roasted chicken; if not, do as on Fridays.

These were, supposedly, highlighted meals, with such staples as bread and milk left aside. Nevertheless, it is worth noting the absence of breakfast, the omission of supper for four of the seven days, and the midweek drop in quantity if not quality. The most likely explanation is that Bernard did not intend to formulate a set menu but, rather, to sketch a sample regimen for maintaining a good appetite and preventing *fastidium.*

Fastidium often served as a comprehensive category that included up to four conditions, namely, abomination, nausea, stomach upset, and vomiting. Compilers attributed the four to closely related causes and, therefore, to treatment with similar purgatives, correctives, restoratives, and so on. Noting that his peers treated the conditions as synonymous, Savonarola decided, "I will summarily dismiss a description or explanation of each, for quibbling about names does not suit the physician." It is ironic that, here as in many other instances, the dismissal of semantics coexisted with a keen awareness of the real differences that were reflected by the terminological spectrum. In fact, the differentiation of *fastidium* was nuanced enough to belie the common assumption that medieval culture lacked any sense for gustatory esthetics. In *abhominatio,* the most acute form of disgust, food became so abhorrent that the very sight of it caused the face or nose to contort; the patient became agitated and, if forced to take it, would vomit or emit smelly, smoky, or sour belching. This was dangerous because it disabled not only the appetitive but also the digestive faculty.

Compilers defined nausea, a second form of *fastidium,* as a nonproductive urge to vomit; they attributed it to corrupt humors that were stuck in the fibers of the stomach. Pregnant women were particularly susceptible, and the notion of corrupt humors (which we have seen applied to *bolismus*) rationalized the universally familiar morning sickness. Other internal causes of nausea included, Bernard taught, an imbalance in the complexion or a defect of the "appetitive, contentive, digestive, or expulsive" faculty of the stomach. Extrinsic factors included sleeplessness and excessive sex as well as satiety and inactivity, and taking food without having an appetite as well as "the frequent eating of geese and the like." Valesco added the impact of "seeing someone vomiting nearby, or a toad, or something foul of which the imagining faculty perceives an abominable form." According to Savonarola, "the disposition is common these days, due to gluttony and indiscipline." Still another variation of *fastidium* was a deeper tendency to be nauseous, called an "upset" (*conturbatio*) or, more descriptively, a "turning" (*subversio*) of the stomach. Affecting the villi of the stomach, it often ended in a violent contraction of the base and ejection of ingested substances.

Vomiting was classified as a fourth form of *fastidium* or, at least, placed on a continuum with nausea. Valesco illustrated the link in a comment that is too pithy to omit—and suggests that frogs' legs and snails were not a French invention. He observed that retching could be caused by

> taking foods which [one's] nature by itself does not enjoy but abhors. This is the case for eating frogs, which Italians freely consume as a kind of food. And if you should try this but you are not Italian, you would barely manage to avoid vomiting.

Valesco gave the impression that even escargots were alien to France, for he added,

> snails are taken as food *in certain regions,* and they may occasionally be useful and beneficial, yet on account of different custom they are disgusting to other nations, for which they trigger *fastidium* and *vomitus.*

These vignettes illustrate the general characterization of vomiting as an extension of disgust and a polar opposite both of appetite and of attraction. The initial impulse of vomiting was allocated to the *os stomachi,* as it was for appetite and disgust. The process itself, however, was allocated to the stomach and associated primarily with stomach function.

The Stomach

With vomiting as a climax, *fastidium* came to overlap with forms of *indigestio*, and the focus shifted from the *os stomachi* to the organ of digestion. This is the appropriate place to review the fundamental scheme of the three digestions that sustained or fueled human life, in a process that was analogous to cooking, distillation, and combustion. A "digestive faculty" (*virtus digestiva*) governed the entire process. Powers or faculties of attraction, retention, and expulsion (*virtus attractiva,—retentiva,* and—*expulsiva*), which were inherent in the principal instrument, governed each of the successive stages. In the first digestion, which began in the stomach and continued through the intestines, food and drink were processed into chyle (*chylus*), a milky liquid akin to plant sap; impurities and superfluities were excreted naturally through defecation or counter-naturally (with room for ambiguity, as we will see) through vomiting. The second digestion, in the liver as the seat of the natural or vegetative faculty, produced blood; two by-products, yellow bile and black bile, were stored, respectively, in the gallbladder and spleen. In the third digestion, blood nourished the entire body with radical or substantial moisture, natural or innate warmth, and vital *spiritus*. The blood was not envisioned as circulating but as receiving steady replenishment from the liver; sweat and urine were eliminated as distillates; and milk, menses, and sperm were generated as superfluities, according to an authoritative doctrine with profound implications.

The importance of superfluity and elimination framed the multiple functions of vomiting as symptom, disorder, and remedy. Savonarola introduced his discussion of vomiting, as an action of the *fundus stomachi*, with the admission that he was omitting other stomach characteristics and, "for a little while, leaving my leader," Avicenna. Indeed, vomiting demonstrated the internal performance of the stomach and, even more impressively, the pivotal role of various *virtutes* in digestion. The *virtus desiderativa* or *attractiva* of the stomach led Bernard to some arresting if convoluted speculation. He posited that the psychic component of this *virtus* resided in the stomach (inferentially, in the nerves), while the vegetative component was diffused through the body. On this premise, he surmised that, whereas "by design of nature, the *psychic* sense should make the stomach *feel* empty" and attract or retain food, the *vegetative* faculty occasionally caused a more automatic result. "This is what we see in Jews in whom food is drawn to the stomach even when they are hung by their feet, which would not happen unless the vegetative faculty attracted it and made something heavy go upward." The casual tone of the remark betrays a harsh side of early 14th-century society. Closer to the medical import, it is worth noting that both Bernard's interpretation of observed fact *and* his emphasis on the attractive power of the stomach ran counter to a near-contemporary report. This was a report of treatment rather than torture, and it illustrated (albeit unwittingly) the force of gravity rather than a faculty of the stomach. A few decades after the *Lilium*, Berthold Blumentrost of Würzburg mentioned that patients who had taken poison were "hung up by their feet so that they might vomit more easily."

This reported practice, which implied that vomiting was a simple mechanical and natural movement, sets in relief the multivalent characterization of the process in the compendia. In medical teaching, it was against nature on three accounts. Ejection from the stomach opposed the appetitive faculty, expulsive force exceeded the essential power of retention, and the normal upward direction was inverted. Some compilers adopted, from Greek sources, a distinction between difficult and easy vomiting. They called the latter "throwing up" (*anastropha*) while, in an ironic twist of nomenclature, *catastropha* or "throwing down" was the term for *easy* downward discharge. Whether easy or difficult, both vomiting and diarrhea were potentially life-threatening and called for decisive remediation. Reinald recalled two successful treatments. In one, "I cured a woman who had moved her bowels at least ten times and vomited as many times, and whom I held for desperate." He prescribed a compress for her stomach, mint syrup, and a potion with sugar water, "all of which she used, and within the space of two days she was liberated." The second case was more memorable, at least on account of the patient. "A young nephew of Pope Alexander [probably IV, reigned 1254–61], had me called when he was near death on account of excessive vomiting which could not be stopped." Reinald ordered two sachets to be filled with mint, myrtle, sumac, and other herbs; to be boiled in water and vinegar; and to be applied repeatedly and alternatingly to the stomach. Further, "I gave aged rose sap and quince jam, and then anointed the stomach with mastic oil, and that same night his vomiting was stopped and he was liberated."

In the introductory quote, we saw another view of Reinald, which he shared with his colleagues, namely, that vomiting, while inherently contranatural, benefited nature by eliminating superfluous or noxious matter. It was widely advocated not only for treatment of ailments but even for the maintenance of health. Compilers cited the dietary recommendation, which Avicenna claimed to adopt from Hippocrates, to induce vomiting twice a month as a purge; they did not give the impression that it was followed, however, and some indicated that it was as controversial as the recommendation of a monthly inebriation. Therapeutically induced vomiting was particularly beneficial for "diverting offending matter" from parts below the diaphragm. It was also "helpful for ailments of the head and stomach," according to Savonarola, "as long as it is done with ease and without distress, otherwise it would be harmful, especially to the eyes." He then applied a distinction we encountered above: "I will give here, to please you, a method for easy and another for forceful vomiting." If the drinking of lukewarm water as a weak emetic had no effect for more than four hours, the practitioner should insert into the throat a feather of which the tip was dipped in common oil or sesame oil; if this did not work, it might be necessary to use the fingers. Whatever the purgative benefits of vomiting, Savonarola reiterated his caution, adding that "it should not be done frequently" because that would make the stomach too empty.

The diagnostic significance of emesis, while more incidental than that of urine or feces, related to anatomical as well as humoral causes of ailments. Savonarola drew up a differentiation based on each of the humors as cause: for example, astringent, burning, or green vomit indicated an excess of warm choler. He added, however,

> be very careful not to be deceived. We should not always conclude from a green color that it is due to choler, for when you see yellow or green vomit with noticeable viscosity, it is better to infer that the matter is cold. Experience proves that green color is also produced by cold, as is seen in lettuce. In addition, we see that nursing babies excrete green stools when they get cold.

He further mentioned the diagnosis of a mechanical cause that, if we may judge from the appearance in several compendia, was not uncommon. "If due to drinking water in which there was a leech, the vomit will contain thin blood and pus from the small ulcer made by its bite."

Savonarola showed a particular concern with the vomiting of blood when, unlike in spitting blood (hemoptysis), it was a direct result and sign of an ailment in the stomach rather than in the lungs, throat, or brain. His interest may have been sparked by the correspondence between a striking statement in the *Canon* and a notable event in his own experience. "Know," he wrote, "that I have seen the Venetian nobleman Petrus Maurocenus vomit a crust of blood that the physicians judged to be flesh. Avicenna says, 'on many occasions, a person ejects a shred of flesh in vomiting.'" The case of Cardinal Pietro Morosini (d. 1424) impressed Savonarola enough to return to it later: "if the vomit is hard, felt-like or fleshy, like a shred of flesh, as it appeared in the case of Lord Pietro Morosini of Venice, and with some blood, it is a sign that it comes from a fistulated ulcer of the stomach, as Avicenna says." Savonarola urged his reader, "heed the words of Francis of Piedmont [Naples, fl. 1310] who said, 'The treatment of this is not for the dull or lazy but for the prudent and solicitous physician.'" He underscored the seriousness of this concern with the authority of Galen's teaching that the loss of blood "usually causes the failure of the spirit that is the substance of every member, so that death follows."

The vital role of the stomach placed it among the principal or noble organs, as Savonarola argued in a masterful summation of the general doctrine and of the practical implications.

The nobility of the stomach is apparent from what is said about its anatomy, because it has affinity with all the principal organs, and it is the first to prepare nourishment for them. It is also susceptible to being affected by an ailment from any of the other organs, as will become evident below. Therefore, we should be most diligent that it be protected, so that I have planned to discuss it and its ailments in detail. Let me add that people seem to be suffering from these more frequently these days, to their utter exhaustion.

Four centuries earlier, however, Petrocellus also noted that the stomach incurs many dangers and "faults" (*culpas*), which he then itemized and discussed. He and several other Salernitan masters omitted anatomy, in noteworthy contrast with Savonarola and other late-medieval authors. Before addressing gastric ailments, Savonarola drew attention to the essence of the stomach, "an organ of cold and dry complexion, situated in the center of the body." He described it, with a catchy comparison with the alchemist's alembic, as "oblong in shape with a round sweep, in the manner of a gourd-retort."

In their descriptions of the stomach, compilers manifested tendencies with which we have become familiar by now. They introduced complexion ahead of location, shape, and construction. In addition, they viewed a name as the first key to understanding, anatomy as learned chiefly from books, and purpose as determining every faculty and function. With a name derived from the Greek word *stoma,* the organ was the mouth of the belly and the real place where the body takes in the food. Galen and Avicenna were explicitly acknowledged as the sources for identifying the major features between the entrance of the *os stomachi* and the narrower exit of the pylorus. Longitudinal villi in the inner layer exerted attraction, "the principal and most natural action of the stomach"; they were interwoven with "transversal villi that aid in retaining the contents"; in the thick external layer, the villi were "latitudinal so that they would achieve the expulsion of harmful contents, which is the secondary but more difficult function of the stomach." This was Valesco's lucid overview of the anatomy that he read in Galen and Avicenna. He also learned from them that the stomach takes a globular shape in the area where the esophagus enters (the fundus), but deeming their explanation lacking in teleology, he added several reasons. He began with a bemusing illustration of the purposefulness of Nature's architecture—while revealing the limited depth of associations between anatomy and afflictions. "The first reason is, because this shape is more resistant to harm, as is evident in a round tower on which the stones of siege engines do not easily have an impact."

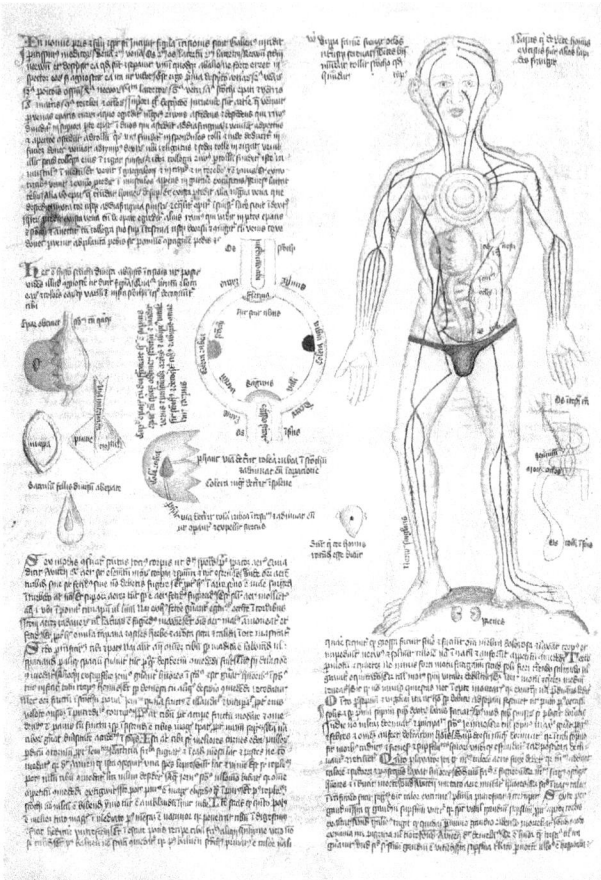

General anatomy, with arteries and intestines; and diagrams of the stomach, liver, and other organs of digestion. Drawing in a 15th-century manuscript of anatomical and medical texts embedded in *Apocalypsis S. Joannis cum glossis*. (Wellcome Library, London. Wellcome Images L0000842)

Stomach afflictions were numerous. In the *Passionarius,* Gariopontus itemized no fewer than 31, ranging from ache to aposteme, wound, and paralysis. It is of interest to note that his inventory listed some Greek labels that were apparently abandoned by his successors, such as "lipothomia id est malfactio" and "pneumatosis id est inflatio"; it included a few items that other authors discussed elsewhere, such as anorexia and vomiting; and it omitted three categories, two of them minor and one major, which occupied considerable space in later compendia. Certain affections, like others we have encountered earlier, received seemingly disproportionate attention: these included ructus or belching, and hiccups. Both were presented as serving the purpose of expelling harmful matters and, therefore, as governed by the *virtus expulsiva*. This had important implications for therapeutics, which often wavered between promoting the expulsive movement and stopping the involuntary spasm. Hiccups, however, did not promote expulsion and therefore needed to be stopped. Platearius claimed, "giving sap of wormwood with sugar and honey is very helpful: believe the expert." For more obstinate attacks, striking "intense fear into patients when they are suddenly told something terrible" might help. Varignana observed the effectiveness of "powerful and sudden impressions," and also of holding one's breath all the way until choking; he further cited a proven recipe of Platearius. Reinald recommended a mixture of castor oil and mint juice in "a tried and true remedy (*experimentum expertum*) of my master."

A bad complexion was the most comprehensive stomach problem. The notion seems to have gained prominence with the influx of translations from Galen and Avicenna. The category branched into stomachache and into malfunctions of the faculties that led to various types of indigestion. All these were so closely related, Bernard taught, that their "cures are almost the same." Nevertheless, he adapted treatments to a complexion's excessive warmth, cold, or dryness. For the latter, he prescribed milk, preferably human and taken directly from the breast, and he added a cross-reference to previous places where he had mentioned the prescription. He also differentiated a dry and humid imbalance of the stomach as leading, respectively, to hectic fever and dropsy. Totally undigested material was "the origin of nearly all diseases, most of them chronic, such as epilepsy, scabies, dropsy, and the like. Therefore, beware." A "good and perfect digestion," on the other hand, was evident when

> someone sleeps well, wakes up feeling tranquil and without disturbance; bowel movements are normal and on the usual hour, and the urine is well digested; there is no feeling of ructus, windiness, corruptions, pains, revulsion, or heaviness in the head; and sleep is without frightful, false, or sad phantasms. This means that the stomach has taken all the food perfectly, that there has been enough quiet time, and that the digestion has been good and complete.

The absence of these conditions indicated a disturbance of the stomach that called for medical attention.

Stomachache was, no doubt, a very common problem. Bernard's recommendation of a particular remedy may even hint at personal experience. After a recipe that contained cloves, aloe wood, and the juices of mint and wormwood, he added, "in long-standing, syncopal, and paroxysmal stomachaches I have not found greater help." The ache could be so sharp "that the patient is unable to speak," according to Gariopontus, or so intense that it caused fainting. The intensity was due, Varignana explained, "to the sensitivity of the stomach on account both of its proximity to the heart and of the two thick nerves that connect it to the brain." The number of internal and external causes was almost limitless. Internal factors varied widely, from excessive food or corrupted humors to an abscess. Platearius stated that an aposteme occurred "sometimes in the cavity, sometimes on the surface, and sometimes in the layers" of the stomach and that it was difficult to diagnose "when it develops between the layers." Reinald recognized that an abscess could cause severe pain, but then he deferred treatments to the section on fevers because he believed that "this could not be in the stomach without fever." The external cause often was some traumatic event, as in the case of Valesco's patient who was "struck in the esophagus by the hind foot of a horse and who, after a long time, became a confirmed stomach patient (*stomaticus*)." The variety of treatments paralleled that of the causes. Varignana mentioned a mild one: "it is written and we have experienced that fennel juice boiled in water marvelously relieves a stomach ache that is accompanied by nausea and hiccups." A more widespread, though more drastic, treatment was by the induction of vomiting, which Platearius called "a vile but excellent remedy."

The Intestines

Many compilers discussed the intestines largely as an extension of the stomach, and they ambiguously applied the term *stomachus* to both the single organ and the entire abdomen. Here is a paradox. First, the pylorus represented a sharp boundary in therapeutics, especially between treatments by upward and downward purges. Moreover, there were marked differences in notions and perceptions, between the relatively organized noble upper digestive tract (still associated with the chest, notwithstanding the diaphragm) and the more chaotic lower windbag or bellows of the "belly" (*venter*). Even when embalming, autopsy, and dissection became more frequent, the intestines were discarded too hastily to increase the opportunities for observation, not only for the obvious physical reasons but also because they were obstructing the view of the liver and spleen, nobler organs. Descriptions of intestinal anatomy and physiology, when they appeared in medical compendia at all, remained markedly more derivative, sketchy, and inconsistent than in surgical manuals. It takes a collation of several compendia to reconstruct the content beyond the major division into the peritoneum, the small or thin intestine, and the large or broad intestine. Several authors presented some list of the segments within these principal areas, but the description of each segment tended to be concise and casual, or simply bypassed, on the way from definition to diagnosis and therapeutics.

The prevalence, extent, and detail of the practical sections suggest that intestinal woes caused daily misery and presented mortal danger. Furthermore, a slightly less conspicuous dependence on written sources and more frequent references to personal experience may imply an increased prevalence—or, at least, awareness—of digestive problems. The discourse covered two major areas, namely, general abdominal complaints and topical ailments. Pain was an encompassing concern, both as an illness per se and as a symptom of windiness, worms, and other problems. The kind and intensity of pain allowed the practitioner to identify such direct and remote causes as a hot humor if the pain was sharp and piercing. Copho pointed out that "intolerable pain" accompanied "inflation of the belly" when the digestive faculty failed and allowed gases to accumulate. If acute, this might prove fatal; if chronic, it might resemble the accumulation of fluid in dropsy, but it was less grave because, as Bartholomeus taught, "it does not compromise the good condition or color of the body." When flatulence was accompanied by intestinal torsion or twisted bowel, it caused even more serious pain, and "piercing distress," Bernard observed. "This ailment," furthermore, "has symptoms so terrible that it is compared to a heart attack." In general, Plateraius and other compilers stated, "growling, gargling, and noise of the intestines" were clues for a diagnosis of windiness. Bernard clarified that "the diverse sounds and melodies" indicated whether thick or thin matter was involved, in broad or narrow passages, and in one site or another. Authors blamed flatulence mainly on diet. Bernard reflected a broad consensus when he warned against "the eating of too many warm foods such as onions and garlic, or cold foods such as melons and gourds." Copho intriguingly singled out "the eating of a certain fish that is called barbel (*barbus*)."

Copho claimed that he treated flatulence without delay: "we immediately boil cow dung in vinegar, apply pieces to the aching site, and renew them frequently." "When windiness begins to develop," Bernard recommended, "the patient should try to expel it upward with a burp or downward with a fart"—*peditu,* origin of the French word *pet.* Persistence flatulence, if caused by excessively warm or cold complexion, was to be countered with suppositories, digestives, purgative syrups, baths, and the application of sachets and ointments. For a cold imbalance, the more common cause, contraries included spikenard, anise, and zedoary; for a warm imbalance, barley, purslane, and pomegranate. "The empirics say," Bernard continued, "that roasted hedgehog and the heel of a pig are very helpful against this ailment." His subject here was torsion, and he supplemented the treatment with a remedy from the *experimentatores* for this ailment that was "difficult because the organs are delicate and the cause is substantial." Torsion was even difficult to diagnose, he believed, because it was concentrated "sometimes in the fundus of the stomach, sometimes in the cooler part of the intestines, and sometimes in both."

Every part of the digestive tract might harbor intestinal worms, which seem to have been a pervasive plague. Their presence in the bowel was consistent with the tenet of natural philosophy, ever since antiquity, that their spontaneous generation occurred in soil, dirt, and decomposing matter. In the humoral scheme, phlegmatic matter was their preferred medium. "The argument, that hot and dry medicine kills them," supported this conventional view, according to Gilbert. In the same vein, he contradicted Copho's opinion that they frequently grew in the stomach, with the argument that they would not survive "the strength of the digesting heat." At the other end of the humoral spectrum, however, Platearius speculated that worms could not develop in intestinal phlegm if it was vitreous or glassy and therefore too cold for giving life. Bernard combined philosophical and medical notions in the proposition that worms were most likely to arise from anything that "produces a crude phlegmatic humor." He sounded almost censorious in citing examples "such as nauseating satiety and sexual intercourse after filling up," and similar preconditions that exist "more frequently in children and gluttons."

Bernard's distinction of three principal kinds of worms echoed that of several other authors who, however, were not always clear or consistent. Long worms, called *lumbrici* for their "lubricity" or slipperiness, grew from "salty phlegm" according to Platearius. They lodged in the upper or small intestine. Petrocellus specified that these were "delicate, of endless measure, and knobby." Copho reported that they were "called belts (*cinguli*)"—and all the descriptions add up to certainty that they corresponded to human tapeworms. Savonarola asserted that they could cross the pylorus and cause a stomachache, "as happens everyday in children." The middle intestine was the normal habitat for the short and broad ascarids, which were produced by natural phlegm, in the humoral taxonomy. They looked like gourd seeds and therefore were also called *cucurbitivi*.

The putrid contents of the rectum generated small round worms that, in Bernard's view, were mercifully "unable to remain there for long, for they grow." He suggested, unappetizingly, that they "resemble those found in cheese." Petrocellus added another peculiar detail to the description of roundworms, as "resembling earth worms but paler, harder, and sharp."

The symptoms of intestinal parasites varied according to their species and location, but diagnostic precision was inconsistent. For Petrocellus, for example, patients with long worms felt "twisting of the intestines and great pricking in the pubic area and the rectum." Other Salernitan masters agreed on the significance of intestinal torsion, but they added other symptoms. Some of these were rather odd. Platearius, among others, mentioned symptomatic itching of the tip of the nose, which he attributed to "the connection between the intestines and the nostrils." He further taught that patients "shout and grind their teeth in their sleep." Identifying more serious symptoms, Bartholomeus noted that patients "suffer insomnia, and they are thin and pale." Gilbert believed that the agony of worms was

> so acute that it sometimes drives the patients out of their mind. As a result, sometimes they seem to be frenetic, sometimes maniacal, sometimes melancholic; sometimes they fall silent like lethargic apoplectics; sometimes they fall down like epileptics; sometimes they faint like in the suffocation of the womb [hysteria]; sometimes they suffer runs like in dysentery; sometimes they grind their teeth and shout like in sciatica; sometimes they beat their belly like in colic.

He listed several criteria for distinguishing these cases from true insanity. Bernard added one distinction, namely, that these patients, unlike the insane, did "not gather grass or suffer a heavy headache." He also repeated the observation of several authors that "the worms are sometimes ejected below, sometimes through the nose and mouth." His credulity was stretched, however, by the report that the worms "sometimes perforate the intestines and come out, but this is an amazing thing to hear if it is true." Gilbert, for one, had written, "it happens that, when they are old, they perforate the stomach so that the tops of their heads stick out; these cases seem incurable."

Both objectives of treatment, to kill and expel the parasites, were served by bitter simples, among which wormwood (*absinthium*) was predictably ubiquitous. Platearius advised to administer the bitter ingredients together with honey in order to bait the worms. Cures filled so many pages that the problem must have been rampant. This impression is reinforced by the compilers' frequent advertisements of their own recipe or nostrum (literally, "ours"). "Salernitan women," Copho reported, take strong wine, grind pepper, cumin, and laurel seed or root, bring this to a medium boil with sea or salt water, then strain it and give it. We, however, give *hieralogodion* [a precious compound] with rain water: there is nothing better." He further specified, "to nursing infants we give powder of southernwood, and they are freed," while "for all patients we make lupin bean paste tempered with wormwood sap, and place pieces on the navel." For worms "around the anus, which are known by the itch there, burned deer horn, with pyrethrum and knotgrass are said to be remedies; however, you should not forget ours, because it is not inferior to any." After endorsing the conventional helminthicides, Gilbert brought the treatment up-to-date by adding, "you should make this electuary of today's practitioners (*electuarium modernorum*)," which was a syrup with more than a dozen ingredients. Bernard showed a more emphatic interest in being current when he observed, about a different recipe, "here is something new that is commonly done now: give ground zedoary seed to drink, with broth or wine, and without doubt it kills all [worms]."

Another problem that dated back centuries—and that advances in the culinary arts may have allayed—was lientery, the partial or complete failure in the processing of food and drink. Compilers attributed this disorder, in principle, to a failure of the digestive and retentive faculties in the stomach. In practice, however, they also associated lientery with the intestines because the most notable manifestation was the excretion of food in the same form and amount as it had been ingested. Underlying causes included ulcers, a bad complexion, excessive phlegm or corrosive bile, and, according to Copho, "eating too many fatty things." If the origin lay in the stomach, "occasionally, you should induce vomiting after a meal, by introducing a feather into the mouth." Even if outright paralysis of the stomach was responsible, it might be remedied, unless the patient had lost all taste and appetite: in this case, Gariopontus admitted, "we give up on the ailment as incurable, because it swiftly leads to the danger of death."

Gilbert assured that, when a cold or warm complexional imbalance prevented food from being processed, "the arsenic troches of the Four [Salernitan] Masters are helpful either way, and even when it is desperate." It bears noting that, after Salerno, chapters on lientery seem to lack personal recipes and to be largely derived from conventional sources. Savonarola, for instance, was actually copying a classic authority when appeared to be addressing his reader directly, "know that lientery should not be underestimated, because it leads the patient to dysentery and dropsy if treatment is delayed. Serapion." It stands to reason that Savonarola also drew on traditional lore when proposing that the disorder "is sometimes caused by pestilential air and evil winds, by the influence or conjunction of the stars, and by the aspect of the Head and Tail of the Dragon [the north and south nodes of the moon's orbit] and of the other planets in their signs."

Savonarola's allusion to an epidemic nexus is of special interest, not only with regard to events of the era but also within the context of the compendia. His remark dovetailed with his treatment of lientery as a type of intestinal flux, rather than as a separate syndrome. It seems significant that most compilers after 1300 shared this taxonomy. Valesco summarized the consensus most lucidly, as he did in so many instances.

> There are many kinds of intestinal flux. However, so that the mind may not be exhausted in a profusion of kinds and may not forget one kind while contemplating another, the authors of medicine have reduced them to three; if there are others, they have named them differently in order to prevent confusion. Hence, there are three kinds of flux, that is, lientery, diarrhea, and dysentery. There is a verse for this: "*lien* is crude, diarrhea simple, and dysentery bloody."

Since treatments varied little, as authors emphasized, Valesco accepted a simplified classification for all the types of *fluxus ventris*.

In the compendia in general, a growing number of pages supplemented the separate chapters on the three major and other kinds of flux. While this development was consistent with an increased concern for organization and comprehensiveness, it also evinced a greater awareness of the issue, and it even suggested a rising threat from the affliction—from one type in particular, as we shall see. Bernard dedicated his most expansive chapter on digestive ailments to "a recapitulation of the intestinal fluxes, containing twenty-two treatises." He surveyed no fewer than 17 types, which he distinguished by the affected site, the external or internal cause, the responsible humor, the involvement of an organ outside the intestines, the collateral effects, the affected patient, and so on. Here again, however, the corresponding treatments varied little, with recurrent mention of theriac, aged cheese, the rennet from a hare's stomach (probably on the authority of Avicenna), and a few other remedies that, "almost without a difference, cure every flux." When Valesco cited Bernard, he objected, "it seems hard to me to propose certain medicines that would cure every kind of abdominal runs," but he supplemented his own expansive chapters on flux with a "repetitio." In this review, he examined various puzzling issues (*dubia*), among which the most notable was the question, "which kinds of flux are most commonly known as pestilential?"

Savonarola began his section on intestinal diseases with a "division of all manners of flux." He promised "a summary treatment of eleven, at least of the simple ones," but the part grew into 17 chapter-length "rubrics," and these were supplemented further by debates of four *dubia*. Throughout these pages, he digressed repeatedly from his base texts in the *Canon*, although he had set out to "follow, for a large part, the leader" Avicenna. In addition, he singled out, more conspicuously than other authors, one type in which flux was combined with vomiting. This was *passio colerica* or *cholerica*, "choleric ailment," the convulsive and complete expulsion of consumed food, in simultaneous vomiting and loose bowel movement. This disorder should neither be equated with cholera, in spite of intriguing parallels, nor confused with *passio colica*, about which more later. Gilbert defined it as "an ailment of the stomach or intestines due to furious yellow bile," and thus "acting faster than any other acute disease." Among the frightening effects, the most ominous was "utter exhaustion of the nerves, which might be followed by spasms leading to speedy death." He urged to "stop the flux as much as we can, prevent the loss of moisture, and boost the patient's strength." The obvious common sense in Gilbert's advice seemed lacking in his counterintuitive suggestion,

> if you observe that the matter is drawn upward, induce vomiting, for as flux is cured by flux, thus vomiting is cured by vomiting: Avicenna agrees in his chapter on the treatment of *colerica*, on the authority of Hippocrates. Similarly, induce a bowel movement with a suppository.

One may also see a contrast between Gilbert's aggressive approach and Savonarola's weak recommendation to "try to make the patients sleep." In fairness, it should be added that Savonarola also recommended, "above all else, try to restore the strength." The discussion of *colerica* brought him, "with the help of Almighty God the Father, the Son, and the Holy Spirit," to the conclusion of "the lengthy matter on fluxes, which everyone should consider carefully because it affects people in our region every year as it were."

Compilers gave special and growing consideration to one type of flux, namely, dysentery. Although feared since antiquity, dysentery apparently became more prevalent in the course of the Middle Ages. The subject seemed submerged in the *Canon*'s diffuse discourse on loose bowels, but it occupied several central "rubrics" in the *Practica* of Savonarola, an avowed follower of Avicenna. In this development, as in other areas, Gilbert appears as a figure of transition. He attested to an intensifying concern in the second half of the 13th century, by the detail of his descriptions, the roster of diverging opinions and his own answers, and the register of extraordinary treatments. "Better than all the others," he claimed, "are the troches that the Salernitan masters prescribed for the Lord King, excellent for patients of dysentery and lientery," and that contained more than two dozen ingredients. For the most amazing remedy, Gilbert instructed the practitioner,

> let the patient's messenger bring, without speaking, two cups of which one contains a little water from a spring. You take the cups and bless the water, "Flesh with the Chalice, confirm the blood of the Israelite." Next, twice say the rosary and the Credo, while pouring the water into the other cup and switching both from hand to hand three times. Then have the messenger drink the water while saying the words above. The patient will be healed within three days, or he will advance towards death; he should, however, make a good confession.

Gilbert stipulated, "this should be done in cases of dysentery and not in others." Gaddesden cited the remedy, nevertheless, as "Gilbert's *experimentum* for every bloody flux."

Although Gilbert demonstrated a heightened preoccupation with cures, he showed no expanded awareness of causes. His passing mention of cold wind as an environmental factor even fell short of Avicenna's reference to seasonal and regional factors. By the early 14th century, compilers alluded with increasing frequency to epidemic aspects in the environment, virulence, episodes, spread, and virulence. Bernard may have been the first to link corrupt air explicitly to dysentery. It was hardly mere coincidence that, after the stricken 14th century, Valesco moved beyond indirect linkage to pestilential flux. An occurrence was signaled, he declared, when "previous or present weather was very warm and dry, beyond the complexion which it should have naturally." This remark may have been close to some of Avicenna's teaching, but he added that the epidemic incidence was "known also, more conclusively, when at that time many in the same region or area are felled by the same disease, and a great number die." The same applied to prognostication: when "there are many cases of dysentery in one area in a time of pestilence, and some begin to have tenesmus, lientery, or diarrhea, you will judge that they are in the grip of the near-terminal disease." With still greater precision, Valesco asked in one of his *dubia* "whether pestilential dysentery and tenesmus are contagious diseases;" he answered that they were indeed, "not only in the same house but also in an entire locale, and with [the affliction] moving from a child of ten or fifteen to a sexagenarian." Savonarola remarked that "Avicenna has said little about the treatment of pestilential fever," and then he assured, "I will not be afraid to repeat or amplify" propositions on dysentery. He argued, as he did for *colerica*, "these days I see so many things in extreme need of plain and clear teaching about treatment, because every year more and more die of this pestiferous disease."

As compilers widened the epidemic dimensions of dysentery, they also deepened their examination of its other causes and its nature, symptoms, and treatment. Bernard elucidated the traditional definition of the ailment as loose bowel movements containing bloody stool and intestinal lining. He added detail and his own thoughts to the traditional division that hinged on the ailing site in the abdomen, the organ where it originated, the amount of discharged blood, and the degree of intestinal excoriation. He opined, for example, in disagreement with Gilbert and other authors, and "with due respect for Galen," that it was possible for undigested food to accompany the excretion of blood. In fact, when followed by lientery, an attack of dysentery would be deadly. A fatal prognosis was also certain to Bernard "when the excreta, upon falling to the ground, boil like vinegar so that the flies shun them." Valesco warned that this disease was so "dangerous that it tolerates neither the ignorance of the physician, the disobedience of the patient, nor the laziness or indifference of the assistants and servants."

Valesco was one of several authors who blamed medical error for cases of dysentery (which would now be called iatrogenic), for example, when "illiterate apothecaries give a strong medicine, with scammony or ellebore, in an unregulated dose." He reinforced this warning with personal reminiscences.

> I know a man who was still alive when this was being written and who, instead of two drams of *dyaturbit* [a powerful laxative], took two ounces as the foolish servant told him. I also know another to whom a foolish apothecary administered a medicine that gave him such loose bowels that he nearly died. It was dysentery in each case, but both recovered by divine permission and with the help of some person.

This person may have been Valesco himself, who often expressed the wish to share his solicitousness with the reader.

> I want you to know one thing. In prolonged dysentery, a person does not have the strength to rise and go to the toilet all the time. Foul as it may be,

I advise to place a sheet under the patient's haunches so that he/she does his/her business there, to remove and change the cloth continuously, and to cleanse the anus with a soft cloth or stupe.

He mused, "for it is better to suffer a little embarrassment than to move suddenly from this world to the ancient Fathers."

When compared with the agonies and danger of lientery and dysentery, "the simple flux," as Copho and others called diarrhea, seemed thoroughly ordinary. It was defined by negatives, as loose bowels "without bloody stool, excoriation of the intestines, or the passing of unprocessed food." Copho observed that it took many forms and afflicted all ages, "but it is more common in the old on account of the abundant cold and humidity." Telltale signs pointed to the humor that was responsible, as thirst and green stool indicated a problem with yellow bile, for example. Although compilers agreed that diarrhea might lead to worse flux and to exhaustion if ignored, they covered it quite casually. Bernard gave it barely a paragraph, before delving into his *clarificatio* on all the kinds of flux. Valesco did not discuss the signs and causes separately, as was the norm, but he combined them "so that the teaching may be understood more easily." He proposed that, when diarrhea came "with tolerance and other good signs, it is not necessary to treat this kind." For the rest, the treatment resembled that of lientery, "and therefore many philosophers have placed both categories in the same chapter and made little distinction between them." The reference to philosophers instead of the usual citation of *phisici*, while possibly due to a scribal error, may indicate that Valesco considered therapeutic differentiation more a theoretical than a practical issue here. In the same vein, Savonarola simply omitted the predictive significance of diarrhea, while referring the reader to the *Pronostics* of Hippocrates, for the sake of brevity.

General abdominal complaints occupied substantial and integrated sections in the compendia, whereas localized disorders were often scattered through the discourse on intestines. Four sites, however, normally served as bases for the organization of the chapters, namely, the ileum, colon, rectum, and anus. The peritoneum was a part of the abdomen that, while drawing serious concern, remained elusive. It remained almost invisible in Salernitan compendia, even though their authors must have been aware of it when they discussed such grave ailments as a supposedly acute form of dropsy, a diffuse inflammation of the colon, and inflation of the belly. Subsequent compilers of medical manuals largely ignored the anatomical precision of Galen and Avicenna, in spite of the expanded access to sources and dissection. They adopted Arabic terminology in Latin transliteration (*mirach* for the parietal or external layer and *sifac* or *cyphac* for the visceral or interior layer), but they often applied either term indistinctly to the peritoneum. Once, Bernard—perhaps in a moment of absentmindedness—inverted their meaning by describing *mirach* as "directly wrapped around the intestines, in the manner of a net," and *siphac* as "the other membrane closer to the skin."

The ileum was the first segment of the intestines to be singled out for separate discussion. There was a vast distance, however, between *yliaca passio* in the compendia and modern ileitis, let alone the form that is now most notorious, Crohn's disease. Compilers differentiated affections of the ileum from those of the colon, but they left much latitude for overlaps in understanding and for inconsistency in treatment. Gilbert pointed out a "contradiction" (*contrarietas*) among some authors on the location of *yliaca*, and even within Constantine's *Pantegni* on the fabric of the ileum. A precedent for confusion was set in the definition, as in the *Viaticum*, "pain of the ileum is a pain *of the intestines* that prevents the feces from coming out below." Some contradicted the effect, including Copho, who attributed bloody flux to at least one type of *yliaca*. Platearius endeavored to tighten the anatomical, etiological, and diagnostic boundaries. He excluded the duodenum and jejunum by arguing that the ailment was not named "for the small intestines, as is claimed falsely by some." He further insisted, in a strict interpretation of the *Pantegni*, that the ailment pertained specifically to "the hard and twisted intestine in which hardened residual feces cause *yliaca*, with pain from the navel downward." Thus, Platearius reinforced a threefold though hardly ironclad proposition that the ileum was the prime location of bowel obstruction called *yliaca* (ileus in modern medicine) and that pain was an essential ingredient and symptom.

Savonarola echoed the *Viaticum* in defining *yliaca* and especially in equating it with pain, but he added his own accents. He qualified the pain as "extremely violent," cleared up the ambiguity by locating it "in the intestine called the ileum," and elaborated that the bowel obstruction caused the feces "to come out above." Authors diverged on the exact location of pain, with Platearius placing it "from the navel downward," Bernard "from the navel upward," and Gilbert "above and around the groin, in front and back up to the kidneys." There was complete agreement, however, on the vehemence of the pain, which was attributed to the sensitivity of the ileum. It hurt "as if the intestines were being pierced by an auger," according to Bernard, or "as much as being in labor, and enough to drive one mad," according to Gilbert. On the whole, Gilbert believed, *yliaca* "is barely curable because of the thinness, vulnerability (*passibilitatem*), and keen sensitivity" of the ileum. He adopted the traditional account that "sometimes phlegm collects and hardens in it," but he added the result, "so that the feces, unable to pass, are forced to exit through the mouth. Therefore, this is the most foul of all ailments."

Gilbert may have been the first to draw attention to fecal vomiting as accompanying *yliaca*. The linkage was apparently still recent enough to impress Bernard. He opened his prognostication on the ailment with a vividly enhanced report, in which he mentioned the phenomenon twice.

> This disease is horrible for the fact that feces are sent upward; it is also accompanied by abominable symptoms such as fainting, spasm, cold extremities, insanity, fetid feces by mouth, and stench of the entire body; all these are lethal, and they are accompanied by continuous vomiting.

The relative newness of the observation is further suggested by an academic question or *dubium* that Bernard raised, "one could reasonably doubt whether it is possible for feces to be expelled upward." After carefully weighing the contrary and supporting arguments, he reached the conclusion that it was difficult but not impossible. The phenomenon still drew unusual attention in Savonarola's time. He cited the claims by Francesco da Piedemonte (d. 1320) and Guglielmo da Brescia (1250–1326) of "having seen some cured among those who vomited feces." Moreover, Savonarola moved from Bernard's speculative question to actual fact by adding "I have [cured] only one whom I had in my care, by the Savior's grace."

The most remarkable aspect of the accounts of fecal vomiting is the suggestion of an epidemic nexus that, here again, seems to have emerged in the latter part of the 13th century. Gilbert did not yet make the connection, but Bernard proposed that *passio yliaca* was distinct from *colica* because it "results more from pestilential air." Valesco described, with clinical precision, the evolution from *yliaca* to "pestilential tenesmus" and, in the end, to dysentery, which "frequently lasts until the causing matter is evacuated, unless the patient dies before." Savonarola provided striking albeit puzzling etiological detail, by indicating that *yliaca* resulted "from pestilential air on account of the proximity of the heart to the stomach, and it moves from person to person and from region to region, in the manner of the disease of pestilence (*ad modum pestilentis morbi*), and it is a contagious disease." He added that the ailment was "called 'have mercy' (*miserere*) by the ancients, because the name is derived from the Greek *eleo* for 'have mercy.'" He offered this clarification as if in a footnote, with a reference to the *Conciliator differentiarum philosophorum et medicorum*, in which Pietro d'Abano (1257–1315) sought to reconcile the legacies of natural philosophy and medicine.

This is a good place for pointing out that it would be anachronistic and misleading to translate *passio yliaca* as "ileitis" and *passio colica* as "colitis" or "colic," since the modern terms designate more specific conditions. Latin compilers repeatedly blurred the diagnostic and therapeutic lines between ailments of the ileum and of the colon, notwithstanding the formal distinctions that they drew in anatomy and, occasionally, in taxonomy. Bernard stated plainly, "about this subject, it should be understood that *passio colica* and *yliaca* coincide in causes, signs, prognostication, and treatment." Bernard and other compilers drew a clearer distinction between ailments of the colon, which they called "the penultimate intestine," and a particular disorder of the rectum or *longaon*. The disorder, "which the Greeks call *tenesmon*," as we learn from Petrocellus, became latinized as *thenasmon* or *tenasmon*. These terms, forerunners of the modern term "tenesmus," designated a strong but ineffective urge to evacuate the bowels. The problem appeared less worrisome than the previously discussed intestinal diseases, and it was ascribed to a variety of more ordinary causes. Platearius explained that yellow bile might be responsible for rectal irritation and phlegm for fecal retention. Gilbert and others suggested the involvement of anal worms, and Bernard the presence of hemorrhoids or ulcers. Tenesmus was also due to such external causes as "sitting on a cold rock, or a cold bath, or cold ointments, or the exposure of a naked anus to the cold air, and the like," according to Bernard. If prolonged, the pain "leads to *colica* and *yliaca*, insomnia, weakness, fainting, poor resistance, and headaches," but not to the danger of death. Treatments naturally ranged from warm baths and aperitive ointments to suppositories, enemas, and suffumigations in which the patient sat above burning medicines in order to absorb their smoke through the anus.

Anal exposure is commonly associated with medieval culture, in a simplified stereotype drawn from fabliaux, marginalia, sculpture, and other evidence. Yet the image seems consistent with the disproportionate attention that compilers devoted to the end of the digestive tract. At the same time, it takes little research to find that factors in the lifestyle, not only nutrition and hygiene but also clothing and seating, must have caused an inordinate amount of anal discomfort and disorders. Petrocellus exemplified a combination of cultural and medical preoccupations, by opening the chapter with the declaration, "the anus has many names," and by

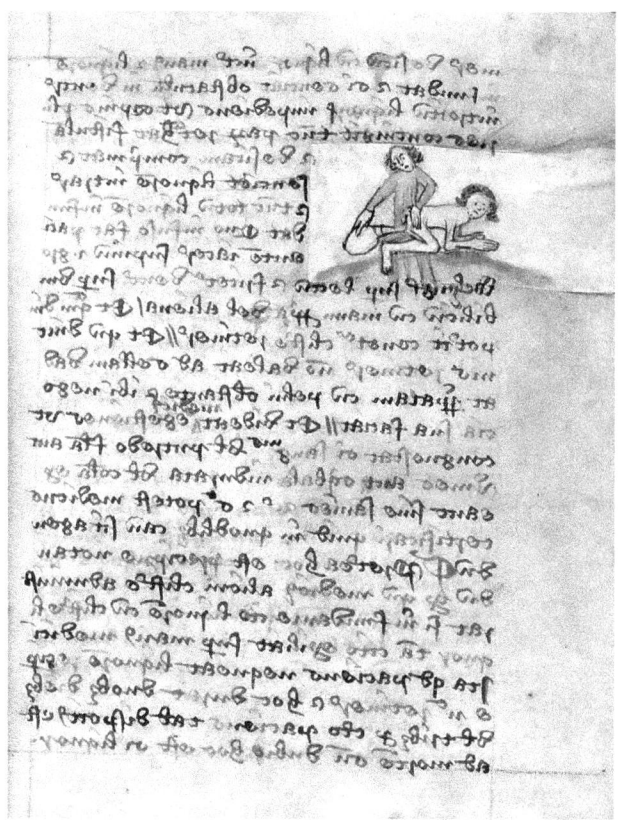

A practitioner administers an enema to a kneeling patient. Drawing in an early 15th-century manuscript of an anonymous *Practica a capite ad pedes*, in *Miscellanea medica*, XXIV, fol. 193v. Note that the drawing was inserted into the page before the text was written. The page (inverted here) offers precise instructions for applying a clyster. (Wellcome Library, London. Wellcome Images L0031725)

including several vulgar ones. After dwelling on etymology and description somewhat more than usually, he itemized a dozen ailments, "all of which need to be remedied." Many patients, however,

> decide not to be treated, because the problem is situated in the most foul and shameful place. And yet, it is not only the anus that swells but also other nearby parts, with filthy and bad wounds of the belly as the result. Physicians, for their part, have not been aiding the patient by examination and treatment if, on account of the foulness or stench, they did not diligently wipe the dirt.

The practitioner's chief concerns extended from itch to pain, from growths to fissures, and from paralysis to extrusion; several of these concerns were routinely deferred to surgery.

Anal itch, Bernard instructed, called for treatment that addressed such causes as worms or ulcers. If it resulted "from sharp humors, the regimen and diet should be turned around, and painkilling suppositories should be administered, as was said in the chapter on tenesmus." Rectal pain and anal itch were most commonly attributed to dietary and humoral causes, but pains in the anus were almost exclusively determined by anatomical factors, growths and faults in particular. Hemorrhoids outranked all the other growths and tumors, not only in captivating the interest of compilers but also in manifesting the power—and ambivalence—of teleology. Since antiquity, they were seen more as natural than as contrary to nature, which may indicate how common they were. In the framework of teleology, hemorrhoids served as emunctories, that is, outlets for superfluous blood and corrupt humors. A growing emphasis on this function in the manuals is evident in successive definitions. Copho described hemorrhoids as "*veins* that protrude from the anus and *often shed blood*," but Bernard defined them as "the *flow of blood from veins* in the anus." The flow was instrumental, to a degree, in maintaining the body's humoral balance; when restricted, it might cause a host of diseases. The list of these diseases was intended less for accuracy than for emphasis, as becomes apparent in a juxtaposition (with some terminological liberty in the translation) that also demonstrates that compilers followed Avicenna closely yet less verbatim than is readily assumed. See Table 7.1. The list was omitted by some authors, and limited by others. Platearius, for example, mentioned "dropsy, phthisis, mania, and melancholy."

Table 7.1 Bleeding hemorrhoids, in the *Canon* and the *Lilium*

Avicenna	Bernard
The flow of blood from the anus protects from herpes estiomenus, mania, melancholy, erysipelas, cancer, excoriation, scabies, ringworm, leprosy, pleurisy, pneumonia, and frenzy . . .	When the flow is moderate, it is greatly helpful and it protects against many diseases from burned and corrupt melancholy, such as mania, melancholy, pleurisy, leprosy, morphew, dropsy, mormal, quartan fever, and ailment of the spleen, and the like. When it ceases, all these diseases occur. When it is excessive, it causes dropsy and phthisis.
When it is retained, the same diseases occur, and there is fear of dropsy and phthisis	

The appearance of hemorrhoids indicated their source: they looked like grapes if blood was the sole humor, like warts if black bile was involved, and like morello cherries if yellow bile; they resembled white blisters if they were due to phlegm, which was unusual. The flow was periodic, regulated by nature in order to help itself, particularly by the evacuation of melancholic blood. Bernard clarified that women, even when purged periodically by menstruation, could have hemorrhoids when the menses were irregular or when melancholic blood was too abundant. This rationale led him to an observation that, while egregious, attested to existing sentiments—and to the common ground between vulgar lore and learned medicine.

> It should be noted that Jews most often suffer a flow of the hemorrhoids for three reasons. They are commonly idle, so that melancholic superfluities accumulate. Second, they are commonly in fear and anxiety, which increases melancholic blood, in accordance with this teaching of Hippocrates, "Fear and timidity, if they last long, produce much melancholy" [*Aphorisms,* 6.23]. Third, it is divine punishment, in accordance with this, "And He struck them in their posteriors, and he gave them everlasting disgrace" [*Psalm* 77:66].

Valesco quoted this excerpt and, while clearly indicating its hearsay character ("Bernard de Gordon says"), he also expanded on it. Jews were idle, he explained, "because they are without corporal labor, for they are neither plowmen nor grave diggers but, rather, they live from moneylending (*ex usuris*) and other mechanical arts, but some from the practice of medicine." They were "in fear about the threats from the Christians to whom they pay taxes."

Such a striking excursus as this, motivated at least in part by the encyclopedist's temptation to include marginalia, should not make us overlook the substance of the discourse on hemorrhoids, in which Bernard and Valesco, like the other compilers, stayed close to the core of medical tradition. A recurrent concern with differentiating anal ailments suggests that complaints were common—and, perhaps, increasing. While Avicenna observed, "one often thinks to have hemorrhoids when having only rectal ulcers," Platearius was more specific. He pointed out that "many who suffer from hemorrhoids are deceived into thinking that they suffer from dysentery or tenesmus, and the reverse," because bleeding was common to all three afflictions. Bernard repeated Avicenna's caveat, but he underscored the importance of an accurate diagnosis.

> It is useful to consider the signs because it often happens that someone believes to have hemorrhoids but it will be tenesmus or fissures or the like; or sometimes one who has them does not believe so because no external swelling appears, but they are inside the anus. It is also beneficial to recognize the responsible humor, so that we know by what method it should be drained.

Draining was imperative, on the authority of Hippocrates, when the natural flow appeared dangerously impeded.

Universal doctrine or, one could argue, dogma dictated that hemorrhoidal bleeding should be allowed, or even brought about in case of plethora. Drainage was especially advisable when the growths were protruding but bloodless, for example, in people who are "sedentary or riding on horseback," as Bartholomeus taught. Once obstructed hemorrhoids were opened, "with a leech or a phlebotome," Bernard believed that the flow should be continued until the patient showed signs of weakening or, in more positive wording, "feels relieved and eats and sleeps better." Copho instructed to stop the flow as soon as these signs turned, by tying off the swelling "with a thread of silk or laurel bark." The least drastic methods included placing the patient in a sitz bath, or over medicinal smoke or steam as recommended by Platearius. He also reported, "it happens sometimes that surgeons burn hemorrhoids that run too much, and these then form scar tissue and become difficult or impossible to open." Bernard prescribed bloodletting from the hepatic vein, cupping with scarification between the shoulder blades, as well as, less drastically—and less counterintuitively—plasters and ointments containing "spider web, very finely cut hare's hair, fish glue and carpenter's glue," and other ingredients.

Aside from the issue of inducing or stemming the flow of blood, hemorrhoids constituted a medical problem to the extent that they caused discomfort, pain, and the risk of complications. They were "generally difficult to treat," as Bernard admitted, for several reasons:

> that part is irregular and wrinkled, and thorough examination is impossible unless it is done by surgeons (*restauratores*), and these are mostly ignorant. In addition, the part is highly sensitive; it is warm, and the path of almost constant wastes; at the same time, it is a "cold" part, devoid of inherent strength. It is situated in the lower body. People are commonly ashamed to bare it.

Even patients who did bare it, Bernard sighed, "are not obedient" to the practitioner. This becomes understandable in the light of his description of some treatment.

Should the hemorrhoid be enlarged, it could be removed with a razor or some caustic agent such as quicklime, atrament, vitriol, or orpiment. It could be pared away with a hair of horsetail, or washed off repeatedly. Ultimately, it may be cauterized with a hot iron, and then we should leave it to the surgeons.

Bernard and other compilers evinced not only an increasing readiness to defer to surgery, but also persistent misgivings about the surgeons' lack of learning, experience, or both. A slight indication of an emerging presence of learned surgeons appears when we compare the *Canon* and the *Viaticum*. In the former, the incision and burning were mentioned without reference to the surgeon, while we read in the latter that, once hemorrhoids became scarred, "they are incurable except by surgery; if the patient is in a place where there is no *master* surgeon, we may apply sharp and cutting medication as if it were iron," that is to say, in lieu of a blade.

The growing acceptance of surgery by physicians may be illustrated, anecdotally, by the changing response to a fig-like anal growth. Bartholomeus noted that hemorrhoids are "commonly also called *ficus*." By Bernard's time, two centuries later, the synonymy was replaced by a distinctive description of *ficus* and the stipulation that "their treatment is relegated to the surgeons," although it was similar to that of hemorrhoids. For various other anal problems, ranging from apostemes and warts to fissures and protrusion, physicians showed little confidence in cure without surgical intervention. Their chief competence lay in providing a differential diagnosis and a reliable prognosis. Their treatment consisted mainly of restoring the humoral balance by diet and medication, slowing down any deterioration, and relieving pain. Fissures and ulcers, described as particularly painful, were sharply distinguished from hemorrhoids, not only because they occurred inside but also because they were entirely against nature and they entailed the double risk of abdominal inflammation and fistula. An accurate diagnosis was equally important when sudden anal or rectal protrusion resulted from trauma because then, Bernard cautioned, "hemorrhoids are sometimes cut carelessly." Protrusion was generally equated with paralysis of the sphincter and considered incurable, unless it was due to the patient's weakness or excess humidity as, most frequently, in children. Copho, after citing what the women of Salerno do for such cases, added "but I tear up rosewood and spread this on the site, or powder from myrtle leaves."

A likely sequela of hemorrhoids and anal fissures and paralysis was fistula, the gravest threat to overall health and to life if feces escaped into the abdomen. For external fecal leakage, Copho recommended the application of leeches and cupping. Once the fistula penetrated a nearby intestine or the bladder, it was beyond cure. Cases of external leakage, Valesco claimed, he had "seen very clearly,"

> most recently, however, in a certain youth who suffered a fistula, after the ulceration and corrosion of one hemorrhoid that was badly treated by unlearned barbers and surgeons. The fistula, too, was badly treated, and virulent pus corroded and penetrated the intestine, for feces came out through an opening away from the anus. I was called too late, [the fistula] was examined, and I judged that he was close to death. This, the Lord permitting, is what happened because he was very weakened by the prolonged illness.

The impersonal phrase, "it was examined" (*fuit visa*), conveys the impression that Valesco delegated the actual examination to an assistant. In the same vein, and notwithstanding his knowledge of inept surgical treatments, he indicated that, if medicinal applications were ineffective and "you wish to operate with iron, once the opening has been enlarged, a well experienced surgeon should cautiously apply actual cautery." A few lines further, however, he offered precise instructions for restorative surgical intervention, with the argument, "although Avicenna and Rhazes present this treatment adequately, modern authors describe it more extensively." Valesco specified what needle and thread to use, how to insert them with a lubricated index finger, how to extract them, "with silver pincers which good operators always have," and how to tie the thread. Bernard displayed a similar ambiguity when he concluded his detailed discussion of fistula with the decision, "from here on, let us leave the treatment entirely to the surgeons." A surgeon indeed, John Arderne (1307–1392), wrote the most famous treatise on anal fistula, *De fistula in ano*.

Liver and Spleen

A section on the instruments of the "second digestion" followed the chapters on the "first digestion" in the Latin compendia, unlike in the *Canon*, where these organs were treated as part of the intestines. By setting apart the instruments that transformed *chylus* into the three primary humors, the compilers led directly into the core of the humoral construct. The liver produced and regulated the blood, the gallbladder stored the yellow bile, and the spleen collected the black bile. These were vital and "noble" organs, yet inaccessible to surgical intervention and to the direct external *or* internal administration of medicine. The paradoxical challenge was matched by a discourse that was more intense but less extensive than the chapters on the intestines. In general, this was the area that depended most patently on traditional doctrine and on conceptual schemes for definitions, diagnosis, and therapeutics. On the other hand, when compilers were preoccupied with concrete practice, they might move directly from stomach problems to kidney stones, as Reinald did in the *Breviarium,* skipping the liver and spleen altogether. After all, the physiology and pathology of these parts remained elusive for several centuries after the Middle Ages. A most remarkable facet of this elusiveness is the minimal knowledge, until the 19th century, of the fabric and function of the gland that the Greek Rufus of Ephesus called "pancreas," or "all flesh"—with the result that, perhaps surprisingly, diabetes will not appear here but in the next chapter.

The liver naturally was the central subject of these chapters, with between 4 and 12 associated diseases, most of which were anatomical or localized, although two systemic ones generated the greatest concern. In covering localized liver afflictions, which ranged from pain to tumors, authors managed to combine a vague notion of anatomy and physiology with a degree of diagnostic precision. Their general outlook is projected in the conventional definition, as abridged by Bernard, "the liver is the first organ and the principle of the production of the humors in the consideration of physicians." The humors, together with complexions and *virtutes,* dominated nosology, etiology, and diagnosis. The domination surged with the expansion of Galen's authority. Chapter-and-verse references to Galen, as well as to Avicenna and Constantine, supported the identification of anatomical features, for instance, by Valesco. Others mentioned such features as the "hump" (*gibbus*) or the "hepatic portal vein" (*porta epatis*), only in passing. Savonarola was a notable exception in sketching the form and composition of the liver, and in hinting at actual dissection. After pointing out that the organ "lies more underneath the ribs in a dead body than in a living one," he invited the student to "pull it down if you wish to see it better." In all compendia, however, conceptual priorities were underscored by the place that a bad complexion held at the head of liver problems. In diagnosis, concepts were responsible for the importance of colored urine as demonstrating the organ's excessive warmth, a livid face as indicating excessive cold, and so on. Even hepatic obstruction and bleeding, unless they were due to trauma or another external factor, were attributed to an imbalanced complexion, the abundance of a humor, or a weakness of the digestive or expulsive faculty.

Humoral etiology led Bernard to dietary concerns when he urged the reader "to understand very carefully that many things injure the liver" by causing obstruction. Among these, he singled out three, namely, foods and drinks that are "intensely sweet," or "coarse and hard to digest," or "softening and moistening" and thus producing watery blood. When he extended the list to "drinking too much cold water, especially in the morning and after vigorous exercise," he came close to suggesting, as Gariopontus and Petrocellus implied, that liver problems might be confused with pleurisy or pneumonia, primarily because they had lateral pain and pressure in common. Bernard's ideas turned more original when he proposed, "the liver is much hurt by one thing to which physicians commonly pay no attention." He explained that, when the patient had a cold stomach or liver, physicians believed that the digestive faculty was fortified by taking a very "warm" confection after eating. The same assumption led to the

> taking of pure wine, or nectar, or Greek wine, or wine from Cyprus, as the rich do immediately after their meal when they enter their bed chambers. These are nothing but poisons, because they make the raw food penetrate into the organs and induce boiling and putrefaction: this is also what Avicenna says; hence these destroy the digestive power of the liver.

Concluding his stern plea against (the pleasure of) a desert wine or after-dinner liqueur, Bernard deemed an aperitif acceptable, "if we wish to fortify the digestive faculty, we may give something before the meal."

Failure of the liver's digestive faculty was a major cause of sclerosis or progressive hardening. This ailment could be diagnosed, Gariopontus taught, "when the hand is placed over the liver, it feels like a stone and does not hurt." As one way to counteract the hardening, "you should order the patients to exercise on an empty stomach, by flexing, that is, kneeling and standing up repeatedly." A related problem was swelling of the liver that, at the onset, could "be cured only with extreme care and adequate diligence." Once the swelling made the liver hard as a stone (a condition which would loosely correspond with the modern category of cirrhosis), Gariopontus believed,

> no medicines can cure it, for I have never been able to or seen anyone able to, because the part is too tender and sensitive to tolerate strong medicines. Some of these patients, however, survive by inertia, prolonging their miserable life; others more quickly reach an end that is preferable to life.

Such fatalism as this did not preclude continued attendance by the practitioner: compilers displayed the same ambivalence here as we have seen for other diseases. Savonarola, for one, asserted that sclerosis, when advanced, "has no cure, and if it has one, it is very difficult," yet he left open the possibility that the advance was slow enough to leave a margin of curability.

A broad disease category that was generally difficult to cure, and that was attributed to hepatic malfunction, was dropsy or *hydropisis,* a term derived from the Greek *hydor,* "water." It is related, though not identical, to the similarly comprehensive category of edema in modern usage, which refers to the swelling of soft tissues from the accumulation of excess water. The category occupied a growing number of folia in the compendia, which makes one wonder whether this was due to an influx of texts—or to a rising incidence of the syndrome and, if so, in which forms and from what causes. Dropsy seems to have been ignored by some Salernitan authors, including Gariopontus and Bartholomeus. Petrocellus mentioned it very casually, as "quite incurable," and he placed the root cause in the prolonged hardening of the spleen. Platearius, however, offered a formal definition, as "an error of the liver's digestive faculty, which causes a swelling of the members." He also clearly listed four kinds, distinguished by the humoral and qualitative imbalance responsible for each. Excessive cold and humidity of the liver caused *leucoflegmantia,* which manifested, predictably, the corresponding marks of white and phlegm; excessive cold and dryness caused *hyposarca* or *anasarca;* warmth and humidity, *ascites;* and warmth and dryness, *timpanites.* Before they became established, the former two kinds were curable, the latter barely; "after confirmation, none of them."

No compiler covered dropsy in greater detail than Gilbert. He began with an amazingly lengthy and philosophical explanation, profusely citing authorities from Aristotle and Pythagoras to Johannitius and Constantine, of the relation between the liver's commutative and digestive faculties in converting the *chylus* or "succus" into the humors. The subject even diverted him into discussions that ranged from "the division of faculties according to physicians" to "the opinion of some that the liver would not be the origin (*principium*) of the blood, except by way of preparation." When at last he returned to the opinions on the kinds of *ydropisis,* he subscribed to the fourfold division. In addition to describing common symptoms, particularly swollen legs and sunken eyes, he provided detailed criteria for a differential diagnosis, beyond the standard recognitions of *timpanites* by abdominal tenseness and of *ascites* by the distention of the abdomen. After devoting many folia to issues related directly and indirectly to dropsy, Gilbert argued a personal thesis, "propria opinio" on the reason why a patient's urine turned livid. In therapeutics, which he also expounded at disproportionate length, he adopted treatments from authors whom he variously identified as ancient physicians, practitioners, and Salernitans.

Bernard equated the true dropsy of *hyposarca* and *leucoflegmantia* as a syndrome identical to swelling of the entire body and as the least malignant. The worst type was *aschitis* or ascites (from *askos,* Greek for water bag; *alchitis* in many manuscripts), which could be diagnosed by the sound of "a bladder half filled with water, as if kwak kwak." In the third kind, *timpanites* or *timpanistes,* the belly was inflated by winds and sounded "like a beaten drum or bladder filled with air." To the Hippocratic aphorism that all dropsy in acute fever is bad, Bernard added, "if dropsy follows chronic fever, patients rarely or never escape." After identifying such signs of impending death as dyspnea and diarrhea, he composed a section of almost 2,000 words on treatment and prevention. Considering the likelihood that many cases of dropsy were due to malnutrition, it seems odd that he ordered that the patients should, "at first, be deprived of food and drink as much as possible." After this, they should follow a special diet and regimen, which Bernard detailed, from chicken soup and parsley to exercise, and to sitting

> in an oven right after the bread has been removed, in order to induce perspiration; or buried in sea sand up to the neck, with the head covered so as not to be harmed by the sun. Or the patient should go to sulfureous or aluminous baths, or heat seawater and bathe in this.

The confidence of one dropsy patient in the cure made a lasting impression on Savonarola. He remembered, "during the time that I was staying at the Baths of Abano with Count Carmignola, I saw someone stay in the bath continuously for ten days; he never left it and he even slept in it, so that all the outer skin of his feet and hands fell off."

Baths constituted a small part of dropsy treatments. Bernard concluded his elaborate therapeutics with remarks that, even if not original, are too illuminating to ignore.

> Ultimately and in despair, and when we see no other way, a two-inch incision should be made for a diagonal opening below the navel; once the first exterior membrane is cut and we reach the interior membrane (*cyphac*), it should be cut below the first wound so that the outer skin covers the opening in the *cyphac* and the water does not come rushing out.

Then, through a carefully introduced tube, the water should be drawn out slowly, a little the first day and so on the next day until all of it was drained; meanwhile, the liver should be fortified with styptic aromatics. The precision of Bernard's instructions becomes most relevant in an afterthought.

> According to Avicenna it would be better to drain this water with medicines that drain by their [entire, inherent or 'occult'] property. It is true that this way life can be prolonged for some time, a month or half a year; afterward, however, the water returns gradually. I have never seen anyone cured completely without dying in the end, and I think that it would be better to administer five or six cauteries below the navel and in the scrotum, so that the watery matter is purged by gradual exudation.

Still not satisfied with his copious prescriptions, Bernard promised to list many more in the pharmacopoeia at the end of his book. His emphasis on medicinal treatment and his reservation toward the draining operation suggest that physicians may have been alarmed by a more widespread and more aggressive recourse to paracentesis.

Savonarola reinforced this suggestion when he expanded Bernard's instructions and added a similar but more involved and risky incision. He vividly recalled the outcome of one actual performance.

> I saw a woman to whom this was done. She was greatly swollen and bloated, and her swelling was reduced in two days. She lived like this for about fifteen days, and she died like this. I certainly think that, because she was a poor wretch, this must have happened to her from a bad regimen and because she was not given help with a restorative regimen. She was around thirty-two years old, but not very robust.

Savonarola (who enlivened this part with enough anecdotes for a separate chapter) informed the reader that the barber who operated on the woman "cured another dropsical woman with his incisions, and thereafter he was called for every case of dropsy." This and other anecdotes illuminate, once more, the ambiguous response to a presumably incurable disease. Valesco attested to the same ambivalence by contradicting skeptics who doubted the effectiveness of some remedies in treating dropsy. "Repudiating their lie, I affirm that, by God's power, I have seen many patients with combined ascites and *hyposarca* cured, most recently a presbyter of thirty-seven who suffered from *timpanistis* and to whom I applied my usual treatment" with a confection and pills that contained the herb mezereum.

Compilers worried less about the curability and lethality—or even about the very issue—of another hepatic problem, namely, *ycteritia,* icterus or jaundice. The latter modern term is derived from "jaune," French for "yellow," in a logical allusion to the agency of yellow bile as well as to the symptomatic yellowing of the skin. However, Copho indicated that there was also a black form of the disease and, by the time of Bernard, the ailment came in three colors: yellow, green, and black. Copho recorded an empirical remedy (*experimentum*) that "a certain woman used for producing a good color," by having the patient inhale the steam of boiling cow milk and fat. Given the importance given to nomenclature by authors, it is significant that the ailment had "many names," as Petrocellus explained,

> but it has two major divisions. One is accompanied by fever, and the Greeks call it *oxites,* the Latins *auriginem* [*auruginem,* from *aurum,* gold]. The other is without fever, and the Greeks call it *comatem,* the Latins *morbum regium.*

It is worth noting that the latter label, "the royal disease," here referred to jaundice, long before it was applied to scrofula, the disease to be cured by the royal touch of English and French kings. This terminological change, in addition to the remark of Petrocellus about many names, reflects the fluid nature of early nosology and the pervasive lack of specificity. The same is true of the hazy identity of black jaundice and, inferentially, the association with black bile and with its reservoir, the spleen.

The constitution, function, and disorders of the spleen received limited attention or, for that matter, understanding from most compilers, the Salernitans in particular. Some saw the spongelike organ as a filter for the blood or as a repository of the black bile that was a by-product of filtration in the liver. Most classified the disorders in the usual scheme of apostemes, obstruction, hardening, weakening, and so on. They attributed spleen ailments to the usual spectrum of external and internal causes, with complexional imbalance again as the dominant factor. Effects were not only physical, such as constipation and other problems of the ileus, but also emotional. Petrocellus, while providing little information about the disorders themselves, claimed, "the patient becomes sad and lazy." Gilbert recommended a confection based on senna for patients who were "melancholic, sad, and forgetful." Among the symptoms, Bernard listed "sadness, fear, worry, frightful dreams, and many similar things that pertain to melancholy." He reiterated the general doctrine that "what benefits the liver benefits the spleen." Nevertheless, he identified several substances that relate to the spleen. He even supplemented these with empirical remedies that "help by their [inherent] property, as Avicenna says: the lung of a fox, of a bat, the spleen of a wild ass, the spleen of a foal, if they are dried and made into a powder." In his clarifying section, Bernard endeavored to explicate the meaning of a celebrated verse as he knew it, "the heart savors, the lung speaks, the gall moves anger, the spleen makes one laugh, and the liver makes one love." He argued, not too persuasively, that the spleen causes laughter to accompany the riddance of the melancholic humor. He was in form, however, when explaining that the liver "makes one love sex" because it produces warmth, one of the three requisites for sex, together with air or *spiritus* from the heart, and moisture from the brain. In this synopsis, Bernard, citing Constantine, captured the essence of what sex meant to the physician, as we will see in the next chapter.

From the Haunches to the Heels, and *Passiones Membrorum Generationis*

The bladder is an innervated organ, like a small sac, composed of nerve-like and ligated fibers, with a fleshy, muscular, and anfractuous neck, supported in men and not in women . . .

Before I proceed to the treatment of diseases of the bladder, be aware that the bladder has considerable connection with royal organs, so that Avicenna says, "Sometimes regal and noble organs, such as the brain, communicate with the bladder." Thus it happens that these suffer intensely from diseases in the bladder, as the brain sometimes suffers vertigo from warm disorders of the bladder, which is an innervated organ with great dependence on the brain, as we have said. Similarly, the liver sometimes incurs dropsy, when cold from a bad complexion of the bladder affects it, because of proximity. Therefore, you should be careful in treating these diseases of the bladder, which usually strike it more in winter, in cold air, and in the North, because a natural complexion makes it prone to falling into a cold imbalance.

In these opening lines of his "Chapter on the conditions of the bladder," Savonarola exemplified the relationship between compilers and their sources, the priority that they gave to practical concerns over theoretical questions, the framework in which they responded to urinary disorders, and the place that they allotted to the bladder in that response.

A word-by-word comparison reveals the derivativeness of Savonarola's lines. Avicenna was the source not only of his acknowledged quotation but also of the more specific ideas about the bladder, including interactions with the brain, the connection with the liver, and the prevalence of problems in winter. This is hardly surprising, since Savonarola was an avowed follower of Avicenna, and he devised his *Practica* as an informal commentary on the *Canon*. And yet, he omitted all six of the invocations with which, in these few lines, Avicenna glorified creation and the Almighty. Savonarola's omission, which can hardly be ascribed to his lack of piety—as will become clear below—was no doubt prompted by his pragmatic objective of making the reader careful in treating. On the other hand, he injected some didactic details into the teaching of the Leader. With regard to the nervous interaction between the bladder and the brain, he emphasized the great dependence of the former on the latter, which was a theme in academic debates about the role of various faculties in urination. With regard to the relationship between the bladder and the liver, Savonarola pointed out the importance of anatomical proximity. His most significant addition was an emphasis on the complexional nature of this relationship and, in particular, on the effect of external cooling factors on an organ that was already cold by its natural complexion.

Kidneys and Bladder

Savonarola was somewhat unusual among compilers in allotting the same number of folios to the bladder as to the kidneys. He was typical, however, in attaching more weight to the construct of complexion than to the concrete intricacies of anatomy and physiology. Before 1300, Gilbert was one of the few compilers to offer a firm, albeit concise or even dense, anatomical description of the kidneys and bladder. He cited Rhazes as his source, but then he seemed to call on observation for proof that constrictive mechanisms prevented urine from flowing back into the ureters or leaking into the urethra. He remarked, "you see that the air does not escape when a bladder is inflated" (he did not mention valves or sphincters, however). In the next chapter, in a subtle play on the varieties of cognition, Gilbert juxtaposed or, rather, interwove rational and empirical learning. He argued,

> insight into the anatomy of the parts is not less useful than the knowledge of doing and helping. Knowledge of anatomy reveals the proper method of treatment and the essence of every internal part. Thus, if through anatomy

we are aware that the lung channels are cartilaginous and the neck of the bladder is innervated, we will at least know how to interpret the information about their ailment.

The "knowledge of anatomy," which Gilbert compared here with apprentice practice, was no doubt primarily conceptual, even bookish. This inference agrees with the explanation, by several compilers, of Galen's tenet that "it is necessary to know anatomy, the *quality* and *essence* of every part." Valesco deduced, "it is good, therefore, to *write* the anatomies of the parts of which we intend to discuss the ailments, in this case, the bladder." Thereupon, he adopted the description from Galen with a reference to "chapter five, towards the end of the fifth column" of the book on *The Usefulness of the Parts of the Body*.

Compilers largely conceived of the urinary system in terms of Galen's teaching, in *The Usefulness of the Parts of the Body* and other treatises, which was neither lucid nor consistent. The general understanding, in any event, was that the watery fluid, which facilitated the passage of freshly produced blood through the veins, became superfluous and burdensome once the entire body was supplied. A "faculty of attraction" (*virtus attractiva*) drew the blood to the kidneys, and these removed the watery residue. The process of this removal left room for confusion, between mechanical filtration as described by Aristotle and extraction or secretion as taught by Galen. It became somewhat easier to imagine Galen's view through analogies with the separation of whey (*serum*) from curdling milk, or with skimming off fat from gravy. In an apparent compromise between the two authoritative notions, Latin medicine adopted the term *colamentum*, "the product of straining"—a translation that is more precise than "the filtrate." The principle that urine was the *colamentum* of the blood supported the position of uroscopy as the most reliable method of diagnosing the humoral status of the entire body, and even of the major organs. The exposition of this rationale was left to the specialized treatises on urines, particularly those by Theophilus Protospatarius, Isaac Israeli, and Gilles de Corbeil. Compilers presented the anatomy and physiology cursorily, if at all; and even those who showed any interest in this subject matter limited themselves to general concepts and to condensing Galen's rationalizations and Avicenna's distinctions.

The crucial role of definitions and explanations, which has become increasingly evident in the preceding pages, makes it easy to see the development of terminology as an organic process with broad implications. Changes in the Latin vocabulary convey a sense of a gradual though not linear movement toward conceptual and thematic precision. Early on, authors hardly distinguished between problems in the lumbar region and in the kidneys. Bartholomeus stated, "pain of the loins (*lumborum*) is called *nefresis* among the Greeks." Limited precision was still evident in the *Breviarium* when Reinald opened his chapter "on the problem of stone in the kidneys and bladder," with the declaration, "In the following pages I intend to deal with ailments of the kidneys, bladder, and testicles, and with [inguinal] hernia." There are also hints of a linguistic shift in Salernitan teaching, or between Salerno and the universities. For instance, Gariopontus kept *nephros,* Greek for kidney, in referring to patients of kidney disease as *nephretici;* later Latin compilers virtually abandoned the term. These compilers similarly discarded *lithiasis* in references to kidney stones, which they called *calculi* or, more commonly, *lapides.* Petrocellus marked the linguistic transition more explicitly when he devoted a chapter "to the treatment of *nefreticorum,* which Latins call 'pain of the kidneys (*renum dolorem*).'"

Already Galen observed that physicians mistook colic pain for renal pain. The difference between both, according to Bartholomeus, was that the former "changes daily from one side to the other," whereas the latter "is stable, and easier to recognize in urine that, unlike in colic, appears sandy, scaly, or bloody." Excess warmth or cold and the accumulation of humors constituted the principal cause of urinary problems, which might actually originate in the liver or spleen. More than half of the treatments of pain, tumors, and ulcers of the kidneys and bladder were based on humoral and complexional allopathy, so that they were too generic to shed light on facets that we have not seen in previous chapters. Most diverse, on the contrary, were "specific" remedies with elusive or occult powers such as resemblance, signatures, or sympathy with the kidneys. Bernard covered the entire therapeutic spectrum, drawing on the vast information that was available in the sources. "Because the noble and the rich frequently suffer pain in the kidneys," he decided, "we will deal with it more in particular and add some factual detail."

Bernard's prescriptions for kidney and bladder ailments were more comprehensive than those for many other complaints, and they ranged from detailed diets to baths and phlebotomy. One of the more curious instructions, for persistent lumbar pain, was to "use a shaking motion, either by running or by riding a horse that jumps and trots." In his dietary and medicinal formulas, he showed a special fondness for one particular item that he mentioned at least a dozen times. "Above all else," he recommended, "use the little bird that is called wagtail, whether fresh or salted, roasted or boiled." Bernard and several other compilers seem to have discovered the medicinal power of the wagtail in the *Canon*. Avicenna, however, depicted the little bird with much greater precision and with delightful details about its plumage, behavior, and habitat. This depiction fascinated the translator of the *Canon,* Gerard of Cremona, enough to make him wonder whether this "bird, which is called *tragulidos* in Greek" matched the one "called *sasuriam* in French." It is not clear when, where, or why the wagtail acquired the reputation of having a "specific" power to cure urinary ailments, particularly stone.

Stone or Calculus

The development of urinary calculi was associated with the kidneys and, secondarily, with the bladder. Authors disagreed, however, about the exact association. Gariopontus reported, "some have said that stone is produced in the urethra, and this is manifestly not true": instead, "it originates and develops in the kidneys," from where it can come down "and contort and close the bladder." Most compilers learned from Galen that calculi, in the general sense, could develop anywhere in the body. Gilbert, who showed a particular interest in lapidary lore, elaborated that stones were also produced in the stomach and in other body parts, "such as the joints of patients with arthritis." Gaddesden illustrated the incidence of calculi in various places with a poignantly personal anecdote.

> I saw a stone, as long as half of the little finger, in my father's mouth, under his tongue. I have shown it in the schools, and I still carry it with me. After treating it with gargles and mouthwashes, I extracted it with a thin knife. In the beginning, I did not know what would come of it; as I found a hard spot there, I believed that it was an aposteme. But because he loved fruits and milky foods all his life, and yellow bile dominated his temperament, I guessed that there was a stone, produced by viscous and milky matter and by complexional warmth.

"An abundance of viscous humors" was the first of "three common causes of calculus which the ancient masters propose," according to Gilbert. The other two were "the closing of pores and meatuses, and the weakness of the expulsive faculty."

"Because of wide pores and the liquidity of the humors," Gilbert believed, "stones occur most rarely in the old." When they did, they were also most resistant to treatment, as Reinald declared on the authority of Hippocrates: "note that it is difficult or impossible to free old patients, past their fortieth year." The effects of aging led Gilbert to propose, in passing, "the old suffer deficiency in three parts in particular, namely the brain, the lung, and the bladder." As their brain grows cold, "they become sleepy as a result of blocked pores; in addition, they abound in rheums, running of the nose, and denseness of the senses." Explanations of disparities according to age and gender, however, were quite inconsistent. Physiology accounted for a lower incidence of calculus in the old, but anatomy explained why women were much less susceptible than men. By long-standing consensus, summarized by Gaddesden, "stone in the bladder rarely occurs to girls and women because, unlike in men, the meatus of their bladder is shorter, wider, and less anfractuous; in short, it expels easily." Extending the role of anatomy, Gilbert further specified, "women suffer from stone in the kidneys but not in the bladder, because the neck of their bladder is short and wide."

Gaddesden cautioned against overestimating the advantage of feminine anatomy. He qualified the consensus with an expression of reserve: "from one woman, however, I saw a stone extracted that was almost as large as a hen's egg." Valesco reported an anecdote more animatedly, as proof that "it is undeniably possible for a stone to be produced in the kidneys and bladder of women." He recalled,

> I saw a woman of almost fifty who was so incontinent that urine was discharged from the neck of the bladder as continuously as it ran through the ureters. This happened because some unlearned surgeon had extracted two stones from her bladder by cutting in the neck of the bladder and, in the process, cutting the muscle that closes this neck. Those stones were whitish, and one was the size of a dove's egg, the other the size of a goldfinch's egg.

It is paradoxical that, in spite of a sustained focus on anatomy in explaining gender difference, Valesco showed limited awareness of the two sphincters controlling urination.

The prostate, too, was unknown until the 16th century. This may raise the question whether an inflammation or growth of the gland, benign or malignant, was ever diagnosed as stone. The compendia offer no support for this possibility, which has profound implications with regard to surgical interventions and stonecutters. Vague clues, which await systematic collection, may lie hidden, for example, in frequent allusions to prolonged, vigorous, or incorrect horseback riding. It seems plausible that prostate problems fell under apostemes around the neck of the bladder that caused "violent pain, like the pain of a woman giving birth," according

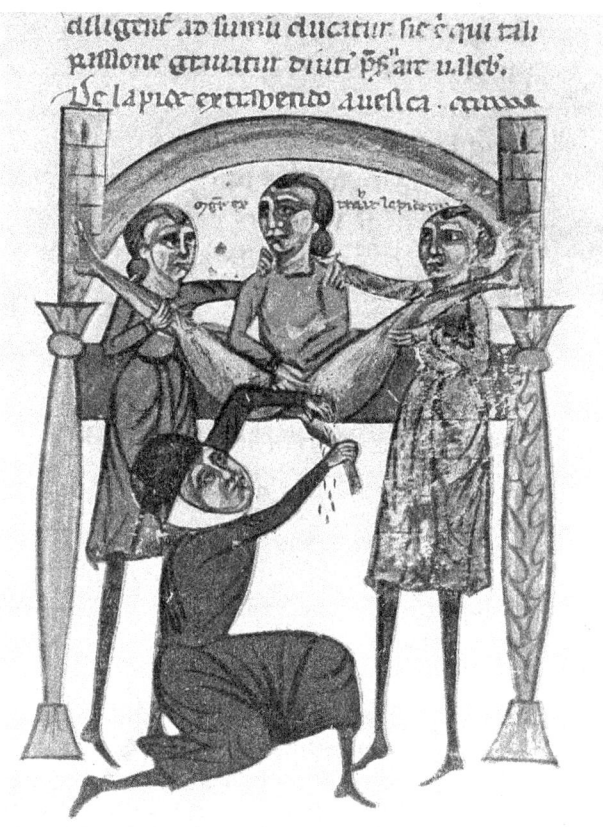

"The master extracts a stone" in "the Celsan operation" for bladder stone, performed from the rear. Miniature in an early 14th-century manuscript of Rolandus Parmensis, *Chirurgia*, fol. 23v. (Wellcome Library, London. Wellcome Images L0011173)

to Bernard. Some authors were aware of possible confusion between stone and an abnormal growth of tissue. Gilbert warned, "one should see that it is not, instead, tissue growing in the neck of the bladder from some wound." He illustrated the point with a case.

> A certain man suffered from this problem, with pain in the urinary passage. When we inserted a probe, we found that there were wounds in that site, for when they were touched by the probe, soon urine was discharged, then a little blood and a bit of flesh. This is relevant to our intention in this book.

The nature of growths in or around the bladder orifice seems to have been the subject of some debate, for Gilbert continued, "whatever the moderns investigate belongs more to dialectic than to reason, since it is of no help to us in medicating. Nothing pertains more to the practice of physicians than knowing with utmost certainty whether obstruction of the urine results from a stone or from coagulated blood."

Careful verification could prevent confusion between calculus and an abnormal growth of tissue. The examination was exceptionally thorough before an attempt to excise the stone, as in Savonarola's instructions for examining the patient before proceeding to surgery.

> Before you commit to an incision, you should consider diligently whether or not a stone is present. While two fingers of the right hand are introduced into the anus, with the left fist you press the abdomen down toward the thigh. If you feel something like a hard lump, you may assume that it is a stone; but if what you find is soft, it is fleshy tissue (*carnositas*) that obstructs the urine.

These instructions may be correlated with Savonarola's observation that cold apostemes of the bladder "occur mostly near the neck," and that these, "particularly the hard ones, sometimes lead to dropsy"—a possible suggestion of systemic deficiency as an ultimate result of cancer?

The compilers also took pains in outlining the differential diagnosis of kidney and bladder stones, and of the developmental stages, with full appreciation of the prognostic and therapeutic ramifications. The major distinction, obviously, lay in the nature and area of pain: for renal stones, stinging in the lumbar region; for bladder stones, pain in the lower abdomen and pubic area, with an urge to urinate. For kidney stone, Gilbert and others added such symptoms as "sleeping of the thighs and formication of the legs, and of the foot on the side" of the affected kidney. It was possible to recognize the provenance of a discharged stone, Bernard taught, because one from the bladder was whiter, larger, and harder, while one from the kidneys was softer, smaller, and reddish. In addition, he claimed that there was a predictive factor, because "kidney stone occurs more in the obese and the old, because their expulsive faculty is weak; bladder stone, in contrast, occurs more in the emaciated, children, and youths, because their expulsive faculty pushes it further along." It was possible to determine the stage in the growth of a calculus, and hence the usefulness of diuretics, by the amount of sand in the urine. Turbid urine signified that a stone was either growing or dissolving while, subsequently, thin and painful urination indicated blockage. This process, too, was debated among the authors. Gilbert contradicted Maurus of Salerno, for example: "it is not true what he [Maurus] said, about sand indicating the formation of a stone, because intensified warmth may be dissolving loosely coagulated matter." The dual therapeutic implication was that diuretics remained effective when sand was present and that "warm" remedies promoted the dissolution of a stone.

Therapeutic chapters on kidney and bladder stones, like those on other ailments, covered the objectives of prevention, pain relief, removal of the cause, and the restoration of health. Although often not clearly separated, the objectives were supposed to be pursued in this Hippocratic order. A preventive regimen was particularly urgent for anyone who had a patient among immediate relatives and who was thereby predisposed to stones. The family connection was so well noted that, at least since Avicenna, calculus was characterized as a hereditary disease. The daily management of the six nonnaturals was a priority not only in prevention but also in remediation. "It would be ridiculous," Valesco stressed, "to begin working with medicines unless the diet is considered first, in due order." The most surprising aspect of dietary instructions, whether preventive or remedial, was the limited concern with sufficient fluid intake, notwithstanding the universal recognition that viscosity was a key factor in the formation of calculi. Guidelines were silent on the quantity of liquids to be taken, but specific on their quality. Wine should be white and light; water, as Bernard instructed, "should be fresh, clear without turbidity, and from a spring that is open and runs eastward." The pea broth or pea juice that was widely recommended as potage must have been different from the proverbially thick and turbid pea soup.

The negative side of preventive regimens contained an extensive range of banned foods. At the head of the list, naturally, stood fatty or salted meats, including beef and goat as well as goose and duck. The ban on fish without scales extended, for Valesco, to "big wild ones, such as whale, dolphin, and tuna; and all those that lack scales, such as eels, dace, lamprey, and ray." Most authors agreed that cheeses should be avoided, although some singled out old cheese and others young cheese. They also frowned on legumes, with the exception of peas. On the positive side of dietary advice, no items ranked higher than radishes, asparagus, celery, sage, and similar vegetables and herbs. Valesco offered a glimpse into his own preferences.

> This is what I usually do when red grains of sand appear at the bottom in the urine flask: first, in the early morning, one should take the decoction of peas, of rue with the leaves, of parsley root, together with spikenard. Next,

one should place about one-fourth handful of parsley leaves in water that is boiling with meats or something, and then take it with vinegar on an empty stomach. This should be continued for ten days: it cleanses the urinary channels and opens small obstructions in the liver.

Valesco here illustrated therapeutic practices that lay on the border between the prevention and the remediation of stone, as was typical for most regimens. Mitigating treatment, in turn, lay in an area between dietetics and medication. Indeed, many powders, poultices, and purges ran on a continuum of targets, from discomfort to acute pain, and from reversible stone formation to critical urinary obstruction.

A "real cure" of stone, Bernard noted, "is extremely difficult, so that no one should take offense if we pursue it with the utmost diligence and in greater detail." Medicinal treatment was two-pronged, with approaches that may be called, with some liberty, allopathic and homeopathic. Cures by contraries were adaptations of the general therapeutic pattern and therefore not very revealing. They consisted mainly of simples and compounds, administered internally or applied externally, to correct a complexional imbalance, purge a harmfully viscous humor, or fortify a weak expulsive faculty. Remedies with an essential or specific affinity for calculus, on the other hand, constituted a cornucopia of pharmaceutical lore. Some seemed to be effective because they were exotic and expensive. "If the patient is rich," Gilbert suggested for one recipe, "a little balsam may be added." Most of the "specific" remedies were herbal, animal, or mineral simples with a God- or Nature-given affinity for kidneys, the bladder, or stone. This specificity might be signified by their appearance, their behavior, or even their name. The attribution of the special power to a substance was often of unknown origin. The reputation tended to grow on itself, boosted by such reports as Reinald's anecdote about goldenrod (*virga aurea*), "I saw an empirical remedy (*experimentum*) in a patient with bladder stone who ate this herb with eggs, every morning for nine days. The calculus was broken, and he showed me his hand full of small stones." No herb was more common in urinary therapies than saxifrage or rock breaker—historians do not agree whether the name once referred to a species that grew in rocky cracks or was simply derived from its common use in prescriptions for lithiasis.

A remarkable group of specific remedies consisted of various stones and forms of petrification, which occasionally also appeared in remedies for dissolving calcium deposits or hard tumors elsewhere in the body. These were items that, in Bernard's words, "marvelously break the stone thanks to their specific property." The most noteworthy were Jews' stone (*lapis judaicus*), a club-shaped spine of a fossilized sea urchin; spongestone or the stone that was described as "found in sea sponge" (a possible confusion with coral); and agate. "Also valuable," Gilbert claimed, "is the stone found in the joints of an old rooster or in the bladder of a pig; or even human calculi, which may be given in warm water, every third day." When Gaddesden recorded the actual application of an apparently traditional treatment for crushing calculus, he raised implications that stretch as far as modern medical ethics—*and* psychology, logic, and sensitivities.

> Avicenna says that fine white glass, burned and pulverized, should be given in white wine or barley water. I have frequently applied this remedy, but I do not tell patients what the powder is made from, because they would not be cured, and they would say that a man wanted to kill them with glass in the same manner as one kills a dog. They are deceived, however, because the glass does not kill dogs except that these ingest it whole and with some grease that then stays in the stomach and cannot be discharged: if it were pulverized it would not harm them except by causing slight dryness.

Therefore, Gaddesden concluded, "the glass given to humans should be minutely pulverized, and be sweetened with sugar so that it does not cause excessive dryness."

More ordinary ingredients, among which saxifrage was omnipresent, made up many pulverized compounds. Bartholomeus praised one such powder with the assurance, "if anyone wishes to prove the efficacy of this antidote, place a stone under the powder in a glass vial, and leave it there for one day and night, and when you come to look for it the second day, you will find it in pieces." There was "the powder proven to break the stone, which was used by Pope Eugenius" according to Reinald. Gilbert, too, advertised this remedy as "the powder of Pope Eugenius." Since this was presumably Eugenius III, pope from 1145 to 1153, it is likely that Gilbert and Reinald drew on a 12th-century source. Reinald recorded prescriptions for several other celebrated types of compounds, including an electuary experienced by the pope's physician, and

> a marvelous syrup compounded for the treatment of the king of the Franks by several masters and philosophers [*sic*]. It breaks kidney and bladder stone, opens the urinary passages, and dissolves clots; in short, it resolves all heaviness of the kidneys, it cleanses, and it expels anything thick or lapideous.

The recipe contained more than three dozen ingredients, in an extreme example of polypharmacy, presumably for the dual purpose of impressing the royal patient and making sure that all possibilities were covered. Gaddesden, on the contrary, needed no exotic substances for a syrup that he advertised as "excellent for breaking and bringing out a stone, and for soothing the pain: I call it 'radish syrup', and it has given me immense honor in a case of stone that others had given up, as I cured the patient with just this remedy."

The most exotic ingredients were compounded in precious oils for liniments. One oil, most highly prized because of Avicenna's approval, was made with scorpions and cantharides. Gaddesden, however, found that such oils are expensive, and he advertised substitutions that he used in treating "a patient with stone whom I had been unable to cure for a long time." He described the treatment in detail.

> I had someone collect many beetles that are found in the dung of cattle in summer, and crickets that sing in the fields. I placed the crickets, after their heads and wings were removed, in a ceramic jar, together with the beetles. After stopping up the jar, I placed it in an oven that had recently contained bread, and I let it sit there for a day and a night. Then I took out the jar and warmed it a little over a fire, squashed everything together, and smeared it onto the kidneys and pubes. In three days the pain ceased and the stone came out, broken and pulverized.

It is of interest to observe that the procedure was clearly Gaddesden's own even though he adopted some such conventional rituals as using an oven from which newly baked bread had been removed. For another recipe, he claimed to have personally verified the effectiveness of fox blood, which Constantine prescribed for an ointment on the pubes: "for proof, place a stone in it and it will be resolved in three days, as I have experienced. I also have made this blood to be dried for a powder, and it has cured patients with calculus."

Medicines for stone were also administered internally, not only by mouth but also by rectum in enemas by clyster, and even through the urethra, by means of a lubricated catheter (*syringa*). Gaddesden prescribed to "put a louse in the opening of the penis, or the bug which is called *cimice* in French and which stinks when crushed, or a flea may be put there"; this would be a most startling method of introducing medication, were it not for indications that "*in* the opening" was an erroneous transcription for "on" or "near," as it occurs in various remedies for provoking urination (mentioned, for instance, by Reinald and Bernard). Some external applications, particularly of plasters, were supposed to loosen or dislodge a stone, but most aimed at alleviating the pain. Bernard recommended applying, to the pubic area, a sponge soaked in water in which sulfur had been boiled, in the event that "sulfur baths were not readily available." Reinald was personally acquainted with taking the waters.

> One should use the bath of Prata, which is on the seashore between Naples and Pozzuoli. The use of this bath is as follows: drinking the water, or taking a syrup that is compounded with this water and sugar, breaks the stone right away. I have seen many who tried this, and I have often seen that they were freed of kidney and bladder stone by the power of this bath.

Two systemic therapies that may seem more drastic, yet that often were part of prevention as well as treatment, were bloodletting and the induction of vomiting.

The most localized interventions were manual, either by dislodging the stone and removing it through the natural passage or by extracting it through an incision. In the most rudimentary manipulation, described by Bartholomeus, "the patient should lie down so that the kidneys are higher than the head, and the abdomen should be moved around the pubic area so that the stone falls from the neck [where it blocks the urine flow] into the bladder cavity." Bernard offered more detail about the occasion and method of this simple—and, literally, inverted—treatment.

> If the patient is unable to urinate, either because the stone is large and obstructs the meatus, or because it is small and has entered the opening of the penis, these are the localized remedies: let the body be positioned so that the head is down; shake, rub, and press the bladder; and then the stone will descend from the passage and he will be able to void. This will be a temporary remedy. Or else, a finger may be inserted into the rectum to squeeze the stone.

When Reinald mentioned the digital rectal insertion, he added, "as is done by those surgeons who cut the patient for stone, and of whom I do not approve, for it is dangerous and deadly, so that any decent physician will not consent to this." Bernard moved from disapproval to denial when, at the end of his section on therapeutics, he noted, "at this time I completely omit the treatment of stone by surgical hand." Learned surgeons did describe and perform such treatment, but they showed awareness of the great risk, and they insisted on proceeding with extreme caution.

Wandering lithotomists, on the contrary, may have been brazen enough to attempt "incision of the iliac region and in the back, which is against reason," as Gaddesden warned.

Diabetes and Other Urination Problems

Surgery was of no avail for diabetes, which the authors recognized as a chronic and deadly disease, but which they understood and treated unevenly. They were divided in the emphasis of their definitions and, somewhat less, in the thrust of their etiologies. One group, which reached from Platearius, Gilbert, and Reinald to Savonarola, adhered to a Galenic outlook that may be called "instrumentalist." They characterized diabetes as, "in sum, a bad disposition of the kidneys," in the words of Savonarola. Half of the disorder lay in a hyperactive renal *virtus attractiva,* which was due to "intemperate warmth and dryness of the loins," and which drew too much urine from the liver to the kidneys. The complementary problem lay with weakened kidneys that exerted insufficient *virtus retentiva* to control the flow of urine. Savonarola explained, "everything that is likely to weaken the kidneys and to dry them too much can be an actual cause of diabetes; this includes excessive sexual intercourse, as I have seen in old Andrea de Anselminis." He dropped this name so casually in making his point, that the libidinous reputation of the Paduan nobleman must have been fully established.

Compilers in a second group, which included Bernard and Valesco, seem to have been more directly influenced by Avicenna in their definitions of diabetes, which emphasized profuse urination and intense thirst as hallmarks. Different accents, however, did not preclude continuity in the authoritative tradition, as Valesco showed by stating, "Avicenna and *we,* the others *who follow Galen* in Book Six, Chapter Three of *De interioribus* ['On the Affected Parts']," compare urinary diabetes with intestinal lientery. From definition to treatment and clarification, Valesco demonstrated greater than usual dependence on Avicenna, who, ironically, discussed diabetes less thoroughly than several other urinary disorders. The limitations, which Avicenna and Valesco had in common, may suggest a broader paradox in medical views of diabetes. Several authors combined a vague understanding of the disease with an awareness of its serious effects. This paradox dovetails with the degree of ambivalence displayed by Salernitan compilers.

Gariopontus spent less than 100 words on "*diapnis,* that is, the ailment of the bladder from a frequent discharge of urine," which made the patient emaciated and pale. *Diapnis* was no doubt a distortion of the labels *dyampnis* and *diamnis* that other authors applied to urinary incontinence. Petrocellus observed that diabetes "has many names: some call it incurable dropsy, others diarrhea, others *diapides,* and others *diapsacoy.*" He further asserted, "this ailment seldom occurs in humans, but when it comes about, they feel an immeasurable weakness in the kidneys." Bartholomeus attributed the "immoderate flow" to an intemperate warmth "of the kidneys and loins," causing a "constant passing or distillation of urine to the bladder, which exhausts the liver and intestines." Platearius similarly placed the liver at the center of his terse account, which led to the therapeutic conclusion, "diabetic patients need to be helped immediately." It is significant that Reinald, while presenting an almost identical account, lumped diabetes together with the far less grave issue of bedwetting.

The crucial symptom for distinguishing diabetes from other forms of abundant urination, was thirst. This thirst was incessant, unlike the thirst that, according to Savonarola, affected big gluttons after too much food and drink. Bernard viewed this unquenchable thirst as analogous to the insatiable hunger of canine appetite, and he added other distinctive signs, including a warm feeling in the kidneys. We are left with the intriguing question, whether any diagnosis in the compendia hinted at the seemingly inevitable association with a sweet taste that, after all, led Thomas Willis in 1675 to designate the disease as *mellitus,* "honeyed." In the earliest printed versions (1492 and 1502) of the *Rosa medicine,* Gaddesden appeared to state that diabetes "is called 'candepisse' in English," which would indicate that common people recognized the sweetness of urine as a distinctive symptom. This is a tantalizing hint, especially since neither Gaddesden nor any other compilers mentioned a characteristic of taste or smell as a diagnostic criterion. The supposed hint in the *Rosa* vanishes, however, and it is replaced by a puzzling incongruity, when we check the manuscripts. In at least three early manuscripts, the original statement referred to what "is called 'chaudepisse' *in French."* This was—or, at least, became—the term for blennorrhea, a mucous discharge (as in gonorrhea) that has nothing in common with diabetes except the point of discharge.

There was general agreement on the dire prognosis of diabetes. Gilbert stated, "this disease is conducive to dropsy or hectic fever because," as he explained further, "the substantial moisture, unable to be restrained, flows out with the urine." Valesco, Savonarola, and others credited Avicenna with the illogical-sounding explanation that the *loss* of liquid led to the body's melting, *liquefactionem* or *liquationem.* In any event, Bernard warned that the disease "wastes and weakens the body and the legs, bringing ruin if it continues without remediation." With excessive warmth as the dominant cause, treatment consisted primarily in cooling the kidneys, the abdomen, or the entire body. For topical treatment, Platearius instructed to "apply to the kidneys a lead sheet, perforated with minute holes so that the resolved smokiness may escape"; this remedy had a long history and more curious applications, as we will see later. For systemic drainage, Bartholomeus ordered to "induce sweating by artifice." Petrocellus cited Rufus of Ephesus, an author of the late-first century, as "confirming that it greatly helps patients to drink and immediately vomit up the coldest water or drink that they are able to find." The conventional character of diabetes treatments, together with the scarcity of personal reminiscences or testimonials, may indicate that success or even experience with the disease was limited. Reinald did not make an exception to this pattern when, in keeping with his earlier mentioned fusion of two ailments, he praised "my master's troches, with which I cured a youth who suffered from diabetes and who involuntarily urinated in bed."

Authors commonly identified three factors as causing incontinence, whether while awake or in sleep. The most obvious cause of occasional incontinence was irritation of the bladder nerves by cold, "as happens to clients (*clientibus*) who are poorly dressed and who walk barefoot on snow and ice in winter." A second factor, more often responsible for chronic incontinence, was the softness of weak bladder muscles, as in infants and the infirm. Valesco threw a harsh light on the effects of this condition on the victims.

> The signs are evident enough, because they urinate without will or awareness, and their bed and clothes smell bad unless they are changed all the time. It is incurable in decrepit persons because their faculties are already weakened, and also because they receive little care: they are resented by their heirs; if they have no possessions they are even more detested by their children, maids, and servants, and even by their spouse and nearest kin.

This poignant observation showed that urinary incontinence, while not a grave disease in itself, could be socially devastating.

A third major cause, particularly of nocturnal incontinence, was imagination. In Bernard's analysis, the sleeping patient "imagines being in the latrine where he or she is used to urinate, and then the imaginative faculty commands the expulsive faculty, so that he or she urinates in bed, intending to be somewhere else." He instructed to "decorate and beautify the room so that, in the daytime, he or she will abhor urinating there." Other compilers added graphic details to their instructions for psychological deterrence. Gaddesden wanted "crucifixes to be hung on the wall." Valesco urged, "place a wooden or iron crucifix there, so that he or she will at least feel shame or fear God and not urinate on the crucifix." Savonarola assured that children would outgrow bedwetting, but "if the patient is a male adult, he should be rebuked with sharp words while being led into the place where he has been urinating; if it is the bed, place the image of some saint in it, or something sacred worthy of such reverence that, when he remembers it, he will be ashamed to urinate."

Allusions to male patients, occupations, and organs further accented the gender bias in chapters on other urination problems. Bartholomeus differentiated *disuria* from diabetes by the cold that a patient felt "in the area of the testicle and penis." He explained that complete or partial urinary blockage could be due to a variety of causes, aside from a stone or tumor, but that it often occurred spontaneously. The worst,

> called suffocation of the bladder, happens to those who, while attending an assembly of nobles, hold their urine longer than they should. The neck, veins, and nerves of their bladder become full and swollen, and the urinary passage becomes obstructed so that afterward, when they want to urinate, they are unable to.

Bernard combined physical and mental explanations in the case of "someone who is in a venerable place and does not want to move; then the bladder fills up, dilating upwards and constricting below," with the result that the urethra locks.

The categories of urinary dysfunction typified the instability of the medical taxonomy and the indistinctness of the nomenclature. Unlike the modern label "dysuria," which refers primarily to painful and burning urination, *disuria* designated temporary difficulty or inability. The "burning sensation (*ardor*) of urine" merited a separate chapter for Valesco. He noted,

> this ailment sometimes comes in the middle of good health, so that men are greatly vexed and kept from their business and activities. Therefore, we must attend to them immediately so that the business is not delayed, and so that they do not lapse into ulceration. When I was a student in Paris, I saw a youth who was burdened by burning urination, and who was cured simply by eating pears from Caluau and drinking spring water.

Valesco then cited a potion that his erstwhile teacher, Jean de Tournemire, obtained from Arnau de Vilanova's *Practica* for Pope Clement. Arnau had treated Clement V (reigned 1305–1314) for stone (and claimed to have cured him of gout). Therefore, Valesco's reference hints at the overlaps between treating such internal ailments as stone, and treating symptoms, in this case urination difficulties, as diseases in themselves. For some of these difficulties, such as the painful drop-by-drop urination of strangury, the underlying problem might not even be mentioned. For another symptom, namely, bloody urination (now called hematuria), Gilbert appeared satisfied with a blurred taxonomy. He reminisced about

> a knight who suffered from diabetes caused by cold, and who had an accumulation of blood with a large tumor in the area of the bladder. I gave a medicine sharpened with scammony: he urinated once between bowel movements, a cupful of blood, and he was cured of the tumor or of whatever ailment or distress.

The Reproductive Organs

In the unlikely event that the gender bias in compendia has not yet become obvious, it will be written large in the following pages on the *membra generativa*. This will be a rather condensed survey because, for one thing, sex is an aspect of medieval medicine that has received ample attention. Moreover, the discussion of reproduction, which usually concluded the head-to-heel sequence of the manuals, expanded substantially over the course of four centuries; it developed toward deeper philosophical contemplation; and it included more citations of Aristotle, Galen, and Avicenna. This development enhanced the prominence of teleology, primary qualities, and *virtutes* or faculties. In particular, it underscored the complexional roles of the brain, heart, and liver, not only in sustaining individual life but also in continuing the species. This emphasis, in turn, found expression in more frequent tributes to the Creator's genius and Nature's ingenuity, warnings about moral implications, and undertones of the traditional gynophobia. Perspectives shifted, substantially if unevenly, between the pragmatic Gariopontus and the prolix Savonarola. Sexual *appetitus,* a stock term for Constantine, and pleasure (*delectatio*), a key notion for Platearius, were eclipsed, first by "desire" (*desiderium*) and then by "concupiscence," a term favored by Savonarola. The organs that were "made for performing coitus" according to Bartholomeus, became "generating parts" for Gilbert, and "instruments of reproduction" for Bernard. Petrocellus focused on problems with "the venereal operation," while Valesco reflected a heightened concern with infertility.

Gilbert's *Compendium,* which was written after an influx of new Latin translations from Greek and Arabic, represented a conspicuous watershed in the development of reproductive medicine. It was the first manual that both incorporated and exceeded the teaching of Constantine in the treatise *On Coitus,* even though this treatise continued to exert a profound influence. Gilbert collated various schools of thought, which he repeatedly introduced as sectarian, with the qualifying phrase, "some claim." He discussed issues of natural philosophy that his Salernitan predecessors had largely omitted but that drew much debate in the university milieu. One of these was the divergent teaching, within the authoritative tradition, about the origin of sperm, which one theory (later called "pangenesis") placed in the entire body and others in more circumscribed sources. Valesco illustrated both the contemporary fascination with this question and his preoccupation with concise comprehensiveness.

> Many arguments can be made for either side, but I omit them for the sake of brevity. It should be known, though, that this question has been debated of old, for the first philosopher posed it. Plato bathed in his bath. Empedocles, in his own opinion, believed to settle the issue but he failed, according to Aristotle who chewed on it a lot. Even Albert [Albertus Magnus, d. 1280] commented on it. For me as a scholar (*michi autem clerico*), however, it is sufficient to refer you to them—and to pass over this like a cat over coals.

Earlier, Gilbert was drawn more deeply into the controversy, although he did not make a clear and unambiguous choice. He did not subscribe to pangenesis, yet he seconded one of its chief premises, namely, the traits shared by progenitors and offspring, when he declared, "this is why we judge scholars (*clericos*) with stout legs to be sons of fullers, and those with thin legs and big shoulders and arms to be sons of soldiers."

Gilbert, as a typical compiler, often refrained from taking sides in controversies of natural philosophy. This resulted in an ambiguous position on one of the most consequential questions about sperm, gender, and conception. He favored Galen's teaching—that men and woman produced sperm—over Aristotle's view of woman as a passive receiver, yet he deemed it necessary to underscore the Aristotelian dichotomy of form and matter.

> Just as in a hen's egg, produced from fat and superfluity, without the rooster's seed there is nothing coagulated, nothing that could make *pepansis* [cake, fruit, placenta]—meaning its like in nature—, or that would have the potential of reproducing. An egg is material only, and so woman's sperm is nothing formal but only material, nourishing and preserving man's sperm.

It is worth contrasting Gilbert's ambiguity with forceful endorsements of the two-seed doctrine by other authors. Valesco, for one, asserted, "physicians say truthfully, with Galen, that both man and woman have sperm, not merely in name but in the same sense." Gilbert, to the contrary, implied male exclusivity in his discussion of the Hippocratic proposition that two juvenile veins behind the ears carry sperm from the brain. Be that as it may, when Gilbert concluded his complex discussion, he proved that he remained conscious of his medical objective. After admitting the possibility that the germ in sperm came "not entirely from the brain, as some claim, but equally from the heart and liver," he decided, "let us set this aside for debate."

Bernard demonstrated, albeit circuitously, the relevance of philosophy to practice in his introduction to Book Seven of the *Lilium,* "On the Ailments of the Reproductive Organs in Both Sexes."

> Everything is complete when it is able to generate its like, thus becoming like a divine and immortal being, according to Aristotle in the second book *On the Soul.* This is why Avicenna, in the *Sixth Book On the Natural Faculties* [also known as *On the Soul*] glorified the reproductive power for allowing to be preserved in its like what could not be preserved in itself. Thus, for the sake of reproduction, blessed and almighty God "created them male and female" [*Genesis* 1:27].

Keeping his philosophical introduction markedly more concise than either Gilbert or Savonarola, Bernard continued immediately with a deft synopsis of basic reproductive anatomy and physiology.

> The instruments of reproduction in the male are the testicles and the penis (*virga*), in the female the womb and its orifice (*os*) and two testicles on the horns of the womb. Three things are necessary for sexual union (*coytus*): warmth, windy spirit, and moisture. According to Avicenna, feeling comes from the brain, spirit and wind from the heart, and blood and desire from the liver. Natural desire comes partly from the kidneys and the liver, with a complement from the heart. Who has all these is fruitful by nature.

This conceptual outline, which contained nothing original, was the basis for an equally conventional depiction of sex that, however, would lead directly into practical applications.

Tightening his focus on the chief target, Bernard summarized the manner of reproduction as follows.

> When the male desires naturally, on account of the accumulated seed, when the digestion in the stomach and liver is completed and the third underway, and when nothing else outside or inside prevents it, then one for whom it is licit should spread his seed into the womb only, and not in any other opening, in accordance with the law of God and Nature. When the sperms join and are retained, this is when conception takes place.

This summary was followed immediately by a schedule of the medical ramifications, which also drew up the contents of the chapters.

> As the combination of all these things causes fruitfulness, so a deficiency causes sterility. If moisture abounds while the rest is lacking, the result is *gomorrea;* if windy spirit abounds but not the rest, satyriasis; if warmth is lacking together with the rest, sterility. Hence a title for this chapter may be "on the cold and bewitched," or "on impotence," or "on sterility from the part of the male," or "chapter on the deficiency of coitus."

This is how Bernard made an almost seamless transition, from reproduction in general to male reproductive disorders, and from the physiology of sex to the taxonomy that guided the organization of the subject matter, not only in the *Lilium* but also in later compendia.

Conditions of the Reproductive Organs in Men

Under this title, Savonarola lined up no fewer than 34 rubrics, which in substance were the equivalent of chapters in other manuals. His coverage is outlined in the right-hand column of Table 8.1. Rather than entering anachronistic translations or crowding the columns with elucidations, I have retained (without adding quotation marks) the authors' original terms, of which the meaning will become clear in the following pages. An elementary purpose of Table 8.1 is to give an idea of the similarities and differences among compilers in discussing male reproductive disorders, and particularly in arranging the aspects—and in inserting the subject matter into the context of their manuals (shown in the first and last lines of each column).

Table 8.1 Contents of sections on the (male) reproductive organs

Gariopontus	Platearius	Gilbert	Bernard	Savonarola
incontinence	involuntary urination	hernia	Dysuria	Hematuria
Gonorhea		aproximeron & natura spermatis	paucitas coitus	*Rubrica. 1* anatomia & complexio membrorum
satyriasis	emissio involuntaria		satyriasis & priapismus	*Rubr. 2–11* testes & vasa
priapismus	erectio involunatria	satyriasis	gomorrea	*Rubr. 12–13* sperma
apoximeron	aproximeron	gomorrea	pollutio nocturna	*Rubr. 14* gomorrea & pollutio
satyriasis & gonorhea	inflatio testiculorum		passiones virge	*Rubr. 15–25* dispositiones virge
satyriasis & gonorhea	pustule in virga		apostemata testiculorum	*Rubr. 26–27* satyriasis & impotentia
				Rubr. 28–33 coitus
				Rubr. 34 hermaphrodita
sciatica	retentio menstruorum	hernia	hernia	muliebria

Table 8.1 also indicates the expanding volume of the discussion; this expansion was, of course, but a small part of much broader developments in medical writing between the 11th and 15th centuries. Nevertheless, Table 8.1 projects a reliable image of a changing purview, from specific disorders to organs and functions. Furthermore, the column for Gariopontus matches the fact that he devoted four times as many lines to satyriasis, priapism, and *gonorhea* (three similar categories in his view) as he allotted to *apoximeron* or *aproximeron,* that is, impotence. On the other hand, the column for Gilbert gives no measure of his fascicle-length philosophical discourse on "the nature of sperm," which is nestled in his chapter on impotence. Similarly, the entries can indicate only indirectly that compilers dedicated a relatively small portion of this section to apostemes, ulcers, warts, and similar afflictions of the penis and testicles, for which they cross-referred to parallel passages in other sections.

Savonarola began his description of the male reproductive organs with praise for the decision of "Divine Providence" to preserve the human species and for accomplishing this "beautifully by creating two testicles as principal organ for producing the seed, one independent of the other." In women, the glands "are minute and, according to several, not called testicles even though according to the physicians they are true testicles." Four centuries earlier, Copho obviously considered only the male organs when he offered the reader a cure for testicular itch—guaranteed, "in case you wish to have cash right away." Similarly, the nomenclature applied only to males when Petrocellus reported that, in addition to the Greek term *cremasteres,* "the testicles have many [Latin] names, such as *didimi, oscelus,* and *orcus.*" Savonarola seemed more ambiguous when he explained that testicles, in a process analogous to the transformation of blood into milk in the mammary glands, whitened the residue from the "ultimate digestion" and turned it into *genitura*. He clarified that the term *genitura* differed, as designating the *product* of the process, from *sperma* and *semen* as the actual *principium* of generation—the ambiguous meaning, of "beginning" and "principle," left (and still leaves) ample room for philosophical debate. Savonarola hastened to add, however, "the physician, and especially the practitioner, should not care about this."

In organizing his section on therapeutics, Savonarola decided to follow a different order than Avicenna ("with all due respect to my Leader") and to begin with the complexion of the testicles. "Every physician should diligently examine and treat" this complexion, "because of the importance of the organ and its connections." The organ's importance was dual: "both in purpose, nothing less than the production of a human; and in substance, which is spongy and thus easily becomes abscessed." In addition, a bad complexion

> prevents reproduction, so that you should be aware that men often come into the hands of physicians to be judged, on the advice of lawyers (*iuristarum*), whether they are capable of intercourse or not. This is because several are found totally unable to have intercourse due to a bad complexion of the testicles and penis, and they say that they are bewitched. Hence, carefully examine their complexion, for cold (*frigiditas*) together with humidity is usually the cause of this.

It seems of interest to note that the adjective "frigid" could once be applied to men.

Savonarola's allusion to medicolegal judgments reveals the lack of clear distinction between impotence and infertility. Bernard confounded both in observing, with a characteristic moral accent, "coitus in public and without shame sterilizes decent men, but some are so evil that, the more something is foul and filthy, the more they enjoy it." He further lumped both together in proposing, "sterility and failure (*paucitas*) of coitus are due to external or internal causes"; inversely, he maintained the confusion by presenting aphrodisiacs that "make a man fecund." Concerns with fertility often led authors to correlate sexual potency and temperament. Bernard proposed such a correlation for diagnostic purposes when, on the basis of various signs in the genitals and characteristics of the semen, he claimed,

> we are able to infer that the sanguine have great desire because of warmth, and great ability because of humidity; the choleric do it very fast and often, and from the slightest cause they desire intensely but can do little; melancholics by nature are neither desirous nor able; phlegmatics are not desirous but all the more able.

Savonarola illustrated the correlation by reporting that he saw a "young man of twenty-four, with a sanguine and slightly phlegmatic complexion," who "fell into a habitual inability to have an erection." This was not a mere academic observation but a real case, for Savonarola continued, "when he consulted me, he said that he sometimes felt a noticeable cold of the heart, and he recovered after receiving a remedy for the heart." Impotence itself, in the literal sense of powerlessness, was in the focus of some compilers, perhaps the early ones in particular. Gariopontus observed that *apoximeron* "happens mostly to the elderly who have the desire but not the ability because nature *denies the power*, and they have an erection but then become flaccid like infants."

There was a wide range of remedies for men who suffered temporary or chronic impotence, which suggests that the problem was particularly frustrating. Gariopontus advised them to "sleep in a soft bed, view and embrace beautiful women, and read love stories." He also recommended, at least according to Bartholomeus, "the sight, conversation, touch, and then the kiss of pretty girls." Petrocellus prescribed "rubbing and ointments" with a salve of laurel and other ingredients, and drinking wine with ground satyrion and arugula. Since antiquity, and with evident input from the Near East, standard aphrodisiacs included sparrow brains, fox testicles, bull penis, and the rennet of a young male camel. These were featured, for example, in a concoction of Constantine's that underwent a startling inversion in the textual transmission. In his treatise *On Coitus*, Constantine prescribed giving seven pills, twice a day and "not more, or the woman will faint under the man." In the *Lilium*, Bernard copied the recipe because "good pals say that it makes the woman faint under the

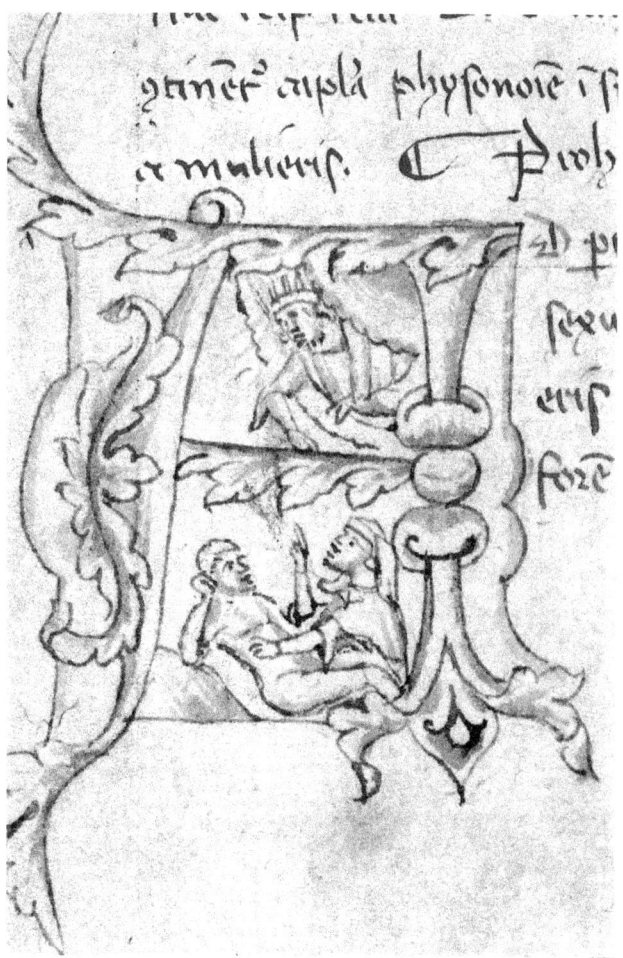

The correlation of *Physionomie*, complexion, temperament, and the planets with sexual function and dysfunction. A master shows a reclining nude male patient the connection between the liver and a winged crowned extraterrestrial. Drawing in an early 16th-century miscellaneous manuscript that contains Michael Scot, *Physiognomia* and ps-Gerard Cremonensis, *Theorica planetarum*. (Wellcome Library Western Manuscript 507, fol. 64v. Wellcome Library, London. Wellcome Images L0032023)

man." He further offered his own "medicament, divinely revealed," with the warning, "do not tell anyone but your sons." For a diet that was both aphrodisiac and fecundating, he recommended such dishes as lamb, dates and almonds, soft-boiled eggs, and fried fish eggs (roe, or caviar?). Reinald underscored the common male bias with his instruction for preparing an ointment, "if you wish to make a woman very enjoyable in coitus, so that she loves you much," and for applying it to the penis and vulva "when you wish to have intercourse, because the woman will join you affectionately and love you."

If the compilers commonly assumed male dominance in prescriptions for female receptivity, they left no doubt that there were (are) two sides to men's preoccupations with potency and power. They paid disproportionate attention to the uncontrollable conditions of satyriasis and priapism, both of which were unanimously termed "shameful and dangerous." They defined the former as a lasting erection accompanied by libido, and the latter as devoid of libido. Further differentiations, however, were not always clear. In cases of priapism, the erection ceased after venery according to Gariopontus, but it continued according to Petrocellus. Although Bernard recognized the distinctive definition of both categories, he tended to interweave their causes and consequences. A blurring of taxonomies is also evident in the strangely diverging combinations in which satyriasis appears in Table 8.1, with "gonorhea" in Gariopontus but with impotence in Savonarola. Priapism received only passing attention, notwithstanding the prognosis that, if prolonged, it might portend tetanus or even death. Satyriasis, on the other hand, stirred universal concern "because it arouses the sex drive incessantly and with the most powerful erection," Gariopontus argued, with the evocative information that it was "named after satyrs whom fame has cast as prone to venery." He further specified, "satyriasis is counted among the acute diseases, even when it is not accompanied by fever."

Treatment of this worrisome condition, while imperative, varied greatly according to the supposedly responsible causes. Petrocellus attributed satyriasis to "the excessive retention of sperm." Bartholomeus claimed, "the sole cause of this ailment is the windy spirit that inflates the nerve channels and erects the penis"; therefore, "helpful things are those which reduce the windiness." Compilers generally adopted both of these physiological etiologies, together with corresponding treatments that ranged from drying diets to phlebotomy. They extended therapeutics into the realm of neurology by adding such inhibitors of sensual stimulation as offensive smells. Platearius cited the verse, presumably of Salernitan provenance, "camphor in the nostrils / castrates males." Salernitan masters occasionally seemed to contradict themselves in this area. Gariopontus, for instance, in one place suggested to "abstain from good scents and from looking at beautiful forms," but in another, he advised to "procure the service of good-looking girls." In either case, this advice pointed to the psychological aspect that gradually eclipsed the physiological interpretation of satyriasis. Bernard concentrated on extraneous causes, among which he singled out "a strong imagination about a certain woman, a reduction in the usual sexual activity, embraces, and the like." As a result, cures as well as causes acquired more explicit moral dimensions, which were not created but reinforced by Christian attitudes toward sex. It is useful to mention here that compilers were silent or, at most, vague on voluntary ejaculations that were dissociated from intercourse.

The chapters on satyriasis in the compendia reflected the expanded medical speculation about correlations between sexual health and disorders, between natural urges and deliberate abstention, and even between chastity and lust. This speculation inspired Reinald's chapter "On extinguishing libido and removing the wish to have sex."

> In various monasteries and religious places, there are numerous [men] who have vowed chastity to God but who frequently and strongly want coitus and have the erections for which this ailment is called "satyriasis." It is due to temptation by the devil, and also because they eat foods that produce a windy spirit and increase libido.

Turning to a personal note, he interjected,

> I have been compiling this book while staying with the monks in the Cistercian monastery of Casanova [near Parma], for the love of the abbot, the prior, and the monks of that place. Therefore, I will say some things here that work to remove coitus, because it is of interest to the religious to preserve a chastity that is more precious than for other men.

This interjection may, at first, be surprising in light of Reinald's other pronouncements; upon closer examination, however, it seems that he was a temporary guest rather than a professed resident of the monastery. If he had been a lifelong Cistercian, he might have been less forthcoming with advice for curing impotence and more reticent on aphrodisiacs. Nevertheless, monk or not, he subscribed—at least in the abstract—to the consensus of "Galen and numerous other authors, philosophers, and wise men" that "coitus is useful and even beneficial in the management and preservation of health, and a temperate man who uses it moderately should live longer."

By Reinald's standard, sex was immoderate when it exceeded a rather generous allowance. "Some have said that once a week is enough, others twice, and others three times, with which I agree." More frequent use is not only exhausting but it even "shortens life," and this is why "the philosopher says that sparrows have a short life because they copulate much."

With an ironic glimmer of compassion, Reinald added, "if someone is too weakened and exhausted by immoderate coitus, let him sit naked in a clean tub in which thirty or forty eggs have been broken, and draw all these eggs in through the anus." Bernard seemed to be more practical and, paradoxically, more moralizing on a healthful sexual regimen. Citing Galen, he proposed that "intercourse is beneficial, by evacuating superfluities and gladdening the soul, at such intervals that the body feels alleviated and one eats and sleeps well enough." He immediately continued, however, with Avicenna's warning that "one coitus in excess is more harmful than forty equivalent bloodlettings," and with Constantine's judgment that "few have sex for the sake of offspring, more for the sake of health, but most for the sake of pleasure." Then, in one of his most forceful censures, Bernard remarked, "Avicenna tells many illicit and improper things about coitus, and he tells them for the sake of treatment; nevertheless, because such things infest the air, I leave them aside."

Remedies for reducing the frequency of intercourse and for diminishing the libido were plentiful. They ran the gamut from medications, with predictably ubiquitous ingredients such as camphor and agnus castus or chaste tree, to a chaste regimen of "fasts, toil, bad food, and bad bedding," as Reinald formulated it. He ended his anaphrodisiac therapeutics with

> the ultimate method, by cutting off the testicles. However, I do not advise anyone to do this. Some kings and princes do this today, having their servants castrated so that they will serve their spouses and ladies.

A far gentler remedy against lust was to walk barefoot, as he learned from Avicenna, who in turn credited the *experimentatores*. This teaching led Savonarola, most likely by way of Gentile da Foligno's commentary on the *Canon,* to claim, "blessed Francis knew very well" why he ordered his followers to be "shoeless" (*discaligati*). Savonarola made much of one particular procedure that was "recommended by many, Galen and others"; indeed, authors from Pliny to Celsus and nearly every compiler mentioned the procedure, and we have encountered it among treatments for diabetes. This was the cooling application to the lumbar region of two lead sheets, with very small perforations, which had been immersed in vinegar. Notwithstanding the widespread reputation of this remedy, Savonarola expanded the warning by Avicenna and earlier authors that it should be applied with care because the lead pressed heavily on the renal area. The remedy could have an adverse effect, as in the case of "a Venetian nobleman in my care, who felt his kidneys become noticeably warm from leaving the sheets on too long."

It is of interest to note that, inferentially, Savonarola was treating the noble Venetian for the involuntary emission of sperm, either while awake, in *gomorrea,* or while asleep, in *pollutio.* Both of these issues carried implications that seemed increasingly complex for physicians—and that challenge the historian's effort to assess medieval medicine on its own terms. Neither the Salernitan authors nor Avicenna mentioned nocturnal pollution as a distinct phenomenon. It appears to have become a special concern for Bernard and subsequent compilers, either because of their personal outlooks or as a sign of the times. By itself, *pollutio* was associated primarily with adolescence and attributed to dietary and humoral causes that paralleled those of *gomorrea.* Erotic stimulation naturally was held responsible for both, but, more notably, it accounted for moral judgment even with regard to nocturnal occurrence. The cause according to Bernard, as he emphasized in his separate chapter on *pollutio nocturna,* was "daytime concupiscence around the inordinate love of a woman," and the power of the imaginative faculty over "the lower faculties." On the authority of Galen he declared, "strong imaginations move [the body's] warmth and spirits, and the mores of the soul are changed by what is seen and looked at, and by evil music." The appropriate treatment of this cause was "to apply the whip (*flagellum*)."

If Bernard's moralization was harsh, it was less explicit than Valesco's admonition that all causes of nocturnal emission were to be remedied by their contraries "so that God and good Nature may not be offended by complacence with this kind of pollution." Still, the expressions of Valesco as well as Bernard were indirect in comparison with Savonarola's verdict that nocturnal pollution, when caused by daytime concupiscence, was "a mortal sin, as some say." The qualifier in this ultimate condemnation becomes more intriguing when we note the paradox between severity and humanity in Savonarola's sex therapy. He followed Avicenna in recommending that the patient sleep on willow leaves, to which he added "the leaves of agnus castus on which, according to Averroes, the Athenians sat on feast days so that it would make them chaste." Yet he also expressed his reservation about such treatments, with a personal reminiscence.

> Listen, in my time a certain great practitioner made a robust youth sleep on willow leaves for this problem, and the youth became ill. Therefore, be careful not to run to those exotic remedies even if they seem useful: unlike

ordinary and domestic things, they give physicians a bad reputation if they do not achieve good results.

Fleabane and chamomile, and seeds of lettuce and rue were among the ordinary and domestic simples that Savonarola and other compilers favored for treating *pollutio.*

A vast cultural distance lies between the medieval and the modern meanings of pollution, while a more precise medical distinction separates *gonorhea* or *gomorrhea* (and variant spellings) in the compendia from gonorrhea in today's vocabulary. *Gonorhea* was defined most broadly, by Gariopontus, for example, as a repeated, copious, and uncontrolled emission of sperm—a disorder analogous to what is now called spermatorrhea. It was commonly mentioned as one of the accidents that accompanied epileptic seizures. Petrocellus traced the origin of the word *gonorhea* to the Greek for "germ" and "flow." Bartholomeus notably modified the first root by stating, "*gonos* means people (*gens*)." The term and etymology metamorphosed further into *gomorrea,* "as if it were, the flux of humankind," by the time of Bernard, who strangely interpreted this as referring to a high mortality. He further inserted an odd allusion to the New Testament, advising that, when excess warmth and moisture caused "this most disgraceful ailment," the patient "should marry in Christ, because it is better to marry than to burn" (1 Corinthians 7:9)—we can only guess whether Bernard was thinking of burning with excess warmth, with desire, or in hell. Valesco seems to have been the only compiler to make a more explicit biblical connection here, one that was probably popular with preachers. He declared, "*gomorrea* is named after the city of Gomorrah (Genesis 18:21) on account of the improper emission of semen which took place in that city."

The causes and cures of *gomorrea* were largely the same as for satyriasis and pollution. Common sense as well as moral injunction concentrated on the role and control of sensory stimulation. Savonarola admonished, more specifically than other compilers, "prudent religious men should not roam through the town or talk to women." This admonition seemed to foreshadow the zeal and puritanism that would triumph in the fiery career of his grandson, the preacher and reformer Girolamo Savonarola (1452–1498). However, the physician's more tolerant side surfaced when Michele Savonarola urged, "you should not prevent the emission of sperm as long as it does not weaken the body," because forcibly retained sperm would become poisonous. He offered a prescription, "from which I have gained honor," for involuntary emissions due to weakened muscles. Indeed, he expressed the long-standing concern that "this ailment must be treated with care" because, if it is prolonged, it weakens the body and eventually results in death. At least as early as Gariopontus, authors claimed that patients occasionally died "because shameful silence prevented them from receiving treatment." Ironically, publicity seems to have surrounded some cases. When Savonarola adopted Avicenna's observation that emission sometimes followed urination, he added, "as we have seen in Mantua." He publicized the individual plight, no doubt posthumously, of a *gomorrea* that was due to a weakened *virtus contentiva*, "as in Lord Gorelus of Sicily" (probably Gurellus Carrafa of Naples, marshal of the kingdom of Sicily, who died in 1401). It is legitimate to contrast the masculinization of *gomorrea* after the 13th century with the egalitarian presentation by such early compilers as Gariopontus and Petrocellus, who called it an ailment that "strikes either gender, men and women." Copho implied a similar equality when he juxtaposed infections of the penis with swelling of the vulva and uterus. It would appear that reproductive issues were often not sharply delineated by Salernitan teachers and that the dichotomy between male and female diseases widened when the *magistri* of medicine became more dominant, as the following pages may demonstrate further.

Conditions of the Reproductive Organs in Women

Medieval gynecology and obstetrics continue to be the subject of such intense scrutiny, keen analysis, and lively debate that it is impossible to do justice here to the perspectives that keep unfolding. In addition, the texts, even within the manuals, are so rich—and so incompletely explored—that their full examination would distract us from the goal of an introductory survey and, beyond, from an overall assessment of the *practica*. The challenge of digesting the entire evidence is compounded by the contemporaneous growth of a literature that paralleled the comprehensive manuals or was excerpted from them, and that covered the spectrum from coitus and conception to sterility, parturition, and care of the newborn. This parallel corpus included works as varied as the compendium of women's medicine called *Trotula*; a group of 14th-century treatises on sterility by physicians of the University of Montpellier; and the *Secrets of Women,* which drew special prestige from being ascribed to Albertus Magnus, "the teacher of everything there is to know." In view of the expanse of medieval women's medicine and of current studies, the only practical approach here is to tighten our focus on diseases of the

Table 8.2 Chapters on female reproductive organs (*muliebria*)

Bartholomeus	Platearius	Gilbert	Bernard	Savonarola
virga et testiculi	virga	hernia	hernia	hermafrodita
retentio menstruorum	retentio menstruorum	retentio menstruorum	passiones mulierum [retentio m.]	*Rubr.1–5* anatomia & complexio matricis
effusio menstruorum	nimius fluxus menstruorum	nimius fluxus menstruorum	nimius fluxus menstruorum	*6–8* menstruorum retentio & fluxus
suffocatio matricis	sufficatio & precipitatio matricis	precipitatio matricis	suffocatio matricis	*9* clausura oris matricis
impedimentum conceptionis	impedimentum conceptionis	excoriatio, apo-stema, vulnera, cancer matricis	apostemata matricis	*10–19* apostema, cancer, ulcera, pruritus matricis
		sophisticatio vulve	vulnera vulve	*20* augmentum & precipitatio matr.
			precipitatio matricis	*21* prefocatio matricis
		impedimentum conceptionis	sterilitas mulierum	*22–26* impregnatio & sterilitas
		generatio & formatio embrionis	regimen pregnantium et aborsus	*27–29* mola matricis & cura pregnantium
		difficultas pariendi	difficultas partus	*30–31* cura em-brionis & aborsus
		secundina intus remanens	retentio secundine	*33–40* retentio secundine etc.
		exitus, sanguis, & dolor matricis	mola matricis	*41–42* fetus mortuus & enixa
sciatica et podagra	artetica passio	cura lapidis per cyrurgiam	podagra, sciatica, artetica	extremitates; *Rubr. 1* ruptura

female reproductive organs, and to consider in passing, or to leave aside entirely, certain areas even though they became incorporated into the compendia. This is the case, most notably, for ideas on reproduction, concerns with fertility, principles of obstetrics, and rules for neonatal care, all of which merit separate inquiry and are receiving the systematic attention of scholars.

As counterpoint to Table 8.1, which outlined the content and context of the coverage of the male reproductive organs in the compendia, Table 8.2 should give at least a sketchy idea of the discussion of the female organs. Table 8.2 shows, first of all, a changing sequence in the overall contents: the two Salernitans (in the left two columns) moved directly from male to female organs, whereas Gilbert and Bernard inserted hernia, and Savonarola hermaphroditism. The change has implications beyond a mere degree of difference among compilers. The placement of hernia, for example, reflected the ambiguous taxonomy, as extrinsic yet linked to male reproductive problems on account of the location, and as predominantly yet not exclusively affecting men. A more important aspect of Table 8.2, which is apparent immediately upon comparison with Table 8.1, is that Bartholomeus has replaced Gariopontus. There are no separate chapters on women in the *Passionarius* of Gariopontus or, for that matter, in the *Practica* of Petrocellus, at least in the extant versions. It is reasonable to propose that these authors could defer to a group of specialized texts that were circulating in Salerno.

A bold dividing line in Table 8.2 sets obstetrics aside from gynecology, although the distinction was not always clear-cut. Here, as earlier, Gilbert marks a striking change between the heyday of Salerno and the rise of the universities. Salernitan masters largely left the management of pregnancy to the midwives (*obstetrices*), while relegating related matters to separate treatises. University-trained physicians, on the other hand, incorporated these matters more and more into their manuals—and, as has recently been demonstrated, into their sphere of authority. Their exercise of this authority, however, may have been more in words than in actions, for the claims of personal success or experience were relatively scarce. Inversely, these physicians acted more and more as teachers (*doctores*) by expounding on gender differences, embryology, and related questions of natural philosophy. From Gilbert on, their teaching was profoundly and increasingly indebted to Avicenna's *Canon* and his commentaries on Aristotle, and to the Aristotelian works themselves. This indebtedness was particularly manifest when such compilers as Valesco and Savonarola followed their regular procedure by introducing the section on the female organs with a methodical description of uterine anatomy and complexion.

As Table 8.2 shows, the discussion itself of the female reproductive organs began consistently with a chapter on menstruation and, more precisely, on "the retention of the menses" (amenorrhea in today's vocabulary). Learned physicians treated menstruation mainly as a natural process, although they were not immune to the traditional ambiguity between curse and flowers or to popular myths and phobias. On the whole, they viewed the diminution or absence of menstruation as a primary concern, which was reinforced by an ulterior issue, as we will see shortly. Bernard and others attributed amenorrhea to "too much exercise, hunger, emotions, obesity, fever, dropsy, vaginal scarring, and similar observable factors." Aside from correcting such extrinsic causes, conventional humoral treatments included letting blood by venesection and cupping, the administration of diuretics and laxatives, and the application of emmenagogues in liniments and pessaries. Bernard urged, "beware that powerful substances such as nigella are applied in small quantity, stay for a short time, and are not kept during sleep, because they sometimes trigger a fever or cause ulcers in the womb. Indeed, when we medicate, let us be cautious in administering stronger remedies, especially to delicate patients."

Among the reasons for caution were the overlaps between emmenagogues and contraceptives as well as abortifacients. These overlaps were more often implied than spelled out—and they continue to fascinate historians. Platearius was quite direct in noting,

> things that induce menstruation also bring out the afterbirth, a dead fetus, and the toad called 'brother of the Salernitans'. Note further that in the beginning of conception, and especially when the fetus is due to become alive (*vivificari*), Salernitan women attempt to kill the said animal (*predictum animal*) by drinking the juice of celery and leeks.

This excerpt calls for more comments than are possible here. Suffice it to point out two details. The phrase *frater salernitanorum* in this version, instead of the more common *frater lumbardorum* or "brother of the Lombards," referred to a uterine mole. This type of mole or *arpia*, Bernard observed, "is allegedly quite common in women of Lombardy." One possible reason was that "they toil more and they are more submissive"; another explanation—with little regard for geography (or cuisine and diet)—blamed it on "spoiled food, as in Apulia, because it is said commonly that Italian women live very poorly, as on fruits and herbs, but that they dress well."

The second part of Platearius's observation calls attention to deeper implications. It brought him to the juncture of emmenagogues with the removal of a dead fetus, morning-after contraception, and abortion. He reported, without criticism, the practice of *mulieres salernitane*, that is, female denizens of Salerno (different from the group of midwives and healers who were often referred to as "the Salernitan women"). Gilbert adopted the report almost verbatim while adding, in similarly factual fashion, the information that a half dozen prescribed remedies "stimulate menstruation, but they also protect public women from conceiving." Earlier, Copho implicitly equated uterine mole or "arpa" with a retained placenta, and he prescribed that, "immediately *after* birth, leek juice be given or a pessary inserted into the vagina." We may note in passing that the nonjudgmental stance of Platearius and Gilbert paralleled that of Avicenna, often overlooked by historians, in his descriptions of abortifacients as well as contraceptives, occasionally even with the admission that they were "sometimes necessary." Gilbert's moral neutrality on this occasion contradicted his attitude in other instances, as we will see. Moreover, it contrasted with Savonarola's decision, in the rubric on a dead fetus, to "go lightly over this matter about which it is dangerous to speak, on account of evil men; what I will say will be said for health and not for perdition, and one who nevertheless makes evil use of these things, will set up the judgment of his soul."

Whatever the potential for unintended applications, the compilers evinced a reasonable confidence in remedies for amenorrhea. This confidence did not extend to the treatment of excessive menstruation, now called menorrhagia. A sense of helplessness in responding to this disorder was suggested by Gilbert's recommendation, in the name of Constantine, of such *empirica* as incantations and talismans "in conjunction with medication." Bernard underscored the seriousness of a grim prognosis, namely, that "excessive menstrual flow leads to consumptive diseases, dropsy, fevers, back ache, stomach ailments such as loss of appetite, and many other things."

The physicians' concerns with menstrual disorders were overshadowed by their preoccupation with a problem that has become identified with prescientific medicine and that continues to generate intense commentary. "Suffocation of the womb" was the subject of a chapter in Constantine's *Viaticum*, with a wide influence that was reinforced by references to Galen and, subsequently, by three chapters in Avicenna's *Canon*. Manifested by swooning and a near-total loss of perceptible breathing and other vital signs, uterine suffocation was defined in two suggestively different ways. The first definition, which had ancient roots (and postmedieval reverberations in the concept of hysteria) and which most closely echoed the *Viaticum*, was literal. Bartholomeus, for example, described a "compression of the respiratory organs" by an expanding womb that was itself choking on accumulated fumes. The second interpretation was probably influenced by descriptions in the *Canon* of uterine movement, "upwards and forwards, left and right." This interpretation dovetailed with the hoary legend of the wandering womb. Valesco rejected the legend as "a notion of the ancients and of some illiterate old women, which Galen dismisses." Bernard combined both interpretations of *suffocatio matricis* by defining it as "the rise of the womb up to the diaphragm, which causes compression of the respiratory organs and fainting."

The principal cause of uterine suffocation, in either definition, was the retention of sperm or menses, and "women who are not using men" were said to be the most likely patients. Therapeutic concerns concentrated consistently—and to the greatest fascination of some historians—on the accumulation of sperm, which in women (unlike in men) turned into poison according to established tradition. Prevention consisted in restricting diets or circumstances that promote sperm production. Medication included drying and purgative agents, particularly such aromatics as sweet flag or balsam that, Gilbert admitted, "one finds around noble women; for common women (*plebeiarum*) you will easily be able to find remedies anywhere." Addressing the root cause raised broader issues, beyond the universal advice. Valesco echoed the consensus that the "patient should acquire a husband" and, if this was impossible or "if she should wish to remain chaste, she should fast and sleep on leaves of agnus castus." More direct treatment may have been viewed as contrary to propriety. However, it caused no misgivings for Platearius when he instructed that the patient,

> if she is bound by a vow of chastity or continence, should apply this remedy: let rock salt and saltpeter be pulverized and mixed in vinegar and salt water; insert a soaked cotton plug into the vulva: this causes slight biting which sometimes causes sperm to be discharged. Or let the woman insert her finger so that by the movement and tickling she is able to produce sperm.

This version of the instruction was but one of many. In fact, the variations from compendium to compendium are so provocative that it is worth tracing their origins.

In the book *On the Affected Parts* (which was translated by Burgundio of Pisa in the 12th century, as *De interioribus*), Galen reported the case of a widowed woman who suffered from

> troublesome and nervous tensions. The midwife said that the womb had turned, and it suited her to apply the remedies that they usually applied to such conditions. Now, when she did so, the warmth and the treatment of the female parts caused contractions, with trembling and pleasure

resembling those in coitus, and in the process, with the discharge of thick and plentiful sperm, the woman was freed from the troubles that burdened her.

In the *Canon,* Avicenna turned the report into an outright and detailed instruction,

> the midwife should insert her hands, lubricated with oil of lily, nard, or laurel, into the patient's vulva and stir the orifice of the vulva and the orifice of the womb with repeated light movement; it is necessary that this cause a combination of pain and pleasure, as happens in coitus. She will probably emit the produced sperm and be healed.

Valesco seems to have been the only compiler to cite both "the teaching of the Fourth Book of the *Canon*" and *De interioribus* with book, chapter, and column, while adding several details. He specified that the midwife "should lubricate her index and middle fingers," and rub the aromatics inside, "with long pauses" and vigorously "because this will increase the good scent," until "perhaps, the corrupt sperm will come out."

The precision of Valesco may be contrasted with the taciturnity of Bernard, an author to whom he deferred constantly. Bernard cut Avicenna's instruction in half, omitting all mention of the vulva, pleasure, coitus, and sperm. It is not clear what motivated the terse abridgment of his citation, but a generation or so earlier, Gilbert left no doubt that some compilers objected, even strenuously, to such methods even if they were sanctioned by authoritative medical tradition. While he accepted the insertion of a soaked tampon for triggering a discharge, he admonished,

> do not listen to the mad lies of masters who teach rubbing with the fingers, and of regulars in the use of venery, who search for wicked things in their books to remove this disease, and who promote things that are alien to Nature or to Holy Scripture. Like outlaws, consumed by the forces of nature into dust and ash, they should be blown away by a rapid wind.

Savonarola took yet another turn that demonstrated the great diversity among compilers. He promoted this method of relieving uterine suffocation to "one of the first to be applied." In addition, he instructed the practitioner directly, "frequently make the woman apply her lubricated fingers to herself," and "let it be your concern to eliminate the cause by means of frequent discharge." As if further elaboration was necessary, he added that "there are some women who contrive to have intercourse with each other with an instrument similar to the male organ, and they derive pleasure and benefit from this."

It is easy to imagine how Gilbert would have reacted to Savonarola's amoral stance. It is ironic that Gilbert borrowed much lore from the earthy *Treatments for Women* (attributed to the Salernitan woman Trota) and that he did so even when it might seem indecorous or improper in "decent" (*honestus*) company. However, he also inserted censure—which some historians have overlooked and others have overstated. The paradox in his position is most striking on methods for feigning virginity. He observed,

> sometimes virgins are corrupted so that their orifice is widened and thus the breach is plain to one who comes in contact. They *deservedly* suffer repudiation and everlasting disgrace; or the men as well as the women wind up in divorce, a danger to both.

The adverb "deservedly" (*merito*) is italicized here in order to underscore the moral inflection, by which Gilbert's observation became more than a mere statement of fact. He continued, while conceding that it was "necessary to remedy this defect," with the admonition

> not to protect one deception with another. The signs of virginity are modesty and shame, with chaste walk and speech, and looking at a man somewhat sideways. Let us address such matters, however, since women who know them have learned to tame unbridled movements and to cover falsehood with an image of truth.

The means for "tricking (*sophisticandam*) the orifice so that they appear to be virgins" ran from distractive perfumes to vaginal constrictives, all of which "help married women as well as wanton women and virgins who are thus impaired." Without disapproval or approval—and, to the modern reader, with a surprising lack of revulsion—Gilbert further mentioned that "some women, in order to appear as virgins, apply a leech to the entrance of the vulva, with care to keep it from entering, one day before having intercourse, so that it draws blood which turns into a crust."

Ulcerations of the vulva, together with several other external and internal female ailments, were treated primarily with adaptations of humoral and abdominal treatments, and with remedies analogous to those for the male reproductive organs. Two conditions, however, caused exceptional concerns. The first of these was *precipitatio matricis,* which is analogous to uterine prolapse in current terminology, the descent of the womb into the vaginal area, although Bernard and others drew a distinction between this, as a "fall" (*lapsus*), and the internal dislocation of the uterus. Many women seem to have foregone treatment, and compendia contained only palliative remedies that ranged from cupping to baths. More active responses were left to the midwife, not only because the condition most commonly affected women after difficult or repeated parturition but also because both an accurate diagnosis and remedial intervention required manipulation. Uterine abscesses constituted a second category of interior diseases that were far more challenging and threatening. In Bernard's prognosis, "every aposteme of the womb is difficult to cure." He diagnosed a cancerous tumor by a discharge that was "virulent, with a heavy odor, and of different colors." In view of his normally comprehensive coverage, it may seem surprising that he did not include uterine cancer in his section on therapeutics where, in any event, he offered little more than palliation. There was a plausible reason, however, for his omission. Gilbert conceded that, "if such cancers do not respond to medications, there is no need to persist. Indeed, Hippocrates says, 'It is better not to treat patients with hidden cancers, for those who are treated perish sooner and the untreated ones complete many more days.'" Savonarola agreed on the incurability of uterine cancer, but he insisted, "it can be treated, that is, medicated palliatively, and you can engage in this, but first notify the relatives; in the end, though, you will not gain honor from this." It may be useful to remind ourselves at this point that compilers, rather than addressing breast cancer among women's diseases, included it in their chapters on the chest, in keeping with the head-to-toe order.

The Extremities

Compilers proceeded from the reproductive organs to the extremities, with the odd exception of Gilbert's excursus to lithotomy (see Table 8.2). Savonarola and some others began their descent with hernia, unlike Gilbert and Bernard, who inserted hernia between their sections on the male and female organs. Both sequences, however, were governed by a shared concentration on inguinal hernia, in which the intestine or other soft tissue protrudes through the lower abdominal wall, and which was known to be most common in men. Bernard distinguished no fewer than seven kinds of hernia. These did not include umbilical hernia, which he relegated to a very brief chapter "on protrusion of the navel, dislocation, varicose veins, and back ache," and which he attributed to a variety of causes that "either do not accept treatment or are treated by surgery, so that I leave them to the surgeons." Savonarola, on the contrary, devoted a separate rubric to "enlargement of the navel," which he equated with *ruptura,* an alternative term for hernia. Another alternative, *crepatura,* was more commonly associated with inguinal hernia that, according to Reinald, "frequently happens to youngsters and robust men who are too eager to jump or run or carry heavy weights, or who throw very big rocks or lift them in a manly fashion (*viriliter*)." Valesco speculated that the milder type of hernia might be hereditary, "coming perhaps already from the father's seed, for it is often seen in fathers and sons, and I have seen it into a third generation."

Diagnostic methods, including the universally known cough-and-palpation, allowed the practitioner to assess the extent of the rupture and the options for treatment. Reinald reported a "good treatment, proven by my teacher who by these means cured all patients with hernia, even if they had been suffering it for thirty years." The procedure hardly differed from the methods that all the compilers described, from laying the patient down with the head lower than the feet and gently pressing the intestines back, to applying a brace or truss and plasters. It is easy to appreciate the distinction between these gentle interventions and the more drastic surgical treatments with cautery or incision. While Reinald admired his teacher's success with conservative cures, Bernard had a less sanguine outlook.

> I have never seen anyone cured except by surgery once hernia is established, even though I have frequently done the many things mentioned in therapeutics. I call hernia established (*antiquatam*) when the internal edges have become hard so that they can no longer join, perhaps after more than *seven days*. Even if we may promise much, we expect little.

He elaborated, a little later,

> even though I have been a painstaking inquirer, I have never been able to cure anyone when the hernia was established and the patient was not a child. But I have seen it done by surgery. I have seen many endangered in the hands of the surgeons (*restauratorum*) because they perforated the intestines, feces came out, and the patients died. Hence, let us beware of false promises.

Reinald, too, noted that he had seen "many perish" in the hands of surgeons, but this left no recourse for the physician, who "should in no way engage in such dangerous treatments."

When and if hernia reached a critical stage and called for intervention, it stood in sharp contrast with the group that followed it in most of the compendia. This was a group of chronic ailments that were all attributed to the running (*rheuma*) or dripping (*gutta*) of a humor, most commonly phlegm, to different parts of the body, particularly the joints (*arthron*). The most likely candidates, Reinald asserted, were

> men who live quietly and in luxury and who neglect purges; also prelates and those who had been poor and then rose to wealth and prosperity, and those who attend only to fattening their bodies; in particular, those who neglect medicines and scorn the advice and help of physicians. This ailment rarely afflicts women except those who lack menstruation and those who live in luxury.

Rheumatismus, gutta, and *arthetica:* any of these three terms normally designated joint inflammations in general, while a special label referred to the location. The common categories began with *ciralgia,* which afflicted the hand (and which is analogous though not identical to the modern "cheiralgia") and to which compilers gave the least amount of their attention, although they noted the nagging pain as well as the resulting distortion of the fingers. They showed greater concern with *sciatica* in the haunches, lower back, and legs (the range was considerably broader than of today's sciatica); Gariopontus noted, "if this ailment last long, patients become crippled and disfigured," but he muddled the picture by adding another inflammation of the haunches that he called "psialga," a rare term that referred more directly to the kidneys and lumbar pain.

The most notorious type of *arthetica* was *podagra,* which affected the foot and which gradually became synonymous with *gutta* or "gout." In an earlier chapter, we have seen that Constantine, in the *Viaticum,* identified gout as "pain of the heel bone (*calcanei*)." Gariopontus explained that *gutta* "begins in the big toe," which then tends to become red. He admitted that patients "may be helped but not cured, because it is utterly chronic, that is, long-lasting. They should abstain from wine, sex, meat and legumes, dainty foods, anger, sadness, and displeasure." Petrocellus provided detailed information on a variety of foot problems, including calluses and plantar inflammation, but he appeared most concerned with pain. He offered remedies for painful heels and for a blister, which "you should rub with soap before it bursts. If it has burst, smear it with pork bile morning and evening, and it will be healed for certain. Also, place a fresh mouse skin over it: this is marvelous."

Thus, the compilers have brought us from head to heel—from head to toe. It seems appropriate to conclude with a testimonial by one of our star compilers to a Master of Medicine who taught the Art of healing, renounced medication, and outlived his patients. When Valesco argued that, at the onset of the inflammation, dietary adjustments could be effective and sufficient, he elaborated,

> to illustrate, let me tell you about the diet observed by our teacher in Montpellier, Bernard Forestier of happy memory, who in his day was greatly tormented by pains in his joints. As soon as he felt the great pains of *gutta,* he immediately placed himself on an extremely light diet, and he imposed such a rein on his mouth that sometimes he stayed for three full days without eating or drinking, intermittently washing his mouth with cold water when thirst became intolerable. With this regimen, the pain ceased, and little by little he returned to a full diet. He claimed that he had not found as good a remedy in any medicine as in this diet and abstinence. He stayed away from all other medication, and with this diet he lived to something like a hundred years.

Chronology of the Collated Latin Medical Manuals

1000–1100

Constantine the African (d. ca. 1090). — *Pantegni*, "The Complete Art," an abridged and very freely adapted translation of Haly Abbas (Ali Abbas al-Majusi, d. ca. 990), *al-Kitab al-Maliki*, "The Complete Art of Medicine."

Constantine the African. — *Megategni*, "The Great Art," adapted from Galen, *Tegni* or *Technē iatrikē*, "The Medical Art."

Constantine the African. — *Viaticum*, "Provisions for the Journey," adapted from Ibn a-Jazzar (d. 980), *Zad Al Mussafir*, "Provisions for the Traveler."

Constantine the African. — *Isagoge Ioannitii*, "Introduction to the *Tegni*," from Johannitius (Hu-nayn ibn Ishaq al-'Ibadi, d. 873), "Questions on Medicine."

Gariopontus of Salerno (fl. ca. 1050). — *Passionarius Galensi*.

Petrocellus of Salerno (fl. ca. 1050?). — *Practica*.

1100–1200

Stephen of Antioch (of Pisa) (fl. ca. 1127).

Liber regalis dispositionis, "The Book of Royal Discourse," a new, complete, and methodical translation of Haly Abbas, *al-Kitab al-Maliki* (see above, Constantine).

Copho of Salerno (ca. first half 12th).

Practica secundum humores.

Johannes Platearius of Salerno ("Johannes Platearius II") (fl. ca. 1150).

Practica brevis.

Archimattheus of Salerno (fl. ca. 1150–1180).

Practica.

Bartholomeus of Salerno (fl. ca. 1150–1180).

Practica.

Johannes de Sancto Paulo of Salerno (fl. ca. 1180).

Breviarium medicine.

Gerard of Cremona (1114–1187).

Canon Medicine, "Canon of Medicine," translation of Avicenna (Abu Ali al-Husayn ibn Abd Allah ibn Sina, 980–1037), (1114–1187). *Al-Qanun fi al-Tibb,* "The Law of Medicine."

1200–1300

Egidius Corboliensis (Gilles de Corbeil) (d. ca. 1214).

Viaticus de signis et symptomatibus aegritudinum.

Gilbertus Anglicus (fl. 1240–1260).

Compendium medicine.

Guglielmo (Guilelmus, William) da Saliceto (1201–1277).

Summa conservationis et curationis.

1300–1400

Bernard de Gordon (ca. 1258–1308).

Practica seu Lilium medicine (1305). Reinaldus ("de Vilanova"). *Breviarium medicine* (after 1300).

Gulielmus de Brescia (Brixiensis, 1250–1326).

Ad unamquamque egritudinem a capite ad pedes practica.

Guillelmus de Varignana (ca. 1270–1339).

Secreta sublimia ad varios curandos morbos.

Niccoló Bertruccio (d. 1347). *Nusquam antea impressum Collectorium totius fere medicine.*

John of Gaddesden. *Rosa anglica practica medicine a capite ad pedes.*

1400–1500

Valesco de Tharanta (1382–1417). *Practica que alias Philonium dicitur.*

Antonio Guaineri (Guaynerius, Antonius) (d. 1440). *Practica.*

Giovanni Michele Savonarola (1385–1466). *Practica medicinae; sive de egritudinibus*

Glossary

accidentia: literally, "things that happen," concomitants; the term covered a broad range, and it was extended to *accidentia anime* (see below) and to everything that accompanied an illness, including symptoms (from *suntoma,* a Greek equivalent of the Latin *accidentia*), signs, effects, and sequelae.

accidentia anime: "things that happen to the soul," that is, emotions.

aposteme: any unnatural swelling or tumor: post-medieval English "imposthume."

Articella: the collective title, the "Little Art," for the core readings of the medical syllabus, was inspired by the Hippocratic characterization of medicine as an art that takes a lifetime to master.

bloodletting: the draining of various amounts of blood from designated locations on the body, with the objective of drawing off what was thought to be excessive or corrupt in the blood or an accompanying humor. Methods included opening a vein (venesection or phlebotomy); making small cuts or scratches (scarification), on which suction cups might be placed (wet cupping; *see* cupping); and applying leeches ("bloodsuckers," *sanguisuge*).

cautery: the application of a hot iron (actual cautery) or a caustic agent (virtual cautery) with the chief purpose of opening channels, and thus closer to phlebotomy and even to acupuncture than to the modern procedure for eliminating abnormal tissue.

complexion: the condition of a body, organ, or substance as a combination of the elements, qualities, and humors. It was balanced in good health or imbalanced ("bad") if dominated excessively by one of these factors. Also *see* nature.

contranaturals: *see* nature.

cupping: the creation of local suction on the skin by the application of heated cups, most often similar to brandy glasses; "dry cupping" aimed at promoting blood flow; in "wet cupping," the skin was scarified, and the amount of blood drawn by suction was less copious and more controllable than in venesection (*see* bloodletting).

etiology: the identification of the causes, in this case, of a disease.

experimentum: literally, "something that has been experienced." The term, which designated a remedy that was proven empirically rather than rationally, frequently implied that effectiveness was due to a specific and hidden ("occult") quality rather than to general mechanics or understood processes. Unlike in the modern "experiment," proof did not rest on repeated, methodical, and controlled testing.

faculty: a key concept in Galenic teaching and in medieval medicine. More comprehensive and fluid than the modern counterpart, the term referred to a power (Greek *dunamis,* Latin *virtus*) or inherent quality that enabled an organ or a substance to perform a certain function and to achieve a definite purpose (*see* teleology). Every human body possessed faculties for perceiving, thinking, and communicating (*animalis*); breathing and maintaining life (*spiritualis*); and nourishing and reproducing life (*vitalis*). A faculty could govern the essential function of an organ (attracting, retaining, expelling) or explain the effect of a substance (laxative, cleansing, cooling) unless this was due to some hidden quality (*see experimentum*). There were separate but overlapping categories for each aspect of life as a process of "digestion" or "combustion."

gnosis: the privileged knowledge that enabled the learned physician to differentiate the meaning of the symptoms (diagnosis) and the portent of the signs (prognosis).

herpes: from the Greek for "creeping" (hence "serpent" and "herpetology"), term for a range of skin afflictions far broader than the viral diseases covered by the modern term.

iatros, iatria: the Greek words for "healer" and "healing," before an explicit distinction was made between knowledge and skill, and before the rise of the specific labels, of *medicus* for one who knows, *physicus* for one who understands and serves nature (*see physica*), and *doctor* for one who teaches.

lepra: the term is kept in Latin in this book, in order to allow for the lack of precision in general medieval usage, which stands in contrast with today's designation of "leprosy" or Hansen's disease. Physicians, nevertheless, were concerned with differential diagnoses and with a classification of variations in a notoriously changeable disease. They labeled the most serious forms *elephantia,* alluding to the "elephantine" thickening of the skin, and *leonina,* for the lionlike deformation of the face; they gave less weight to *tyria,* named for the glossy skin, resembling snake skin, which covered the sites where sensation was lost; the fourth and most open-ended category was *alopecia,* for the patchy hair loss that resembled the mange of a fox (*alopex*).

nature: the term had even more meanings in medieval medicine than in current usage, including that of essence, norm, and inherent design. The elements, qualities, humors, organs, faculties (*see* faculty), operations, and spirits were the "naturals" that constituted the body's essence. The environment, diet, and other factors that were necessary but not part of the essence were called nonnaturals and conventionally listed as six; they governed the first phase of therapeutics, and they provided the structure to many a "guide of health" or *Regimen sanitatis*. Diseases were "contranaturals," outside or against the norm of nature. Nature was considered intelligent in directing every norm toward a purpose (*see* teleology).

nonnaturals: see nature.

nosology: the classification of diseases.

pestilence: widely spreading disease with high fatality rate, therefore also called "mortality."

phlebotomy: *see* bloodletting.

physica: the knowledge of nature (*physis*), which was based in Aristotle's "natural philosophy," and which included an understanding not only of the workings but also of the "ingenious" purposes of Nature (*see* nature).

Res naturales, res non naturales, res contra naturam: see nature.

sanies: bloody matter.

scarification: see bloodletting.

spiritus: a capital concept inside medicine as well as beyond, with meanings that exceeded "spirit" in current usage and that extended from inhaled air to an immaterial emanation and a "pneumatic" force. *See also* faculty.

sternutatory: a substance that induces sneezing.

teleology: the fundamental doctrine, promoted by the influence of Aristotle and Galen and reinforced by Christian theology, that every part, faculty (*see* faculty), form, and function exists for a specific purpose that is determined by the will of God and the intelligence of Nature.

temperament: literally, a "temperate state" or balance of the humors, of which one was dominant. A temperament was "sanguine" if blood dominated, "choleric" if yellow bile (choler), "melancholic" if black bile (melancholy), and "phlegmatic" if phlegm.

venesection: *see* bloodletting.

Bibliography of Sources

Note that the language of all the listed sources is Latin and that, as is the norm for Latin writings, authors are listed by their first names (spelled as they occur most frequently).

This book could not have been written without access to the principal sources in digitized manuscripts, early prints, and modern editions. Web pages and websites that proved particularly rich and user-friendly are cited in the bibliography for ready access—with the understanding that many other digitized sources are available, and that their number is growing daily.

Anon. *Summa Medicinae (Mad. Esc. M.II.17): Estudio y edición crítica,* ed. Cristina de la Rosa Cubo. Tesis de Doctorado, Universidad de Valladolid, 2000. http://www.cervantesvirtual.com/obra/summa-medicinae-mad-esc-m-ii-17-estudio-y- edicion-critica—0/.

Antonius Guaynerius (Antonio Guainerio). *Practica.* Venice, Italy: Locatellus, 1497. http://gallica.bnf.fr.

Antonius Guaynerius (Antonio Guainerio). *Practica.* Lyon, France: Gabiano, 1534. http://books.google.com.

Arnaldus de Villanova (Arnau de Vilanova), *see* Reinaldus.

Avicenna. *Avicennae Canonis libri V.* Munich, Bayerische Staatsbibliothek (BSB) manuscript 13017, 1264 CE, 338 fols. (Beautifully illuminated, parchment). http://daten.digitale-sammlungen.de.

Avicenna. *Canon medicinae (latine): a Gerardo Cremonensi translatus.* Venice, Italy: Bonetus Locatellus, 1490. http://books.google.com.

Avicenna. *Liber canonis Avicenne: revisus & ab omni errore mendaque purgatus summaque cum diligentia impressus [translatus a Bernardo Cremonensis ab arabico in latinum]*. Venice, Italy: Bonetus Locatellus, 1505. http://gallica.bnf.fr.

Bartholomeus Salernitanus. *Practica*, in *Collectio Salernitana*, IV, ed. Salvatore de Renzi. Naples, Italy: Filiatre-Sebezo, 1856, 321–406. http://archive.org/.

Bernardus de Gordonio (Gordonius; Bernard de Gordon). *Practica seu Lilium medicine*. Venice, Italy: Bonetus Locatellus, 1496/97. http://daten.digitale-sammlungen.de.

Bernardus de Gordonio (Gordonius; Bernard de Gordon). *Practica seu Lilium medicine*. Paris, France: Jean Foucher, 1542. http://babel.hathitrust.org/cgi/pt?id=ucm.5316545825. http://gallica.bnf.fr.

Bertrucius Bononiensis (Niccolò Bertruccio). *Nusquam antea impressum Collectorium totius fere medicine*. Lyon, France: Claudius Davost, 1509. http://gallica.bnf.fr.

Claudius Galenus (Galen of Pergamum). *Galeni opera omnia*, 19 vols, ed. K. G. Kühn, Leipzig, Germany: C. Cnobloch, 1821–1833. http://www.bium.univ-paris5.fr/histmed/medica.htm.

Constantinus Africanus (Constantine the African). *Liber Pantegni*, in Isaac Isreali, *Opera* [*see* Isaac Israeli], I-CXLIV [in the second set of foliation]. http://www.bium.univ-paris5.fr/histmed/medica.htm.

Constantinus Africanus (Constantine the African). *Megategni*, in Isaac Isreali, *Opera* [*see* Isaac Israeli], CLXXXIXv-CCVIII [in the second set of foliation]. Lyon: [Trot]. http://www.bium.univ-paris5.fr/histmed/medica.htm.

Constantinus Africanus (Constantine the African). *Opera*. Basel, Switzerland, 1539. http://www.bium.univ-paris5.fr/histmed/medica.htm.

Constantinus Africanus (Constantine the African). *Theorica Pantegni*. Facsimile and Transcription of the Helsinki manuscript (Codex EÖ.II.14). Edited by Outi Kaltio, in collaboration with Heikki Solin and Matti Haltia. National Library of Finland 2011. http://www.doria.fi/handle/10024/69831.

Constantinus Africanus (Constantine the African). *Viaticum*, in Isaac Isreali, *Opera* [*see* Isaac Israeli], CXLIV-CLXXII [in the second set of foliation]. http://www.bium.univ-paris5.fr/histmed/medica.htm.

Copho (Copho Salernitanus). *Practica secundum humores*, in *Collectio Salernitana*, IV, ed. de Renzi, 439–505. http://archive.org/.

Egidius Corboliensis (Gilles de Corbeil). *Viaticus de signis et symptomatibus aegritudinum*, ed. Valentin Rose. Leipzig, Germany: Teubner, 1907. http://books.google.com.

Galen *see* Claudius Galenus.

Gariopontus. *Passionarius Galeni*. Lyon, France: Trot, 1526. http://gallica.bnf.fr.

Gilbertus Anglicus (Gilbert the Englishman). *Compendium medicine*. Lyon, France: Portonaris. 1510. http://gallica.bnf.fr; http://books.google.com.

Guilelmus de Saliceto (Guglielmo da Saliceto). *Summa conservationis et curationis*. [n.p.], 1476. http://gallica.bnf.fr.

Guilelmus de Saliceto (Guglielmo da Saliceto). *Summa conservationis et curationis.* Venice, 1490. http://www.digital-collections.de/index.html?c=digitale_sammlungen&l=en.

Guillelmus de Varignana (Guilelmus, Gulielmus, Guglielmo de Varignana). *Secreta sublimia ad varios curandos morbos.* Lyon, France: Johannes de Cambray, 1526.

Guillelmus de Varignana (Guilelmus, Gulielmus, Guglielmo de Varignana). *Ad omnium interiorum exteriorum partium morbos remediorum praesidia.* Basel, Switzerland: 1575. http://www.digitale-sammlungen.de/

Gulielmus Brixiensis (William of Brescia,). *Ad unamquamque egritudinem a capite ad pedes practica.* Basel, Switzerland: Schott, 1508. http://books.google.com.

Isaac Israeli (Isaac Judeus). *Opera omnia.* Lyon, France: Trot, 1515. http://www.bium.univ-paris5.fr/histmed/medica.htm.

Johannes de Gaddesden (John of Gatesden). *Rosa anglica practica medicine a capite ad pedes.* Pavia, Italy: Girardengis and Birreta, 1492. http://books.google.com.

Johannes Platearius. *Practica,* in *Practica Jo. Serapionis* (*see* Johannes Serapion).

Johannes de Sancto Paulo. *Breviarius.* In *Viaticus de signis et symptomatibus aegritudinum* (*see* Egidius), ed. Rose, 103–107. http://books.google.com.

Johannes Serapion. *Breviarium medicinae.* Venice, Italy: Rinaldo de Novimagio, 1479. http://gallica.bnf.fr.

Johannes Serapion Senior. *Practica studiosis medicinae.* [n.p.], 1525. http://books.google.com.

Michael Savonarola (Giovanni Michele Savonarola). *Practica medicinae: sive de egritudinibus.* Venice, Italy: Bonetus Locatellus, 1497. http://daten.digitale-sammlungen.de; http://gallica.bnf.fr.

Niccoló Bertruccio *see* Bertrucius.

Petrocellus. *Practica,* in *Collectio Salernitana,* IV [see Copho], ed. de Renzi, 185–291. http://archive.org/.

Reinaldus (Reinaldus de Villanova). *Breviarium pratice* [sic]. [n.p.], 1485. (The author is cited in catalogs as "Arnaud de Villeneuve"). http://gallica.bnf.fr.

Valesco de Tharanta. *Practica que alias Philonium dicitur.* Lyon, France: Huss, 1490. http://gallica.bnf.fr.

Valesco de Tharanta, *Practica que alias Philonium dicitur.* Lyon, France: Wolff, 1500. http://www.bium.univ-paris5.fr/histmed/medica.htm.

Selected Bibliography

This bibliography is limited, with a few exceptions, to recent publications in English that bear directly on aspects of the medieval physician's manual.

Arrazibalaga, Jon. *The Articella in the Early Press, c. 1476–1534.* Cambridge, UK: Cambridge Wellcome Unit for the History of Medicine, and Barcelona, Spain: CSIC Barcelona, 1998.

Arrizabalaga, Jon, ed. *Articella Studies: Texts and Interpretations in Medieval and Renaissance Medical Teaching. Number 2* [Papers of the *Articella* Project Meeting, Cambridge, December 1995]. Cambridge, UK: Cambridge Wellcome Unit for the History of Medicine, 1998.

Biller, Peter and Ziegler, Joseph, eds. *Religion and Medicine in the Middle Ages.* Woodbridge, UK: Boydell & Brewer, 2001.

Cadden, Joan. *Meanings of Sex Difference in the Middle Ages. Medicine, Science, and Culture.* Cambridge, UK and New York, NY: Cambridge University Press, 1993.

Crisciani, Chiara and Zuccolin, Gabriella, eds. *Michele Savonarola: medicina e cultura di corte* (Micrologus' Library 37). [Papers presented at the International Conference on Michele Savonarola, Pavia, 2005]. Florence, Italy: SISMEL/Edizioni del Galluzzo, 2011.

Demaitre, Luke. *Doctor Bernard de Gordon, Professor and Practitioner.* Toronto, Canada: Pontifical Institute of Medieval Studies, 1980.

Demaitre, Luke. *Leprosy in Premodern Medicine. A Malady of the Whole Body.* Baltimore, MD: The Johns Hopkins University Press, 2007.

Demaitre, Luke. "The medical notion of 'withering' from Galen to the fourteenth century," *Traditio* 34 (1992): 259–307.

Demaitre, Luke. "Medieval notions of cancer: Malignancy and metaphor," *Bulletin of the History of Medicine* 72 (1998): 609–37.
Demaitre, Luke. "Scholasticism and compendia of practical medicine, 1250–1450," *Manuscripta* 120 (1976): 81–95.
Demaitre, Luke. "Skin and the City: Cosmetic Medicine as an Urban Concern," in *Between Text and Patient: The Medical Enterprise in Medieval & Early Modern Europe,* ed. Florence Eliza Glaze and Brian Nance. Florence, Italy: SISMEL/Edizioni del Galluzzo, 2011, 97–120.
Demaitre, Luke. "Straws in the Wind: Latin Writings on Asthma between Galen and Cardano," *Allergy and Asthma Proceedings* 23 (2002): 61–92.
Demaitre, Luke. " 'Vita brevis, Ars autem prolixa': forging a medical language," in *Petrarca e la medicina. Atti del Convegno di Capo d'Orlando 27–28 giugno 2003,* ed. Monica Berté, Vincenzo Fera, Tiziana Pesenti (Biblioteca Umanistica 8). Messina, Italy: Centro Interdipartimentale di Studi Umanistici, 2006, 123–43.
Dols, Michael W. *Medieval Islamic Medicine: Ibn Ridwān's Treatise "On the Prevention of Bodily Ills in Egypt."* Translation, with an Introduction. Arabic Text edited by Adil S. Gamal. Berkeley, CA: University of California Press, 1984.
Freedman, Paul. *Out of the East: Spices and the Medieval Imagination.* New Haven, CT: Yale University Press, 2008.
García-Ballester, Luis, et al., eds. *Practical Medicine from Salerno to the Black Death.* Cambridge, UK and New York, NY: Cambridge UniversityPress, 1994.
Getz, Faye Marie. *Healing & Society in Medieval England: A Middle English Translation of the Pharmaceutical Writings of Gilbert Anglicus.* Edited with an Introduction and Notes. Madison, WI: University of Wisconsin Press, 1991.
Getz, Faye Marie. *Medicine in the English Middle Ages.* Princeton, NJ: Princeton University Press, 1998.
Glaze, Florence Eliza. "Prolegomena: Scholastic Openings to Gariopontus of Salerno's *Passionarius,*" in *Between Text and Patient,* ed. Glaze and Nance, 57–86.
Green, Monica H. *Making Women's Medicine Masculine: The Rise of Male Authority in Premodern Gynaecology.* New York, NY: Oxford University Press, 2008.
Green, Monica H. "Moving from Philology to Social History: The Circulation and Uses of Albucasis's Latin *Surgery* in the Middle Ages," in *Between Text and Patient,* ed. Glaze and Nance, 331–72.
Green, Monica H. *The Trotula: An English Translation of the Medieval Compendium of Women's Medicine.* Philadelphia, PA: University of Pennsylvania Press, 2002.
Hunt, Tony. *Anglo-Norman Medicine.* Vol. 1. *Roger Frugard's Chirurgia, The Practica brevis of Platearius.* Cambridge, UK: Brewer, 1994.
Jones, Peter Murray. "Mediating Collective Experience: The *Tabula Medicine* (1416–1425) as a Handbook for Medical Practice," in *Between Text and Patient,* ed. Glaze and Nance, 279–308.

Jones, Peter Murray. *Medieval Medicine in Illuminated Manuscripts*. London, UK: British Library, 1998.
Ketham, Johannes de. *The Fasciculus medicinae of Johannes de Ketham Alemanus*. Facsimile edition of the first (Venetian) edition of 1491 with English translation by Luke Demaitre. Birmingham, AL: Classics of Medicine Library, 1988.
Maclean, Ian. "The Reception of Medieval Practical Medicine in the Sixteenth Century: The Case of Arnau de Vilanova," in *Between Text and Patient*, ed. Glaze and Nance, 493–512.
McVaugh, Michael R. "Cataracts and Hernias: Aspects of Surgical Practice in the Fourteenth Century," *Medical History* 45 (2001): 319–40.
McVaugh, Michael R. *Medicine before the Plague. Practitioners and Their Patients in the Crown of Aragon, 1285–1345*. Cambridge, UK and New York, NY: Cambridge University Press, 1993.
McVaugh, Michael R. "Medicine in the Latin Middle Ages," in *Western Medicine: An Illustrated History*, ed. Irvine Loudon (New York, NY: Oxford University Press, 1997), 54–65.
McVaugh, Michael R. "The Nature and Limits of Medical Certitude at Early Fourteenth-Century Montpellier," *Osiris* 6 (1990): 62–84.
McVaugh, Michael R. *The Rational Surgery of the Middle Ages*. Florence, Italy: SISMEL/Edizioni del Galluzzo, 2006.
McVaugh, Michael R. "Surface Meanings: The Identification of Apostemes in Medieval Surgery," in *Medical Latin from the Late Middle Ages to the Eighteenth Century: Proceedings of the European Science Foundation Exploratory Workshop in the Humanities, organized under the supervision of Albert Derolez in Brussels on 3 and 4 September 1999*, eds. W. Bracke and H. Deumens, Brussels, Belgium: Koninklijke Academie voor Geneeskunde van België, 2000, 13–29.
McVaugh, Michael R. "Who Was Gilbert the Englishman?" in *The Study of Medieval Manuscripts of England*, eds. George Hardin Brown and Linda E. Voigts. Turnhout, Belgium: Brepols, 2010, 295–324.
Montford, Angela. *Health, Sickness, Medicine and the Friars in the Thirteenth and Fourteenth Centuries*. Aldershot, UK and Burlington, VT: Ashgate, 2004.
Nutton, Vivian. "The fortunes of Galen," in *The Cambridge Companion to Galen*, ed. R.J. Hankinson. New York, NY: Cambridge University Press, 2008, 355–389.
Nutton, Vivian. "Pseudonymity and the Critic: Authenticating the Medieval Galen," in *Between Text and Patient*, ed. Glaze and Nance, 481–92.
O'Boyle, Cornelius. "The Art of Medicine." *Medical Teaching at the University of Paris, 1250–1400*. Leiden, Netherlands: Brill, 1998.
O'Neill, Ynes Violé. "Giovanni Michele Savonarola: an atypical Renaissance practitioner," *Clio Medica* 10 (1975): 177–193.
O'Neill, Ynes Violé. "Michele Savonarola and the Fera or Blighted Twin Phenomenon," *Medical History* 18 (1974): 222–39.
Pesenti, Tiziana. "The Teaching of the *Tegni* in Italian Universities in the Second Half of the Fourteenth Century," *Dynamis* 20 (2000): 159–208.

Rawcliffe, Carole. *Medicine & Society in Later Medieval England.* Stroud, UK: Alan Sutton Pub., 1995.

Salmón, Fernando. *Medical Classroom Practice: Petrus Hispanus' questions on* Isagoge, Tegni, Regimen Acutorum *and* Prognostica *(c. 1245–50) (MS Madrid B.N. 1877, fols. 24rb–141vb). Articella Studies: Texts and Interpretations in Medieval and Renaissance Medical Teaching. Number 4.* Cambridge, UK: Cambridge, UK: Cambridge Wellcome Unit for the History of Medicine, 1998.

Schalick, Walton O. *Add One Part Pharmacy to One Part Surgery and One Part Medicine: Jean de Saint-Amand and the Development of Medical Pharmacology in Thirteenth-Century Paris.* PhD dissertation, The Johns Hopkins University, 1997.

Siraisi, Nancy G. *Avicenna in Renaissance Italy: The Canon and Medical Teaching in Italian Universities after 1500.* Princeton, NJ: Princeton University Press, 1987.

Siraisi, Nancy G. *Medieval and Early Renaissance Medicine. An Introduction to Knowledge and Practice.* Chicago, IL: University of Chicago Press, 1990.

Voigts, Linda E. and Michael R. McVaugh. *A Latin Technical Phlebotomy and Its Middle English Translation,* in *Transactions of the American Philosophical Society,* Volume 74, Part 2. Philadelphia, PA, 1984.

Wack, Mary Frances. *Lovesickness in the Middle Ages: the Viaticum and its commentaries.* Philadelphia, PA: University of Pennsylvania Press, 1990.

Wallis, Faith. *Medieval Medicine: A Reader.* Toronto, Canada: University of Toronto Press, 2010.

Index

Abnormal cooling, 115
Acid reflux, 43
Affliction (*passio*) of heart, 38
Allusions, 172
Al-Qanun fi'l-Tibb, 10. *See also* Canon medicine
Amenorrhea, remedies for, 317
Amnesia, 130
Anachronism, 241
Anus, 268–74; exposure, 268–69; fistula, 273–74; hemorrhoids, 270–72; itch, 270
Anus, torn, 96
Anus, worms, 260
Anatomia, 14
Anthology (*Synagogae* or *Collecta*), 9
Aphorisms, 1
Aposteme, 79–84. *See also* Cold apostemes from phlegm and black bile; Warm apostemes from blood; Warm apostemes from yellow bile
Appetite, 241–48; corrupted, 244–46; failing, 244; loss, 246–47; source, 242
Apprentice healers, 2
Aromatic medicines, 65

Asthma, 211–14; "bloodsucking," 211; breathing difficulty, 211; domestic remedies, 214; doubled panting, 213; dyspnea, 211; long-term survival, 213–14; orthopnea, 212; phlegm stuck in lung, 211; retention of breath with strangulation, 213
"A Thousand and One Nights," 10
Authors and authority of tradition, 6–8; "The Little Art" or *Articella*, 8; "The Medical Art," 8; parchment, 6, 8; stardom of writers of books, 6

Bad breath, 191–92
Baldness, 115–16
Basilisk, 74–75
Bee stings, 75
Bleeding hemorrhoids in *Canon* and *Lilium*, 270
Blindness, threat of, 174
Blister beetles, 68, 97
"Bloodsucking," 211
Blows, 122
Book of the Eyes, 154

Brain malfunctions, temporary, 130–33; amnesia, 130; congelation, 130; dietary excess, 132; disorders of senses, 130; drunkenness, 132–33; insomnia or watchfulness, 130–31; scotoma, 130; stimulating remedies, 131; transitory problems of perception and memory, 130
Breathing difficulty, 211. *See also* Asthma
Breviarium, 100, 239

Cancer, 98–102; *cancrena*, 99; and crab, connections between, 99–100; definition, 99; diagnosis, 100–1; treatments for early stages, 101
Cancrena, 99
Canine or voracious appetite, 244–45
Canon medicine, 77, 111
Canterbury Tales, 6
Capilli (appendages of head, *caput*), 115
Cataracts, 164–69; couching, 168; dietary and pharmaceutical prescriptions, 167; knowledge and skill, 169; notion of moisture, 165; stages of development, 166; "treatment by instrument," 167
Causon, 44–45, 49
Chest: heart attacks, 204–5; lungs and respiration, 204
Clarificatio, 37
Cold apostemes from phlegm and black bile, 95–98; blister beetles, 97; fistulation, 95–96; phlegm or black bile, 95; scrofulas, 96–97; surgery for fistula, 96; surgical operations, 98
Compendium, 198
Compendium about the Epidemic, 65
Compendium or *Collectorium* to poisons, 70

"The Complete Art" (*Pantegni*), 12
Compound fever, 40
Concupiscence, 300
Congelation, 130
Conjunctivitis, 159–61
Consilium contra pestilentiam, 65
Constantinus Africanus, 11–12
Consumption: an ulceration of lung, 221; diagnosis and prognosis, 224; *humidum radicale*, concept of, 221; milk in treatment, 228–30; nonnaturals, 227–28; nutritional deficiency or malfunction, 222; ptisis, 221; season, clime, and air, 228
Continuous and interpolated fever, 39–40
Contranaturals, 13
Couching, 168
Cough, 214–20; coughing up blood, 219; treatments for hemoptysis, 220

Dead flesh, 119–20
Deafness at birth, 183
"De decoratione," 109, 161
Delusions, 136–37
De medendi methodo, 80
Dental problems, 192–93
Diabetes and urination problems, 296–300; "instrumentalist" view, 296; occasional/chronic incontinence, 298–99; prognosis, 297–98; thirst, 297
Diarrhea, 251, 265
Dichotomy between hand and head, 78–79
Dietetics, category of, 23–24
Diet or regimen: management of nonnaturals, 23–26; category of dietetics, 23–24; Chaucer's *parfit practisour*, 24; culinary recipes, 25; emotions, 24; golden rule, 24;

prevention and maintenance of health, 23; "specific" and "occult" virtue, 25; therapeutics, 24
Diet, in fever treatment, 53
Digestive faculty, 249–50
"The Disease Book" (*Passionarius*), 31
Diseases: against nature: dogmatist, 22; empiricists, 21; Hippocratic-Galenic tradition, 22; ideal physician, 21; methodists, 22; "pro-gnosis," 22; rationalist medicine, 21; rationalists, 22; "roots" of diseases, 22
Disfigurement, 105
Dogmatist, 22
Doubled panting, 213
Drainage, 271
Dropsy. *See Hydropisis*
Drugges, 25
Drunkenness, 132–33
Dubium, 156–57
Dysentery, 262–64
Dyspnea, 211

Ears and hearing: deafness at birth, 183; eardrops, 179; inner ear, 179; "Pain of the Ears," 179; penetration in to ears, 181; prevention and remediation, 184–85; remediation, 184; rural setting on ear health, 180; ulcers/abscesses/bleeding/discharge, 182; wormwood and bitter simples, 180
Elephantiasis, 103. *See also* Leprosy
Emotions, 24
Empirical fever remedies, 56–58
Empiricists, 21
Encyclopedias, 28
Ephemeral fever, 43
Epilepsy, 141–43, 146; animal ingredients in, 143–45

Esophagus, anatomy and function of, 241
Experience, 51–55
Experience, misleading, 6, 16, 38
Experimentum, 55–56. *See also* Experience; Occult remedies
External leakage, 274
Extramission, 157
Extremities, 321–24; critical stage of hernia, 323; hernia, kinds of, 321–22; joint inflammations, 323; *podagra* affecting big toe, 323; "psialga," 323
Eyes, 155–78; cataracts, 164–69; concept of "visual spirit" or "spirit of sight," 156; descriptions of eye, 157; extramission, 157; instrument of sight, 155; neoplatonic concept, 156; sketches of eye anatomy and nosology, 155; social responses and responsibility, 158; vision disorders, 169–78
Eye diseases, 159–64; abnormal appearances, 162; abnormal growths, 162–63; conjunctivitis, 159–61; "De decoratione," 161; diseases of eyelids, 161; injuries, 162; manual treatment with surgery, 163; opening in tear sac, 160; topical applications, 163–64

Face and senses: ears and hearing, 178–85; eyes, 155–78; mouth, taste, and touch, 191–95; nose and smell, 185–90
Facial spasm, 150
Fastidium, forms of, 248–49
Fecal vomiting, 267
Fever(s), 37–39; affliction (*passio*) of heart, 38; burning, 39; *Causon*, 40; classification, 39–40; compound, 40; continuous and interpolated, 39–40; course, 39; hectic, 40–41;

impressions and qualitative judgment, 38; juxtaposition, 41; in medical teaching, 36; organization of chapters on, 41; perception of elevated temperatures, 38; pestilential, 60–66; putrid, 38; Q fever (Query fever), 39; "quotidian," 40; simple, 40; tertian, 40; warmth, 38–39; withering of malnourished children, 40
Fevers, causes of, 42–44; "accompanying particulars," 43; acid reflux, 43; ephemeral fever, 43; extrinsic causes of hectic fever, 44; hints at tuberculosis, 44; overheating, 43; physical and emotional condition, 42; quartan, 43
Fevers, signs and symptoms, 44–50; appearance of urine, 45; attention to, 50; causon, 44–45, 49; complexity of fevers, 48–49; "critical days," 49; hectic fever, 45; interpretation fluid, 45–47; offending humor, 48; palpation, 44–45; patient's appearance, 47–48; pulse reading, 45; unnatural warmth, 44; uroscopy, 45–47
Fevers, treatment of, 50–60; bathing, 58; "bizarre," 56; conservative continuum, 51; drying agents, 52; empirical fever remedies, 56; external applications, 58; Guglielmo's manual, 56–57; helplessness, 55; induce vomiting before and after meals, 53; learned by experience, 55; massages, rubs, and unctions, 59; mixtures, 54; nourishment, 53; occult remedies, 51–52; overlaps, 54; phlebotomy or venesection, 59–60; prescription of human milk, 54; primary qualities, classification, 51; putrefaction, 52; "Sublime Secrets," 57

First Circle of Dante's *Inferno*, 10
Fissures of the lips, 192
Fistulation, 95–96, 274; surgery for, 96
Flower of Medicine, 160
Fluid terms, 129

Gaseousness (*ventositas*), 80
"Gilbertin," 27
Glasses, 177
Glaucosis, 172
Goiter, 203
Golden rule, 24
Graying, 116–17
Gullet, throat, and neck: affliction, 204; "the almonds" (*amigdale*), 199; goiter, 203; hoarseness, causes of, 202; impaired voice, 202–3; infections of tonsils, 199; phlebotomy from saphenous vein, 201; throat, affliction of, 200–1; uvula, five uses of, 199; uvulectomy, 200
Gynophobia, 300

Hair, patterns of study, 113–14
Hansen's disease, 102. *See also* Leprosy
Head, 115–20; abnormal cooling, 115; baldness and color, 115–16; *capilli* (appendages of head, *caput*), 115; graying, 116–17; lice, presence of, 117–18; ringworm, scabies, dead flesh, or morphew, 119–20; treatments of lice infestation, 118
Headache, 120–29; blows and wounds, 122; cooling substances, 125; diet and medication, 124; disorder, 123; drying effect of bad odors, 126; fluid terms, 129; humors, 123; internal causes, 122–23; map of brain, faculties, and senses, 128; narcotics, 125;

nomenclature and taxonomy, 121; severity of suffering, 121; symptomatic headaches, 122; terms and graphic descriptions, 122; venesection, 126

Healing: apprentice healers, 2; authors and authority of tradition, 6–8; connecting with textual tradition, 8–12; diet or regimen: management of nonnaturals, 23–26; diseases: against nature, 21–22; *Edwin Smith Papyrus*, 2; Hippocratic tradition, 3; "liberal arts," 3; managing information, 26–30; medicine by book, 4–6; nature and naturals, 15–21; organizing manual, 31–33; structure of learning as foundation of practice, 13–14; superhuman healing powers, 2; transmission process, 2; trivium (grammar, rhetoric, and logic), 3

Heart, 230–38; accidents of heart, 231; bloodletting, 237; complexional conditions, 234; complexional imbalance, 235–36; heartburn, 231; incidence of syncope, 237; recourse to cordials, 238; threats to, 236; weakening of the, 234–35

Heart attacks, 204–5

Hectic fever, 40–41, 45; extrinsic causes of, 44

Hemlock (*cicutam*), 66

Hemorrhoids, 270–72

Herbal antidotes, 72–73

Herbal concoction, 68

Hernia: critical stage of, 323; kinds of, 321–22

Herpes, 91–94

Hiccups, 255

Hoarseness, causes of, 202

Horrifying vision, 104. *See also* Leprosy

Hot and cold poisons, 69

Human milk, prescription of, 54

Humors, 123; combined effects of, 17; humoral constructs, 149–50

Hydropisis, 277–78

Ileum, 266

Imprecision, risk of, 37

Incurable disease, therapeutic sections for, 146

Insanity, 259, 267. *See also* Mental disorders

Insomnia or watchfulness, 130–31

Intestines: anal exposure, 268–69; anal itch, 270; anatomy and physiology, 256; bleeding hemorrhoids, in *Canon* and *Lilium*, 270; cold or warm complexional imbalance, 260–61; diarrhea, 265; drainage, 271; dysentery, 262–64; external leakage, 274; fecal vomiting, 267; fistula, 274; general abdominal complaints, 257; hemorrhoids, 270–72; ileum, 266; intestinal diseases, 262; intestinal parasites, 259–60; intolerable pain, 257; lientery, 260; *passio colica*, 268; rectal pain, 270; surgery, 273; tenesmus, 268; topical ailments, 257; torsion, 258; worms, 258–59

Intolerable itching, 108

Intolerable pain, 257

Intuition and contemplation, 113

Isagoge Ioannitii, 12

Jaundice or icterus, 280

Joint inflammations, 323

Joy, antidote to depression, 139

Juxtaposition, 41

Kidneys and bladder, 284–300; colic pain and renal pain, 286; diabetes and other urination problems,

296–300; humoral and complexional allopathy, 286; medicinal power of wagtail, 287; stone or calculus, 287–96

Learning, structure of: *Anatomia*, 14; contra-naturals, 13; naturals, 13; nonnaturals, 13; scholastic anatomy, 13–14; theoretical and practical, 13
Leprosy, 102–9; causes, 104; definition, 103; "dia-gnosis," 104–5; dietary factors, 104; disease of skin and flesh, 107; disfigurement, 105; elephantiasis, 103; Hansen's disease, 102; horrifying vision, 104; intolerable itching, 108; phlebotomy, 106; section on therapeutics, 107; skin infections, 107–8; treatments, 106; vocabulary, 102–3
Lesions, corrosive or caustic recipes, 68
Letuaries or electuaries, 25
Libellus de epidemia, 63
"Liberal arts," 3
Liber regalis dispositionis or "The Book of Royal Discourse," 12
Lice, presence of, 117–18
Lientery, 260
Lilium, 159
"Lily of Medicine," 28
"The Little Art" or *Articella*, 8
Liver: dropsy or *hydropisis*, 277–78; dropsy treatments, 278–79; form and composition, 275; humoral etiology, 276; jaundice or icterus, 280; sclerosis or progressive hardening, 276; second digestion, 274; spleen, 280–81
Lovesickness, "heroic love," 137–39
Lung(s) and respiration: anatomy and physiology, 205–6

Lupus, 91–95; cutaneous, 92; herpes, hot apostemes, 94; *medici* and *cura*, 92; skin infections, 95; as type of cancer, 93

Magna chirurgia, 79
Managing information, 26–30; accumulated learning, 29; authoritative texts collection, 27; encyclopedias, 28; "Gilbertin," 27; "Lily of Medicine," 28; limitations, 28; logical structuring of subject matter, 29–30; medical encyclopedia, 30; memory, 29; study material, 26. *See also* Organization of subject matter
Mania, 135–38
Manual, organizing: advertisement of manuals, 33; Avicenna's influence, 31; compilers, 31; "The Disease Book" (*Passionarius*), 31; *Euporiston* of Theodorus Priscianus, 31; purpose and utilization, 31; start with fevers, 32
Manual treatment with surgery, 163
Marasmus. *See* Withering
"The Medical Art," 8
Medical encyclopedia, 30
Medici and *cura*, 92
Medicine and poison, 68
Medicine by book, 4–6; books/manuscripts, 4; depiction of instruments, 5; NLM of United States, 5; "trademark," 5; university-trained practitioners, 4; workshops (*scriptoria*), 4
Melancholy or black bile, 16, 135–38
Memory, faculty of, 129–30
Mental disorders, chronic, 133–40; cooling remedies, 134; delusions, 136–37; extreme measures, 134; imbalance, 139; joy, antidote to depression, 139; mania, 135–38;

melancholy, 135–38; nightmare, 133; promiscuity, 139; sanguine imbalance, 140; transitory and chronic disorders, 133
Method of Healing, 12, 79
"Miasma," concept of, 35
Milk, 227–30; human, 25, 101, 170, 181; and leprosy, 104
Morphew, 119–20
Mouth, taste, and touch, 191–95; bad breath, 191–92; dental problems, 192–93; digestion, role of tongue, 195; fissures of lips, 192; pomander, 191; rinsing mouth, 191; softening or heaviness of tongue, 194; speech, 194; tongue, 193; tooth extraction, 193

Narcotics, 125
Nasal stench, 189–90
National Institutes of Health in Bethesda, Maryland, 5
National Library of Medicine (NLM) of the United States, 5
Natural human condition of health, definition, 15
Nature and the naturals, 15–21; air, 16; choler, 16; combined effects of humors, 17; fire, 16; four elements and qualities, 17; macrocosm of universal nature, 15; melancholy or black bile, 16; natural human condition of health, definition, 15; nutritional digestion, 20; phlegm, 16; physiology, 18–19; processes of life, 18; prominence of blood and bile, 16–17; second digestion, 18; *spiritus*, 20; teleology, 16; third digestion, 19
Nerves and disorders of motion, 140–51; charms and rituals, 142; differentiation between ages, 146; epilepsy, 141–46; facial spasm, 150; humoral constructs, 149–50; petit mal, 149; sacred texts, 142; semantics and practice, 147; therapeutic sections for incurable disease, 146
Night blindness or nyctalopia, 171
Nightmare, 133
Nonnaturals, 13
Nose and smell: blood from nose, 187; dietary correctives/treatments, 186–87; mechanism of olfaction, 188–89; nasal stench, 189–90; phlegm, 185–86; running nose, 186–87; sneezing, 188
Numbing or stupefying drugs, 68–69
Nutritional digestion, 20

Occult remedies, 51–52, 126, 286
Odors, drying effect of bad, 126; medicinal effect of good, 65
"Old Ypocras," 7
On Disease, 159
"On Medicine" (*De Medicina*), 7
On Moral Characters, 165
On the Affected Parts, 318
On the Differences of Fevers (Galen), 35, 63
On the Sacred Disease, 148
On Unnatural Tumors, 79, 99
Opening in tear sac, 160
Organization of subject matter, 31–32
Orthopnea, 212
Overheating, 43

"Pain of the Ears," 179
Palpation, diagnosis from, 44–45
Pangenesis, 301
Pantegni, 77, 154
Parasites, intestinal, 259–60
Parchment, 6, 8
Perception and memory, transitory problems of, 130

Perverted appetite, treatment of, 246
Pestilential fevers, 60–66; aromatic medicines, 65; aromatics in manuals, 65; category of, 61; collocation of epidemics with fevers, 61; "corrupt times," 62; epidemics, 62–63; "Great Mortality" ("Black Death"), 62; *Lilium medicine*, 61; role of vapors, 63; seasonal criteria and cosmic predictions, 64
Pestregiment, 65
Petit mal, 149
Phlebotomy or venesection, 59–60, 106
Phlegm or black bile, 16, 95, 185–86, 211
Physicus, 3
Pneumonia and pleurisy, 207–10; dietary recipes, 210; infection of lung, 207; prognostic signs, 208; respiratory epidemic, 208; symptoms of *pleuresis*, 208; treatment, 209
Podagra affecting big toe, 323
Poisonous potions and bites, 66–76; basilisk, 74–75; blister beetle, 68; compendium or *Collectorium* to poisons, 70; corrosive or caustic recipes for lesions, 68; direct threat of spiders/scorpions, 73–74; hemlock (*cicutam*), 66; herbal antidotes, 72–73; herbal concoction, 68; hot and cold poisons, 69; magical properties, 71; medicine and poison, 68; numbing or stupefying drugs, 68–69; potions, deadly and beneficial, 67; power of sapphires and other precious stones, 71; preventive measures, 70; protection against poison, 71–72; purgation and cleansing, 68; rabies, 75–76; saffron, 67–68; "sardonic grin," 67–68; set of signs, 69; theriac, antidote, 72; wasp and beestings, 75
Pomander, 191
Precious stones, power of, 71
Presbyopia, 174
Priapism, 308
Promiscuity, 139
"Psialga," 323
Ptisis, 221
Pulse reading, 45
Putrefaction, 52
Putrid, 38

Q fever (Query fever), 39
Quartan, 43
"Quotidian," 40

Rabies, 75–76
Rectal pain, 270
Reflection and refraction, 175–76
Regimen of Health, 171, 247
Remedies for Love, 139
Reproductive organs in men, 303–13; contents of sections on, 304; description of, 305; dual importance, 305; erotic stimulation, 311; frequency of intercourse, 310; "gonorhea," 308; *Gonorhea*, causes and cures, 312–13; impotence and infertility, 305–6; involuntary emission of sperm, 311; libido, 308; priapism, 308; remedies for impotence, 306–8; satyriasis, 308–9; sex therapy, 311
Reproductive organs in women, 313–21; abortifacients, 316; chapters on female reproductive organs (*muliebria*), 314–15; emmenagogues and contraceptives, 316; obstetrics aside from gynecology, 315; relieving uterine suffocation, 318–19; sterility, 313; the retention of menses, 315–16;

ulcerations of vulva, 320; uterine abscesses, 321; uterine cancer, 321
"Rhazes" or "Rasis," 10
Ringworm, 119–20
Rosa medicine, 158
Ructus or belching, 254–55

Sacred texts, 142
Saffron, 67–68
Sanguine imbalance, 140
Sapphires, power of, 71
"Sardonic grin," 67–68
Satyriasis, 308
Scabies, 119–20
Scarification, 59, 75, 145, 272, 329
Scholastic anatomy, 13–14
Sclerosis or progressive hardening, 276
Scotoma, 130
Scrofulas, 96–97
Second digestion, 18, 274
Semantics and practice, 147
Senses, disorders of, 130
Simple fever, 40
Skin, 78; infections, 95, 107–8
Smallpox and measles, 84–87; blood and bile, 85; infancy and childhood, 86; role of blood, 86
Sneezing, 188
Spectacles and eyeglasses, 175
Speech, 194
Spiders/scorpions, direct threat of, 73–74
Spiritus, 20
Spleen, 280–81
Stomach: descriptions of, 253–54; dietary recommendation, 251; digestive faculty, 249–50; ejection from, 251; hiccups, 255; ructus or belching, 254–55; stomachache, 255–56; superfluity and elimination, 250; therapeutically induced vomiting, 251–52; throwing up (*anastropha*), 251
Stone or calculus, 287–96; allopathic and homeopathic treatment, 292; diagnosis of kidney and bladder stones, 290; diet, 291; digital rectal insertion, 295–96; dislodging stone, 295; effects of aging, 288; feminine anatomy, 288; fox blood, 294; Jews' stone, 293; polypharmacy, 294; precious oils for liniments, 294; preventive regimens, 291; prostate, 288; turbid urine, 290
"Sublime Secrets for the Treatment of Various Diseases," 56–57
"Suffocation of the womb," 317–18
Superfluity and elimination, 250
Superhuman healing powers, 2. *See also* Occult remedies
Surgery, 26, 96, 163, 273
Surgical manuals, xiv, 79
Sweating, skin afflictions, 109
Symptomatic headaches, 122

Teleology, 16, 154
Tenesmus, 268
Terapeutica, De ingenio sanitatis, 80
Tertian, 40
Textual tradition, connecting with, 8–12; *Al-Qanun fi'l-Tibb*, 10; anthology (*Synagogae* or *Collecta*), 9; Arabic grammar, 10; "A Thousand and One Nights," 10; Avicenna, 11; Constantinus Africanus, 11–12; encyclopedic works, 10; First Circle of Dante's *Inferno*, 10; Galenic medicine, 10; Haly Abbas, 11; ibn Rushd, 11; Rabbi Moshe, 11; "Rhazes" or "Rasis," 10; Unani healing, 10–11
Theriac, antidote, 72
Third digestion, 19

Throat to stomach, 240–49; anachronism, 241; anatomy and function of esophagus, 241; canine or voracious appetite, 244–45; concept of *appetitus*, 242–43; dietary rules, 247; *fastidium*, forms of, 248–49; "light vomiting," 246; treatment of perverted appetite, 246; vomiting, 249
Throwing up (*anastropha*), 251
Tongue, 193; role in digestion, 195; softening or heaviness of, 194
Tonsils, infections of, 199
Tooth extraction, 193
Topical ailments, 257
Torsion, 258
"Treasure of the Poor" (*Thesaurus pauperum*), 56
"Treatment by instrument," 167
Trinity in Orthodox Christianity, 20
Trivium (grammar, rhetoric, and logic), 3
Tuberculosis, 44
Tumors and humors: Avicenna's humoral scheme of tumors, 81; and external ailments, associations between, 82–83; humoral classifications, 83–84; qualitative-humoral construct, 82
Two-seed doctrine, 301–2

Unani healing, 10–11
University-trained practitioners, 4
Unnatural warmth, 44
Uroscopy, 45–47
The Usefulness of the Parts of the Body, 232, 285

Uterine mole, 316–17
Uvula, 197–98

Venesection, 126
Viaticum, 77, 112
Vision disorders, 169–78; allusions, 172; catalog of threats, 170; corruption or malfunction of perception, 177; failing and weakening of, 171; glass eyepieces, 177; glaucosis, 172; loss, weakness, and corruption, 170; night blindness or nyctalopia, 171; physician Rhazes, 176; preoccupation with sharp vision, 174–75; presbyopia, 174; recipes, 173; reflection and refraction, 175–76; remedies, 173; spectacles and eyeglasses, 175; threat of blindness, 174
"Visual spirit" or "spirit of sight," 156
"Vita brevis, ars longa," 1
Vomiting, 240–249

Warm apostemes from blood, 87–89; bloodletting, 88–89; phlegmon and inflammation, 87–88
Warm apostemes from yellow bile, 89–91; bile, 90; combustion, 91; hot eruptions, 91; humoral categories, 90; sacred fire and Persian fire, 90; skin affliction, 89; skin ailments, 91
Warmth, 38–39
Wasp and bee stings, 75
Wateriness (*aquositas*), 80
Withering of malnourished children, 40
Worms, 258–59
Wounds, 122

About the Author

LUKE DEMAITRE, PhD, is a visiting professor in the Center for Biomedical Ethics and Humanities, University of Virginia, Charlottesville, Virginia. His research, which is focused on premodern medical teaching and practice, has resulted in the publication of numerous papers and several books. He has written on early concepts of embryology, childhood, and aging; on diseases such as asthma, cancer, and insanity; and on the efforts of medieval physicians in the areas of diagnosis, prognosis, and care.

Demaitre's first book was *Doctor Bernard de Gordon: Professor and Practitioner* (1980); his latest was *Leprosy in Premodern Medicine: A Malady of the Whole Body* (2007). Professor Demaitre is currently preparing an inventory and analysis of the iconography (depicted symptoms and symbols) of leprosy before it became known as Hansen's disease. He is a member of the American Association of the History of Medicine, the Medieval Academy of America, the International Leprosy Association, and the international study forum *Historia Leprosorum*.

Praeger Series on the Middle Ages

Jews and Judaism in the Middle Ages
Theodore L. Steinberg

Materials, Methods, and Masterpieces of Medieval Art
Janetta Rebold Benton

Islam in the Middle Ages: The Origins and Shaping of Classical Islamic Civilization
Jacob Lassner and Michael Bonner

Mythology in the Middle Ages: Heroic Tales of Monsters, Magic, and Might
Christopher R. Fee

Rethinking Chivalry and Courtly Love
Jennifer G. Wollock